Biochemistry
Illustrated

To our families with thanks for their support and encouragement.

Addendum
We dedicate this book to Peter Campbell who died while it was at press. His passion for biochemistry and his great energy in promoting the subject will be sorely missed.

Commissioning Editor: Timothy Horne
Project Development Manager: Hannah Kenner
Project Manager: Frances Affleck
Designer: Judith Wright
Illustrators: Chartwell, Sue Harris, Jane Templeman, Peter Cox

Biochemistry Illustrated

Biochemistry and molecular biology in the post-genomic era

Peter N. Campbell DSc

Emeritus Professor of Biochemistry
University College London, UK

Anthony D. Smith PhD

Emeritus Reader in Biochemistry
University College London, UK

Timothy J. Peters DSc FRCP FRCPath

Professor of Clinical Biochemistry
King's College London, and
Honorary Consultant Physician and Chemical Pathologist
King's College and Maudsley Hospitals, London UK

FIFTH EDITION

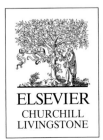

ELSEVIER
CHURCHILL
LIVINGSTONE

EDINBURGH   LONDON   NEW YORK   OXFORD   PHILADELPHIA   ST LOUIS   SYDNEY   TORONTO   2005

ELSEVIER
CHURCHILL
LIVINGSTONE

© Harcourt Publishers Limited 2000
© 2005, Elsevier Limited. All rights reserved.

Fifth edition 2005

ISBN 0443 10034 9

British Library Cataloguing in Publication Data
A catalogue record for this book is available from the British Library

Library of Congress Cataloging in Publication Data
A catalog record for this book is available from the Library of Congress

Note
Medical knowledge is constantly changing. Standard safety precautions must be followed, but as new research and clinical experience broaden our knowledge, changes in treatment and drug therapy may become necessary or appropriate. Readers are advised to check the most current product information provided by the manufacturer of each drug to be administered to verify the recommended dose, the method and duration of administration, and contraindications. It is the responsibility of the practitioner, relying on experience and knowledge of the patient, to determine dosages and the best treatment for each individual patient. Neither the Publisher nor the authors assumes any liability for any injury and/or damage to persons or property arising from this publication.

The Publisher

 ELSEVIER your source for books, journals and multimedia in the health sciences

www.elsevierhealth.com

The
publisher's
policy is to use
**paper manufactured
from sustainable forests**

Printed in China

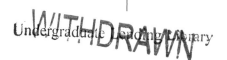

Preface

The first edition of this book was published in 1982; the object was to produce a succinct summary of biochemistry with numerous illustrations, providing an introduction to biochemistry in an easily assimilable form. In the following two editions we included additional text while retaining the organization of the subject matter. The fourth edition represented a major change in layout and organization, providing a much more continuous text while retaining the high proportion of illustrations. The most important change was the introduction of elements of gene structure and function at an early stage, immediately after a chapter on amino acids and proteins, because these concepts should permeate all aspects of modern biochemistry. In the final chapter, we briefly outlined some topics that we thought likely to be of particular significance in the future.

For this fifth edition we have carefully revisited the text and the figures and edited down some of the more detailed biochemistry. The original authors are very pleased to welcome Timothy Peters, a distinguished Clinical Biochemist, as a third author. He has helped to include many more examples of clinical relevance. Our restructuring for the fourth edition has borne fruit, as the impact of the human genome project has become increasingly apparent in what has become known as the 'post-genomic' era of biological and medical research. A knowledge of the structure of the human genome – and influence of the environment on its expression – will surely come to permeate and possibly dominate all aspects of current and future medical practice. The text has been revised to enlarge on this important area.

All the text provides a foundation to a study of medicine; paragraphs that have a particular relevance to the clinic are highlighted with a 'Clinical Implications' heading. This edition should be of benefit not only to medical students but also postgraduates in clinical biochemistry and for those requiring knowledge of the biochemical basis of their medical specialties. Science students should enjoy the medical bias while accepting that the text provides a sound introduction to biochemistry and molecular biology.

We are most grateful for suggestions from those who have been engaged in producing the many foreign language editions and for the careful attention of Hannah Kenner of Elsevier and the Commissioning Editor, Timothy Horne, for his guidance.

PNC
ADS
TJP

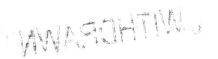

Acknowledgements

The authors are pleased to acknowledge the source of illustrations that have been based on illustrations published elsewhere, and to acknowledge the assistance of those who have helped in the preparation of various illustrations. Our acknowledgements have been grouped as follows:

a. The authors and publishers of books and original reports in journals. Permission to make use of this material has been sought and granted by copyright owners. The list may be of value to those who wish to extend their reading.

b. Those persons who have provided material from their own sources, or who have helped in other ways.

In all cases the numbers in [ ] refer to the number of the illustration in the present book. The other numbers refer to the original source.

a.   References to books and journals

1   General textbooks

1.1   *Basic Biochemistry for Medical Students* (Campbell, P.N. & Kilby, B.A., eds)
Academic Press, London.
Apart from the editors, the authors were J.B.C. Findlay, H. Hassall, R.P. Hullin, A.J. Kenny and J.H. Parish.
Figs 2.6 [2.8], 2.10 [2.7], 2.15 [2.5], 4.10 [4.2], 4.16 [2.15], 4.18 [2.12], 5.24 [6.40], 12.3 [3.17], 12.12 [3.41], 12.16 [3.46], 12.23 [3.49], 12.27 [3.52], Table 2.8 [Table 2.1]

1.2   *Biochemistry with Clinical Correlations*, 2nd edn (Devlin, T.M., ed.)
J. Wiley, New York.
Figs 3.6 [6.31], 6.39 [6.46], 6.50 [9.28], 6.51 [9.29]

1.3   *Biochemistry* (Stryer, L.)
W.H. Freeman, Oxford.
2nd edn, Figs 4.2 [4.22], 4.3 [4.23], 4.6 [4.24], 4.20 [4.21], 30.21 [3.29]
3rd edn, Figs 2.45 [2.20], Fig. 3.16 [2.8], 29.24 [3.63], 29.29 [3.57]

1.4   *Principles of Biochemistry*, 6th edn (White, A., Handler, P., Smith, E.L., Hill, R.L. & Lehman, I.R.)
McGraw-Hill, New York.
Figs 36.1 [5.27], 36.2 [5.28], 36.4 [5.31], 36.5 [5.33], 36.9 [5.32]

1.5   *Molecular Biology* (Freifelder, D.)
Jones and Bartlett, Boston.
Figs 4.32 [3.5], 21.27 [3.30]

1.6   *Biochemistry for the Medical Sciences* (Newsholme, E.A. & Leech, A.R.)
Wiley, Chichester.
Figs 7.9 [13.16], 11.5 [13.10]

1.7   *Biochemistry* (Mathews, C.K. & van Holde, K.E.)
Benjamin Cummings, Redwood City, CA.
Figs 11.1 [6.16], 28.35 [3.79], 28.36 [3.80]

1.8   *Essential Immunology* 6th edn (Roitt, I.M.)
Blackwell Scientific, London.
Fig. 7.10 [5.19]

1.9   *Gray's Anatomy* 37th edn (Williams, P.L., Warwick, R., Dyson, M. & Bannister, L.H., eds)
Churchill Livingstone, Edinburgh.
Fig. 1.75B [15.49]

1.10   *Harper's Biochemistry*, 21st edn (Murray, R.K., Granner, D.K., Mayes P.A. & Rodwell, V.W.)
Prentice-Hall, New York.
Fig. 55.2 [2.13]

1.11   *Principles of Biochemistry* (Lehninger, A.L., Nelson, D.L. & Cox, M.M.)
Worth Publishers, New York.
Fig. 2-24 [1.8]. This figure was adapted from *Molecular Biology of Cells*, 2nd edn, pp.165–166, Garland Publishing Inc., New York.

1.12   *Biochemistry*, 2nd edn (Voet, D. & Voet, J.G.)
John Wiley & Sons, Inc., New Jersey.
Fig. 29-37 [3.58]

1.13   *Biochemistry*, 4th edn (Stryer, L.)
W.H. Freeman and Company, Oxford. Used with permission.
4th edn Figs 15.4 [5.29], 15.9 [5.30], 15.33 [5.34], 15.42 [5.35], 37.35 [3.68]

1.14   *Biochemistry and Molecular Biology* (Elliott, W.H. & Elliott, D.C.)
Oxford University Press, Oxford, with permission.
Figs 25.5 [5.10], 25.7 [5.11], 25.8 [5.12]

1.15   *Biochemistry, Molecules, Cells and the Body* (Dow. J, Lindsay, G. & Morrison, J.)
Addison-Wesley Longman Ltd., Harlow. Reprinted with permission.
Figs 16.17 [5.17], 16.19 [5.18]

1.16   *Biochemistry* (Mathews, C.K. & van Holde, K.E.)
Benjamin/Cummings, Redwood City, CA.
Fig. 25E.1, p. 955 [3.25]

2   Books on special topics

2.1   *Open University Course Book* S322 Units 1-2 (1977)
Open University Press, Milton Keynes.
Fig. 3, p. 14 [2.19]

2.2   *Cells and Organelles*, 2nd edn (Novikoff, A.B. & Holtzmann, E.)
Holt, Rinehart & Winston, New York.
Fig. 1.25 [1.10]

2.3   *Enzyme Structure and Mechanism*, 2nd edn (Fersht, A.)
W.H. Freeman, Oxford.
Figs 1.12 [6.8, 6.9], 10.3 [6.30], 12.13 [6.10]

2.4   *Chance and Necessity* (Monod, J., Trans. by Wainhouse, A.)
A.A. Knopf, New York, and William Collins, London.
p. 47, Fig. 4 [3.62]

2.5 *The Structure and Function of Animal Cell Components* (Campbell, P.N.)
Pergamon Press, Oxford.
Fig. 5.2 [8.22]

2.6 *Advancing Chemistry* (Lewis, M. & Waller, G.)
Oxford University Press, Oxford.
p. 311 [9.22]

2.7 *Supplement to DNA Replication* (Kornberg, A.)
W.H. Freeman, San Francisco.
Frontispiece [3.20]

2.8 *Molecular Basis of Antibiotic Action*, 1st edn (Gale, E.G., Cundliffe, B., Reynolds, P.E., Richmond, M.E. & Waring, M.J., eds)
Wiley Interscience, New York.
Cundliffe, E., p. 278 [3.32]
Waring, M.J., p. 173 [3.53]

2.9 *Structure of Mitochondria* (Munn, E.A. ed.)
Academic Press, London.
Kroger, A. & Klingenberg, M., p. 282 [9.18]

2.10 *A Guided Tour of the Living Cell* (Christian de Duve)
Scientific American Library.
Illustration © 1982 Neil Hardy, p. 272 [3.73], p. 344 [3.61]

2.11 *Molecular Biology of the Cell* (Alberts, B., Bray, D., Lewis, J., Raff, M., Roberts, K. & Watson, J.D., eds)
Garland, New York.
1st edn Fig. 8.24 [3.10]
2nd edn Fig. 11.35 [15.41]

2.12 *Immunology* (Eisen, H.N.)
Harper & Row, New York.
p. 132 [5.16]

2.13 *Principles of Gene Manipulation*, 3rd edn (Old, R.W. & Primrose, S.B.)
Blackwell Scientific, Oxford.
Figs 1.3 [3.84], 1.4 [3.85]

2.14 *From Cells to Atoms* (Rees, A.R. & Steinberg, M.J.E.)
Blackwell Scientific, Oxford.
Figs 10.1 [4.6], 11.2 [5.9], 26.1 [3.9], 40.2 [5.20]

2.15 *Recombinant DNA. A Short Course* (Watson, J.D., Tooze, J. & Kurtz, D.T.)
Scientific American Books.
Fig. 5.4 [3.24]

2.16 *Immunology*, 1st edn (Roitt, I.M., Brostoff, J. & Male, D.K.)
Churchill Livingstone, Edinburgh, and Gower, London
Fig. 7.8 [5.21]

2.17 *Separation of Plasma Proteins* (Curling, J.M., ed.)
Pharmacia Fine Chemicals AB, Uppsala.
Fig. 39 [2.18]

2.18 *Albumin, An Overview and Bibliography*
Miles Laboratories, TN.
Physiological transport functions of albumin [5.2]

2.19 *The Ultrastructural Anatomy of the Cell* (Allen, T.D.)
Cancer Research Campaign, London.
[1.4, 1.5, 1.6, 1.7]

2.20 *Biochemical Messengers* (Hardie, D.G.)
Chapman and Hall, London.
Figs 6.6 [15.18], 8.43 [6.34]

2.21 *Molecular Biology and Biotechnology* (Smith, C.A. & Wood, E.J., eds)
Chapman and Hall, London.
Figs 4.4 [3.51], 4.12 [3.50], 7.8 & 7.19 [3.65]

2.22 *Gene Regulation* (Latchman, D.)
Unwin Hyman, London.
Figs 7.9, 7.10 [3.64, 3.66]

2.23 *The New Genetics and Clinical Practice* 3rd edn (Weatherall, D.J.)
Oxford University Press, Oxford.
Fig. 79 [3.86]

2.24 *Introduction to Protein Structure* (Branden, C. & Tooze, J.)
Garland Publishing, New York & London.
Figs 2.6 & 2.7 [4.4]

2.25 *Molecular Biology of Oncogenes and Cell Control Mechanisms* (Parker, P.J. & Katan, M., eds)
Ellis Horwood, Chichester.
p. 85, Fig. 5 [6.22], p. 89, Fig. 7 [6.23], p. 90, Fig. 8 [6.24]

2.26 *Gene Structure and Transcription* 2nd edn (Beebee, T. & Burke, J.)
IRL Press, Oxford. With permission of Oxford University Press.
Fig. 4.9 [3.67]

3 Reviews

3.1 *Companion to Biochemistry* (Bull, A.T., Lagnado, J.R., Thomas, J.O. & Tipton, K.F., eds)
Longman, London.
Campbell, P.N. (1979) *2*, Fig. 8.1 [3.71]

3.2 *FEBS Symposium* Vol. 53 (Rapoport, S. & Scherve, T., eds)
Pergamon Press, Oxford.
Grant, M.E., pp. 29–41 [5.8]

3.3 *The Plasma Proteins* (Putnam, F.W., ed.)
Academic Press, London.
Putnam, F.W., vol. III, p. 14 [5.13]

3.4 *The Enzymes*, 3rd edn (Boyer, P.D., ed.)
Academic Press, London.
Dickerson, R.E. & Timkovich, R., vol. XI, p. 441, Fig. 8 [6.44]

3.5 *Essays in Biochemistry* (Campbell, P.N., Greville, G.D., Dickens. F., Marshall, R.D. & Tipton, K.F., eds)
Academic Press, London.
Williamson, A.R. (1982) *18*, p. 24, Fig. 13 [3.60]
Sekiguchi, K., Maeda, T. & Titani, K. (1991) *26*, p. 41, Fig. 2 [15.52], p. 40. Fig. 1 [15.53]
Hall, L. & Campbell, P.N. (1986) *22*, p. 3, Fig. 1 [4.9], Table 1 [4.10]
Grant, P.T. & Coombs, T.L. (1970) *6*, p. 76, Fig. 3 [3.38]

3.6 *Current Topics in Cell Regulation* (Horecker, B.L. & Stadtman, E.R., eds) Academic Press, London.
Masters, C.J. (1977) *12*, p. 77, Fig. 2 [6.29]

3.7 *Trends in Biochemical Sciences*
Elsevier/North Holland, Amsterdam.
Huber, M. (1979) *4*, p. 271, Fig. 7 [5.15]
Spiegel, A.M., Backlund, P.S. Jr, Butrynski, J.E., Jones, T.L.Z. & Simonds, W.F. (1991) *16*, p. 339, Fig. 1 [15.6]

3.8 *Seminars in Hematology*
Grune and Stratton, New York.
Rachmilewitz, E.A. (1974) *11*, p. 453, Fig. 5 [4.16]

3.9 *Annual Reviews of Biochemistry*
Annual Reviews, CA.
McIntosh, J.R. & Snyder, J.A. (1976) *45*, p. 706, Fig. 1 [15.43]
Klee, C.B., Crouch, T.H. & Richman, P.G. (1980) *49*, p. 496, Fig. 1 [6.25]
Ferguson, M.A.J. & Williams, A.F. (1988) *57*, p. 292, Fig. 1 [15.7] modified
Strynadka, N.C.J. & James, M.N.G. (1989) *58*, p. 962, Fig. 1 [6.26]
Edelman, G.M. & Crossin, K.L. (1991) *60*, pp. 158, 159, Fig. 1 [15.50]
Kaziro, Y., Itoh, H., Kozasa, T., Nakafuku, M. & Satoh, T. (1991) *60*, p. 361, Fig. 5 [15.24]
Dohlman, H.K., Thorner, J., Caron, M.G. & Lefkowitz, R.J. (1991) *60*, p. 662, Fig. la [15.11]

3.10 *Scientific American*
Grobstein, C. (1977) July, p. 30 [3.82]
Brown, M.S. & Goldstein, J.L. (1984) Nov., p. 55 [230], p. 56 [15.10]
Rothman, J.E. (1985) Sept., p. 86 [3.74]
Lodish, H.F. & Dautry-Varsat, A. (1984) May, p. 51 [15.10]
Gallo, R.C. (1987) Jan., p. 46 [3.31].

3.11 *Biochimica et Biophysica Acta*
Elsevier/North Holland, Amsterdam.
Lotan, R. & Nicolson, G.L. (1979) *559*, p. 239 [15.5]
Kagawa, Y. (1978) *505*, p. 47 [15.46]
Small, D.M., Penkett, S.A. & Chapman, D. (1969) *176*, p. 178, Fig. 7 [12.13]

3.12 *Biomedicine*
Springer International, Berlin.
Maclouf, J., Sors, H. & Rigaud, M. (1977) *26*, p. 362 [14.19]

3.13 *Haemoglobin and Red Cell Structure and Function* (Brewer, G.J., ed.)
Plenum Press, London (1972).
Brenna, O., Luzzana, M., Pace, M., Perrella, M., Rossi, F., Rossi, F.,
R. Bernardi, L. & Roughton, F.J.W., p. 20, Fig. 1 [4.26]

3.14 *Advances in Protein Chemistry*
Academic Press, New York (1981).
Richardson, J.S. *34*, p. 262, Fig. 73, p. 263, Fig. 74, p. 266, Fig. 77
[4.6]

3.15 *Advances in Enzyme Regulation*
Pergamon Press, Oxford.
Saggerson, D., Ghadiminejad, I. & Awan, M. (1992) *32*, p. 286,
Fig. 1 [13.19]

3.16 *Biochemistry*
American Chemical Society, Washington, DC.
Stroud, R.M., McCarthy, M.P. & Shuster, M. (1990) *29*, p. 11013,
Fig. 3 [15.15]
Huber, R. & Carrell, R.W. (1989) *28*, modified from p. 8960,
Fig. 2 [4.8]

3.17 *Cell*
MIT Press, Cambridge, MA.
Cantley, L.C., Auger, K.R., Carpenter, C., Duckworth, B.,
Graziano, A.
Kapeller, R. & Soltoff, S. (1991) *64*, p. 282, Fig. 01 [15.34],
p. 285, Fig. 4 [15.35]

3.18 *Bioessays*
The Company of Biologists Limited, Cambridge.
Dustin, M.L (1990) *12*, p. 422, Fig. 1 [15.51]

3.19 *Journal of Cell Science*
The Company of Biologists Limited, Cambridge.
Grinnell, F. (1992) *101*, p. 3, Fig. 1 [15.54]

3.20 *BioEssays*
Wiley-Liss Inc.N.Y., New York.
Pruss, D., Hayes, J.J. & Wolffe, A.P. (1995), *17*, p. 163, Fig. 2
[3.10B]

3.21 *Trends in Biochemical Sciences*
Elsevier/North Holland, Amsterdam, reprinted with permission
from the publisher.
Schwabe, J.W.R. & Rhodes, D. (1991) *16*, p. 292, Fig. 1 [3.69]
Lane, D.P. & Hall, P.A.(1997) *22*, p. 373, Fig. 2 [16.4]

3.22 *Advances in Protein Chemistry*
Academic Press, New York.
Carter, D.C. & Ho, J.X. (1994) *45*, p. 195, Fig. 21 [5.3]

3.23 *International Reviews in Experimental Pathology*
Academic Press, New York.
Arends, M.J. & Wyllie, A.H. (1991), *32*, p. 223, Fig. 1 [16.1]

3.24 *Current Opinion in Cell Biology*
Current Biology Ltd, London.
Viel, A. & Branton, D. (1996) *8*, p. 52, Fig. 5 [15.39]

3.25 *Biochemical Society Transactions*
Portland Press, London, reprinted with permission © the
Biochemical Society.
Printz, R.L., Osawa, H., Ardehali, H., Koch, S. & Granner, D.K.
(1997) *25*, p.109, Fig. 1 [6.38]
Holness, M.J., Fryer, L.G.D. & Sugden, M.C. (1997) *25*, p. 2,
Fig. 1 [13.3]

3.26 *Biochemical Journal*
Portland Press, London, reprinted with permission © The
Biochemical Journal.
Iynedjian, P.B. (1993) *293*, p. 232, Fig. 1 [6.40], p. 239, Fig. 4 [13.12]
Hufton, S.E., Jennings, I.G. & Cotton, R.G.H. (1995) *311*, p.
359, Fig. 4 [8.20]

3.27 *FASEB Journal*
The Federation of American Societies for Experimental Biology.
Chiang, P.K., Gordon, R.K., Tal, J., Zeng, G.C., Doctor, B.P.,
Pardhasaradhi, K. & McCann, P.P. (1996) *10*, p. 472, Fig. 1 [8.16]
Patel, M.S. & Harris, R.A. (1995) *9*, p. 1166, Fig. 3 [13.17]

3.28 *Advances in Genetics*
Academic Press, New York.
Eisensmith, R.C. & Woo, S.L.C. (1995) *32*, p. 201, Fig. 6.1
[8.19]

3.29 *Biochimica et Biophysica Acta*
Elsevier Science, Amsterdam, reprinted with permission from the
publisher.
Meister, A. (1995) *1271*, p. 37, Fig. 2 [9.35], p. 40, Fig. 9 [9.34]

3.30 *Journal of Nutrition*
American Institute of Nutrition.
Gray, G.M. (1992) *122*, p. 173, Fig. 1 [11.4]
Gurney, A.L., Park, E.A., Liu, J., Giralt, M., McGrane, M.M.,
Patel, Y.M., Nizielski, S.E., Savon, S. & Hanson, R.W. (1994) *124*,
p.1535S, Fig. 1 [13.14], p. 1536S, Fig. 2 [13.15]

3.31 *Nature, London*
Macmillan, London.
Goldstein, J.L. & Brown, M.S. (1990) *343*, p. 425, Fig. 1 [13.21],
p. 427, Fig. 3 [13.22] (Reprinted with permission from
NATURE. © (1990) Macmillan Magazines Limited).

3.32 *Journal of Diabetes and its Complications*
Elsevier Science, reprinted with permission from the publisher.
Kahn, C.R. & Goldfine, A.B. (1993) *7*, p. 93, Fig. 1 [15.13], p. 95,
Fig. 2 [15.12], p. 97, Fig. 4 [15.14]

3.33 *EMBO Journal*
Oxford University Press, Oxford.
Smith, C.J., Grigorieff, N. & Pearse, M.F. (1998) *17*, p. 4946, Fig.
5 [15.38]

3.34 *FEBS Letters*
Elsevier Science, B.V., Amsterdam.
Heldin, C-H. (1997) *410*, p. 18, Fig. 1 [15.33]
Cohen, P., Alessi, D.R. & Cross, A.E. (1997) *410*, p. 5, Fig. 4
[13.4]

3.35 *Gastroenterology*
W. B. Saunders, Orlando.
Lowe, M.E. (1994) *107*, p. 1538, Fig. 3 [11.5]

3.36 *American Journal of Pathology*
American Society for Investigative Pathology
Alexander, N., Wong, C.S. & Pignatelli, M. (2002) *160*, p. 390,
Fig. 1 [16.7]

4 Papers in journals

4.1 *Journal of Molecular Biology*
Academic Press, London.
Josephs, R., Jarosch, H.S. & Edelstein, S.J. (1976) *102*, p. 409,
Fig. 6d [4.17]
Sigler, P.B., Blow, D.M., Matthews, B.W. & Henderson, R. (1968)
35, p. 143, Fig. 6 [6.5]
Rich, A. (1961) *3*, p. 483, Fig. 2 [5.7]

4.2 *Biochemical Education*
International Union of Biochemistry and Pergamon Press,
Oxford.
Hall, L. & Campbell, P. N. (1979) *7*, p. 57 [3.56, 3.83]
Henderson, J.F. (1979) *7*, p. 52, Fig. 2 [6.57]
Smith, I. (1980) *8*, p. 1 [3.39]

4.3 *Science*
American Association for the Advancement of Science.
Baulieu, E.-E. (1989) *245*, p. 1352, Fig. 2 [3.70]

4.4 *Cell*
MIT Press, Cambridge, MA.
Lai, E.C., et al (1979) *18*, p. 834, Fig. 6 [3.55]

4.5 *Proceedings of the National Academy of Sciences, USA*
The National Academy of Sciences, Washington, DC.
Palade, G.E. (1964) *52*, p. 617, Fig. 2 [9.18]
Siverton, E.L. (1977) *74*, p. 5142, Fig. 3 [5.14]

4.6 *Philosophical Transactions of the Royal Society B*
The Royal Society, London.
Evans, P.R., Farrants, G.W. & Hudson, P.J. (1981) *293*, p. 53,
Fig. 2B [6.33]

4.7   *Journal of Cell Biology*
        The Rockefeller University Press, New York.
        Fernandez-Moran, H., Oda, T., Blair, P.V. & Green, D.E. (1964)
        22, p. 73, Figs 6, 7 [9.25]
        Alexander, C.A., Hamilton, R.L. & Havel, R.J. (1976) *69*, p. 260,
        Fig. 14 [11.21]
        Osborn, M., Webster, R.E. & Weber, K. (1978) *77*, R.29 [15.42]

4.8   *Nature, London*
        Macmillan, London.
        Arnone, A. (1972) *237*, p. 148 [4.21]
        Poorman, R.A. et al (1984) *309*, p. 468 [6.32]
        Ungewickell, E. & Branton, D. (1981) *289*, p. 420, Fig. 3 [15.38]
        Barford, D. & Johnson, L.N. (1989) *340*, p. 609, Fig. 1 [10.9]
        Benesch, R. & Benesch, R. (1969) *221*, pp. 618-622 [4.25]

4.9   *Biochemical Journal*
        The Biochemical Society.
        Andrews, P. (1964) *91*, p. 222 [2.17]

4.10   *Journal of Biological Chemistry*
        American Society of Biological Chemists.
        Rosenberg, L., Hellmann, W. & Kleinschmidt, A.K. (1975) *250*, p.
        1877, Fig. 1 [7.11]

4.11   *Immunology Today*
        Elsevier, North Holland, Amsterdam.
        Brodsky, F.M. (1984) *5*, p. 350, Fig. 4 [15.37]

4.12   *Médecine Sciences*
        CDR Centrale des Revues/John Libby Eurotext, Montrouge.
        Hue, L. & Rider, M.H. *3*, p. 569, Fig. 2 [13.9]

4.13   *Cell Motility and the Cytoskeleton*
        Alan R. Liss, New York.
        Lawson, D. (1987) *7*, p. 371, Fig. 2 [15.40]

4.14   *The Plant Journal*
        Blackwell Science, Oxford.
        Traas, J.A., Beven, A.F., Doonan, J.H., Cordewener, J. & Shaw, P.J.
        (1992) *2*, p. 729, Fig. 6 [5.25]

4.15   *Nature, London*
        Macmillan, London.
        Raff, M. (1998) *396*, p. 119, Fig. 1 [16.2]
        Clurman, B. & Groudine, M. (1997) *389*, p.123, Fig. 1 [16.3]
        (Reprinted with permission from NATURE, © Macmillan
        Magazines Limited).

4.16   *Science*
        American Association for the Advancement of Science.
        Editorial (1997) *276*, p. 701 Tree of Life [1.1]

4.17   *Biochemistry*
        The American Chemical Society.
        Joshi, A.K., Witkowski, A. & Smith, S. (1998) *37*, p. 2522, Fig. 4
        [11.15]

4.18   *American Journal of Human Genetics*
        The University of Chicago Press, Chicago.
        Sinden, R.R. (1999) *64*, p. 347, Table 1 [Table 3.7]

b.   Personal acknowledgements

We wish to thank the following for detailed help with the figures
    indicated, or for allowing us to use figures already prepared.

5.1   Beatriz S. Magalhaes, Department of Biochemistry and
        Molecular Biology, University College London [2.14]

5.2   Professor J.S. Hyams, Department of Biology, University College
        London [3.12]

5.3   Professor K.R. Harrap, Cancer Research Campaign Laboratories,
        Sutton [3.23]

5.4   Dr D.F. Steiner, Howard Hughes Medical Institute, University of
        Chicago [3.38, 3.39]

5.5   Dr T.R. Dafforn, Cambridge Institute for Medical Research,
        University of Cambridge [4.1, 4.5, 4.7, 4.11, 4.12, 4.13, 4.14]

5.6   Professor R. Carrell, Cambridge Institute for Medical Research,
        University of Cambridge [5.4, 5.5]

5.7   Dr Stephen D.R. Harridge, Department of Physiology, Royal
        Free & University College Medical School, London [5.26]

5.8   Dr Norman Taylor, Principal Biochemist, Kings College Hospital
        [14.23, 14.25, Table 14.1] and help with the steroid hormone
        metabolism section

5.9   Dr E. Hounsell and Mr D. Renouf, Department of Biochemistry
        and Molecular Biology, University College London [14.28]

We also thank Professor E.D. Saggerson, Department of Biochemistry and
Molecular Biology, University College London, and Professor F. Vella,
Department of Biochemistry, University of Saskatchewan, Saskatoon, for
many helpful comments. The *Oxford Dictionary of Biochemistry and
Molecular Biology*, of which we are numbered among the editors, has
proved a valuable source of information and nomenclature. For scientific
names, the recommendations of IUPAC and IUBMB have been adopted.
Otherwise British spelling is used.

Key to the references

The table below shows how the figures relate to the references.

Fig. No.	Ref. No.	Fig. No.	Ref. No.	Fig. No.	Ref. No.	Fig. No.	Ref. No.	Fig. No.	Ref. No.	Fig. No.	Ref. No.
1.1	4.16	3.41	1.1	4.5	5.5	5.19	1.8	7.11	4.10	15.6	3.7
1.4	2.19	3.46	1.1	4.6	3.13	5.20	2.14	8.16	3.27	15.7	3.9
1.5	2.19	3.49	1.1	4.6	2.14	5.21	2.16	8.19	3.28	15.10	3.10
1.6	2.19	3.50	2.21	4.7	5.5	5.25	4.14	8.20	3.26	15.11	3.9
1.7	2.19	3.51	2.21	4.8	3.16	5.26	5.7	8.22	2.5	15.12	3.32
1.8	1.11	3.52	1.1	4.9	3.5	5.27	1.4	9.18	4.5, 2.9	15.13	3.32
1.10	2.2	3.53	2.8	4.10	3.5	5.28	1.4	9.22	2.6	15.14	3.32
2.5	1.1	3.55	4.4	4.11	5.5	5.29	1.13	9.25	4.7	15.15	3.16
2.6	1.1	3.56	4.2	4.12	5.5	5.30	1.13	9.28	1.2	15.18	2.20
2.7	1.1	3.57	1.3	4.13	5.5	5.31	1.4	9.29	1.2	15.24	3.9
2.8	1.3	3.58	1.12	4.14	5.5	5.32	1.4	9.34	3.29	15.33	3.34
2.12	1.1	3.60	3.5	4.16	3.8	5.33	1.4	9.35	3.29	15.35	3.17
2.13	1.10	3.61	2.10	4.17	4.1	5.34	1.13	10.9	4.8	15.37	4.11
2.14	5.1	3.62	2.4	4.21	4.8, 1.3	5.35	1.13	11.4	3.30	15.38	4.8, 3.33
2.15	1.1	3.63	1.3	4.22	1.3	6.5	4.1	11.5	3.35	15.39	3.24
2.17	4.9	3.64	2.22	4.23	1.3	6.8	2.3	11.15	4.17	15.40	4.13
2.18	2.17	3.65	2.21	4.24	1.3	6.9	2.3	11.21	4.7	15.41	2.11
2.19	2.1	3.66	2.22	4.25	4.8	6.10	2.3	12.13	3.11	15.42	4.7
2.20	1.3	3.67	2.26	4.26	3.13	6.16	1.7	13.3	3.25	15.43	3.9
3.5	1.5	3.68	1.13	5.2	2.18	6.22	2.25	13.4	3.34	15.46	3.11
3.9	2.14	3.69	3.21	5.3	3.22	6.23	2.25	13.9	4.12	15.49	1.9
3.10 A	2.11	3.70	4.3	5.4	5.6	6.24	2.25	13.10	1.6	15.50	3.9
3.10 B	3.20	3.71	3.1	5.5	5.6	6.25	3.9	13.12	3.26	15.51	3.18
3.12	5.2	3.73	2.10	5.8	3.2	6.26	3.9	13.14	3.30	15.53	3.5
3.17	1.1	3.74	3.9	5.9	2.14	6.29	3.6	13.15	3.30	15.54	3.19
3.20	2.7	3.79	1.7	5.7	4.1	6.30	2.3	13.16	1.6	16.1	3.23
3.23	5.3	3.80	1.7	5.10	1.14	6.31	1.2	13.17	3.27	16.2	4.15
3.24	2.15	3.82	3.10	5.11	1.14	6.32	4.8	13.19	3.15	16.3	4.15
3.25	1.16	3.83	4.2	5.12	1.14	6.33	4.6	13.21	3.31	16.4	3.21
3.29	1.3	3.84	2.13	5.13	3.3	6.34	2.20	13.22	3.31	Table	5.8
3.30	1.5	3.85	2.13	5.14	4.5	6.38	3.27	14.19	3.12	14.1	
3.31	3.10	3.86	2.23	5.15	3.7	6.40	1.1	14.23	5.8		
3.32	2.8	4.1	5.5	5.16	2.12	6.44	3.4	14.25	5.8		
3.38	5.4	4.2	1.1	5.17	1.15	6.46	1.2	14.28	5.9		
3.39	5.4, 4.2	4.4	2.24	5.18	1.15	6.57	4.2	15.5	3.11		

Contents

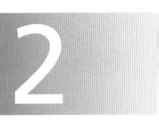

The post-genomic era and its impact on the future of biochemistry and molecular biology

The cellular basis of biochemistry

Three families of living cell can be identified: the Bacteria, the Eukarya and the Archaea. Bacteria are denoted as prokaryotes, and animal cells and fungi as eukaryotes. The eukaryotes are characterized by the presence of a nucleus that retains most of the DNA and by the presence of many membrane-limited organelles. After defining exocytosis and endocytosis, which are characteristic of eukaryotes, the structure of the nucleus, mitochondria, lysosomes, peroxisomes, the endoplasmic reticulum and the cytoskeleton are briefly described. The subcellular components can be studied by electron microscopy and isolated by differential centrifugation after disruption of the plasma membrane. The morphological constituents of the isolated fractions can be determined by analysis for nucleic acids and proteins and by the presence of marker enzymes. This is achieved either by isolation of the organelles or by in situ methods. The total metabolism of any particular cell is subdivided among the various organelles, and the distribution of activity within the cell is briefly described.

TYPES OF LIVING CELL

Three families, also called domains, of living cells can be characterized: namely the Bacteria, the Eukarya and the Archaea. The evolutionary tree of these families and their offspring is shown in Fig. 1.1. The oldest cells in evolutionary terms appear to be the hyperthermophiles, which are able to live in extremely hot conditions. In terms of structure and biochemical activity, the Bacteria and Eukarya differ markedly, and it is usual to denote the Bacteria as prokaryotes and the Eukarya as eukaryotes; the Archaea occupy an intermediate position closer to the Eukarya than to the Bacteria.

It can be seen from Fig. 1.1 that animals occupy a position at the top of the chain of the eukaryotes, not far from the plants and fungi (which include the yeasts). Elaborate mechanisms exist to protect animals from invasion by the prokaryotic bacteria and other eukaryotes. We know of no instance where members of the Archaea invade animals, and thus we will be concerned in this book only with the biochemistry of eukaryotes, as represented by the higher eukaryotes, and the prokaryotes that cause disease in man.

All living cells reproduce in a similar manner and have the same basic metabolism for the synthesis and interconversion of biochemicals. On this basis, biochemists and molecular biologists experiment with many different species of living cells in their search for clues leading to an understanding of the metabolism of multicellular animals such as man. Bacteria,

particularly *Escherichia coli*, have been a major source of discovery but more recently other models, such as the yeasts (budding and fission), the nematode worm, the fruit fly, the zebra fish and the mouse, have proved to be rich sources for our better understanding of human metabolism.

THE STRUCTURE OF PROKARYOTIC AND EUKARYOTIC CELLS

Figure 1.2 shows some of the major structural features of the two types of cell. It can be seen that most of the DNA in eukaryotes is surrounded by the nuclear membrane, which is not present in prokaryotes. The non-nuclear part of eukaryotic cells is known as the cytoplasm, although the term is often used to describe the cell other than the nucleus and mitochondria. That part of the cell in which organized components cannot be detected is known as the cytosol. This term should be confined to the description of the intact cell and should not be confused with the soluble supernatant that results from the centrifugation of disrupted cells. In prokaryotes, the chromosomes are circular, in contrast to the linear chromosomes of eukaryotes. The cytoplasm of prokaryotes is largely undifferentiated, whereas in eukaryotes it contains various membrane-bound organelles such as mitochondria (also chloroplasts in plants), lysosomes, peroxisomes and the Golgi apparatus.

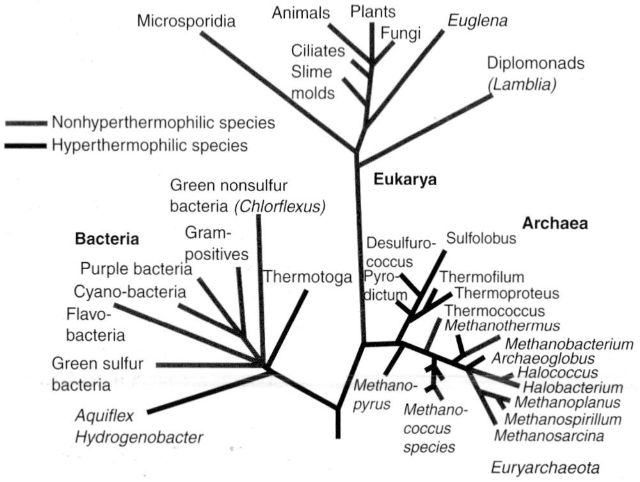

Prokaryotes are protected by a cell wall, which is more substantial than the plasma membrane of animal cells. In prokaryotes, reproduction is by binary division, in eukaryotes by mitosis.

ENDOCYTOSIS AND EXOCYTOSIS THROUGH THE PLASMA MEMBRANE

Endocytosis is the process whereby cells take up macromolecules, particulate substances and, in the case of some particular cell types, even other cells. The material to be ingested is enclosed by the plasma membrane, which invaginates and then pinches off to form an intracellular vesicle, as shown in Fig. 1.3. If the ingested material is fluid in nature, the process is called pinocytosis ('cellular drinking'); phagocytosis ('cellular eating') is the term given when the ingested material consists of large particles such as cell debris or microorganisms. The latter process involves the formation of phagosomes. The reverse process is known as exocytosis. These processes are peculiar to eukaryotes and do not occur in prokaryotes.

THE NUCLEUS

The nucleus of eukaryotes contains the DNA organized into separate chromosomes. (Mitochondria also contain a small amount of DNA, which is therefore known as non-chromosomal DNA.) There are 23 pairs of chromosomes in a human diploid cell, giving a diploid number of 46, with half as many in a haploid cell. Cells with more than the normal complement of DNA are said to be polyploid when they contain more than the usual number of standard chromosomes. The nucleolus is a region within the nucleus, as shown in Fig. 1.4, in which the genes for three of the ribosomal RNA molecules are located. The nuclear membrane is double layered with a perinuclear space. Transfer of substances between the cytoplasm and nucleus is through the nuclear pore, which is a complex of proteins in an octagonal array with a central hole. The proteins synthesized in the cytoplasm (see p. 46) move into the nucleus, whereas the RNA synthesized within the nucleus moves out to the cytoplasm. The structure that surrounds the inner nuclear membrane is the lamina; it contains three proteins: lamins A, B and C. The lamina interconnects the chromosomes.

Fig. 1.1 The tree of life. The Woese family tree shows that most life is one-celled and that the oldest cells were hyperthermophiles.

Animal Cell

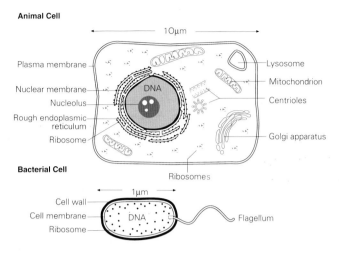

Bacterial Cell

Fig. 1.2 Comparison of the cell structure of a eukaryote (e.g. animal cell) and a prokaryote (e.g. bacterium).

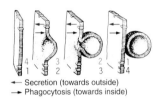

← Secretion (towards outside)
→ Phagocytosis (towards inside)

Fig. 1.3 The processes of exocytosis (secretion) and endocytosis (uptake).

MITOCHONDRIA

Mitochondria are unique organelles within the cytoplasm and lack any direct interaction with other organelles. Although they contain some DNA, which is expressed to produce some mitochondrial protein, most of their protein is derived from the cytoplasm (see p. 46). Besides being a major source of energy in the form of adenosine triphosphate (ATP) produced

by the respiratory chain, mitochondria are also involved in fatty acid catabolism and help to control the level of Ca^{2+} in the cytoplasm.

Mitochondrial membranes are about 6.5 nm thick and the inner membrane is folded to form cristae, thereby substantially increasing the total membranous surface of the organelle. The inner surfaces of the cristae are closely packed with 8.5-nm diameter particles, the site of oxidative phosphorylation (see p. 140). The central part of the organelle is known as the matrix. The major features of mitochondrial structure are shown in Fig. 1.5.

LYSOSOMES

Lysosomes are membrane-bound vesicles that contain a wide range of hydrolytic enzymes, which break down the various types of macromolecules. Lysosomes are

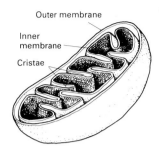

Fig. 1.5 The structure of a mitochondrion.

important in terms of the intracellular digestive system, so that, for example, substances and components of the cell that are to be degraded form phagosomes, which fuse with the lysosomes to form secondary lysosomes (see p. 48).

PEROXISOMES

These organelles were formerly called microbodies. They contain predominantly catalase, urate oxidase, fatty acid oxidases and D-amino acid oxidase and are surrounded by a single membrane. The oxidases generate hydrogen peroxide which is removed by catalase (see p. 46).

THE ENDOPLASMIC RETICULUM

The endoplasmic reticulum is a network of membranes that runs throughout the matrix of the cytoplasm. These membranes form a complex arrangement of connecting vesicles and tubules or large flattened sacs. The membranes run parallel to each other, creating channels called cisternae. The interior of the cisternae is known as the lumen, and the proteins within it are known as the luminal proteins. Large areas of membrane are thus created and it is estimated that the surface area of the endoplasmic reticulum in 1 ml of cytoplasm is $11 \, m^2$. The surface might bear ribosomes (rough-surfaced endoplasmic reticulum, RER) or might not (smooth-surfaced endoplasmic reticulum, SER). The ribosomes are the site of protein synthesis (see p. 35). The RER is the site of synthesis of proteins, which are secreted (see p. 45), whereas the SER is important as a site of synthesis of complex lipids (see p. 186). A cartoon of the endoplasmic reticulum is shown in Fig. 1.6.

THE CYTOSKELETON

The high resolution obtained with the electron microscope shows that there is a

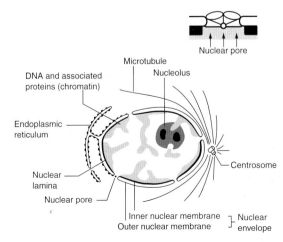

Fig. 1.4 The fine structure of the eukaryotic nucleus.

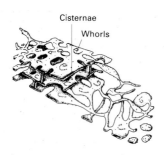

Fig. 1.6 The architecture of the endoplasmic reticulum.

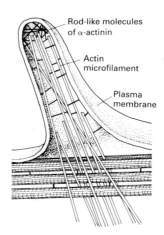

Fig. 1.7 Components of the cytoskeleton.

structural lattice even within the cytosol. This lattice is generally composed of three types of filament: microfilaments (which are multimers of the protein actin; see p. 211), microtubules (which are multimers of the protein tubulin; see p. 212) and a heterogeneous group called intermediate filaments (see p. 212). Cell surface extensions are commonly supported by a core of microfilaments to produce an increase in the surface area; this can be seen in Fig. 1.7, which shows the main features of the cytoskeleton as exemplified by the lining of the small intestine.

SUBCELLULAR FRACTIONATION

The structure and biochemical activity of the various organelles contained within the eukaryotic cell can be determined in various ways but the method commonly used by biochemists is to disrupt the cells and separate the constituents by centrifugation. The principles are shown in Fig. 1.8. The cells are disrupted as carefully as possible so as to minimize the damage to the organelles. The rather harsh Waring blendor can be employed but more often a Potter homogenizer, which comprises a glass tube with a rapidly rotating pestle

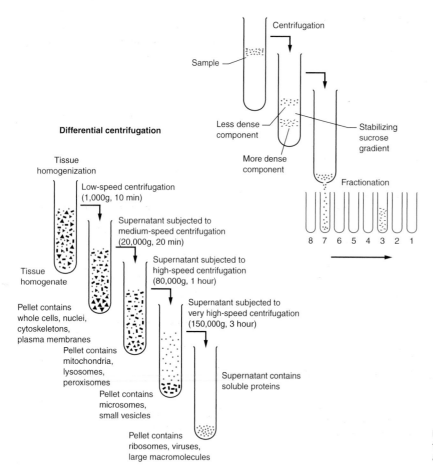

A

HYPOTHETICAL CELL
resembling hepatocyte

Fig. caption labels: Rough endoplasmic reticulum, Ribosomes, Mitochondrion, Plasma membrane, Smooth endoplasmic reticulum, Nucleus, Cytosol (the aqueous phase between organelles), Lysosome, Peroxisome

B

Isopycnic (sucrose-density) centrifugation

Centrifugation

Sample

Less dense component

More dense component

Stabilizing sucrose gradient

Fractionation

8 7 6 5 4 3 2 1

Differential centrifugation

Tissue homogenization

Low-speed centrifugation (1,000g, 10 min)

Supernatant subjected to medium-speed centrifugation (20,000g, 20 min)

Supernatant subjected to high-speed centrifugation (80,000g, 1 hour)

Supernatant subjected to very high-speed centrifugation (150,000g, 3 hour)

Tissue homogenate

Pellet contains whole cells, nuclei, cytoskeletons, plasma membranes

Pellet contains mitochondria, lysosomes, peroxisomes

Pellet contains microsomes, small vesicles

Supernatant contains soluble proteins

Pellet contains ribosomes, viruses, large macromolecules

Fig. 1.8 The fractionation by centrifugation of the morphological components of disrupted animal cells.

made either of glass or of Teflon, is used. The product is often loosely referred to as a 'homogenate'. Three methods can be used to obtain fractions enriched with respect to the various organelles based on the differences in their size and density. In differential centrifugation (seen on the left in Fig. 1.8), the pellets obtained are never homogeneous with respect to the morphological constituents because the homogenate is initially dispersed throughout the tube. In isopycnic centrifugation (shown on the right of Fig. 1.8), the homogenate is layered on the top of a sucrose density gradient and the centrifugation proceeds until an equilibrium is reached. Because this takes a long time, a third, compromise, method is used in which the homogenate is layered on the top of the gradient but the tube is spun for a shorter time. In this case, the main role of the gradient is to provide stability, particularly when the contents of the tube are being collected.

Irrespective of the method of separation, it should be remembered that the morphological characteristics of the pellets or fractions will differ according to the tissue under study. Thus it is essential that all fractions are examined either by microscopy or by analysis of the marker enzymes (see below).

THE MICROSOME FRACTION

As an example of the separation of the components of a disrupted cell, Fig. 1.9

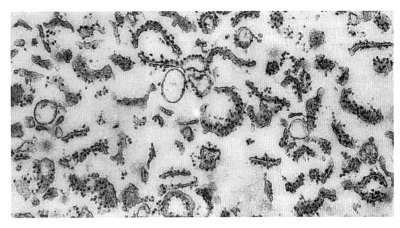

Fig. 1.9 The morphological constituents of a typical microsome fraction from liver as revealed by electron microscopy.

shows an electron micrograph of the microsome fraction from rat liver. It is common to define the microsome fraction as that which sediments more slowly than the mitochondrial fraction but that is particulate. As can be seen, the pellet is far from homogeneous but consists predominantly of fragments of the endoplasmic reticulum and even the plasma membrane. As indicated above, such a fraction from another tissue might contain only membrane-free ribosomes.

MARKER ENZYMES

Confirmation of the morphological constituents of the various subcellular fractions can be obtained by biochemical analysis. Thus the DNA/protein ratio or RNA/protein ratio can be determined. Enzymic analysis is also useful, based on the principle that usually (but not always) one particular enzyme is associated only with one particular morphological constituent of the cell and that the enzyme make-up of a particular cell constituent is unique (e.g. all mitochondria are identical – probably almost true). Such enzymes are known as marker enzymes. Examples are 5'-nucleotidase for the plasma membrane, glucose-6-phosphatase for liver endoplasmic reticulum, galactosyltransferase for Golgi membranes (see p. 45) and succinate dehydrogenase for mitochondria (see also p. 140).

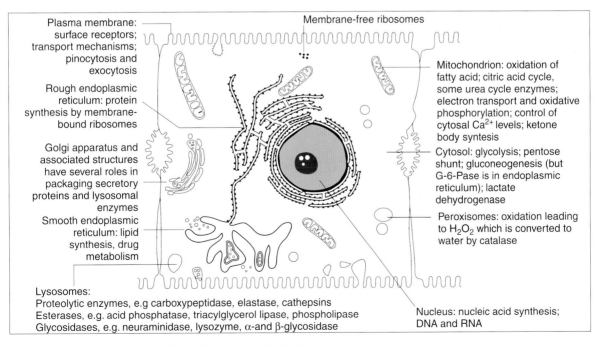

Plasma membrane: surface receptors; transport mechanisms; pinocytosis and exocytosis

Membrane-free ribosomes

Rough endoplasmic reticulum: protein synthesis by membrane-bound ribosomes

Golgi apparatus and associated structures have several roles in packaging secretory proteins and lysosomal enzymes

Smooth endoplasmic reticulum: lipid synthesis, drug metabolism

Mitochondrion: oxidation of fatty acid; citric acid cycle, some urea cycle enzymes; electron transport and oxidative phosphorylation; control of cytosal Ca^{2+} levels; ketone body syntesis

Cytosol: glycolysis; pentose shunt; gluconeogenesis (but G-6-Pase is in endoplasmic reticulum); lactate dehydrogenase

Peroxisomes: oxidation leading to H_2O_2 which is converted to water by catalase

Lysosomes:
Proteolytic enzymes, e.g carboxypeptidase, elastase, cathepsins
Esterases, e.g. acid phosphatase, triacylglycerol lipase, phospholipase
Glycosidases, e.g. neuraminidase, lysozyme, α-and β-glycosidase

Nucleus: nucleic acid synthesis; DNA and RNA

Fig. 1.10 The metabolic function of organelles within a typical animal cell.

METABOLIC FUNCTIONS OF ORGANELLES

Although an extensive description of metabolism is given in the following chapters, it might be useful at this stage to indicate briefly the main features of the distribution of the metabolic activities in a cell such as a hepatocyte. This is illustrated in Fig. 1.10, which is self-explanatory.

A common approach used by biochemists has been to experiment on disrupted cells and examine their contents. However, biochemists also realize that the conditions in these in vitro experiments might be very different to those pertaining in intact cells, which complicates the interpretation of the results. A common way of overcoming this problem has been to use isotopes, sometimes stable (e.g. ^{15}N) but usually radioactive (e.g. ^{14}C, ^{3}H, ^{35}S, ^{131}I). Autoradiography can be used to locate the labelled metabolite within the cells. There are now many other ways of visualizing the molecules of living cells, which are mainly based on optical microscopy and the use of fluorescent tags and indicators. An example is aequorin, a luminescent protein that emits light in the presence of calcium ions and responds to changes in their concentration. The green fluorescent protein (GFP), also isolated from the jelly fish *Aequoria victoria*, can be linked to other proteins to reveal the location and activity of the modified proteins within the cell.

An introduction to proteins and peptides

The fundamental component of a protein is the polypeptide chain composed of amino acid residues; twenty different residues are involved in protein synthesis. These residues might be modified after the synthesis of the polypeptide chain. The other components of proteins are called prosthetic groups. The structure of the amino acids and their characteristic property as amphoteric molecules is described, followed by a description of asymmetry and chirality. The way in which amino acid residues interact within proteins is explained. The ionic properties of proteins are important in such interactions and in their electrophoretic separation. Proteins can also be separated on the basis of their size. After mentioning how the order of the amino acid residues in polypeptides can be determined, the hierarchies of protein structure are briefly described. The tertiary structure of proteins can be destroyed by denaturation. Finally, it is shown that even small peptides can possess biological activity, for example as hormones and transmitters.

THE ROLE OF AMINO ACIDS IN THE CELL

Amino acids are a fine example of the versatile roles performed by the cell constituents. Amino acids contain, among other functional groups, two that are common to all amino acids: an amino (or imino) group and a carboxyl group. The ability of an amino acid to condense with other amino acids to form a peptide is dependent on the chemical properties of these two functional groups. Certainly, a most important role for amino acids is to serve as the monomeric subunits of proteins, but they have other important roles. For example, the tripeptide glutathione has an important function and other small peptides serve as hormones and, in some organisms, as antibiotics; glutamic acid acts as a neural transmitter. Amino acids are the precursors of a wide variety of biomolecules (e.g. nitric oxide from arginine, histamine from histidine). Some amino acids are metabolized and utilized for the production of glucose (gluconeogenesis). As there is no store of amino acids, apart from those involved in protein structure, proteins have to be broken down to free amino acids when the latter are required for gluconeogenesis.

STRUCTURE OF AMINO ACIDS

All the common amino acids, except for proline, have the same general structure in that the α-carbon atom bears a $-COOH$ group, an $-NH_2$ group and an 'R'-group, which is responsible for the different properties of the various amino acids. A general formula for amino acids is shown in Fig. 2.1. The structures of the 20 common amino acids are shown in Fig. 2.2, grouped according to the nature of their R-groups. The internationally-approved three-letter and single-letter abbreviations for each amino acid are also indicated.

The α carbon is optically active in α-amino acids other than glycine. The two possible isomers are termed D and L. All naturally occurring amino acids found in proteins are of the L-configuration (see p. 9).

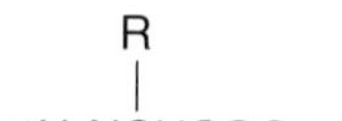

$$\underset{\text{+}H_3NCHCOO^-}{\overset{R}{|}}$$

Fig. 2.1 General formula of an amino acid.

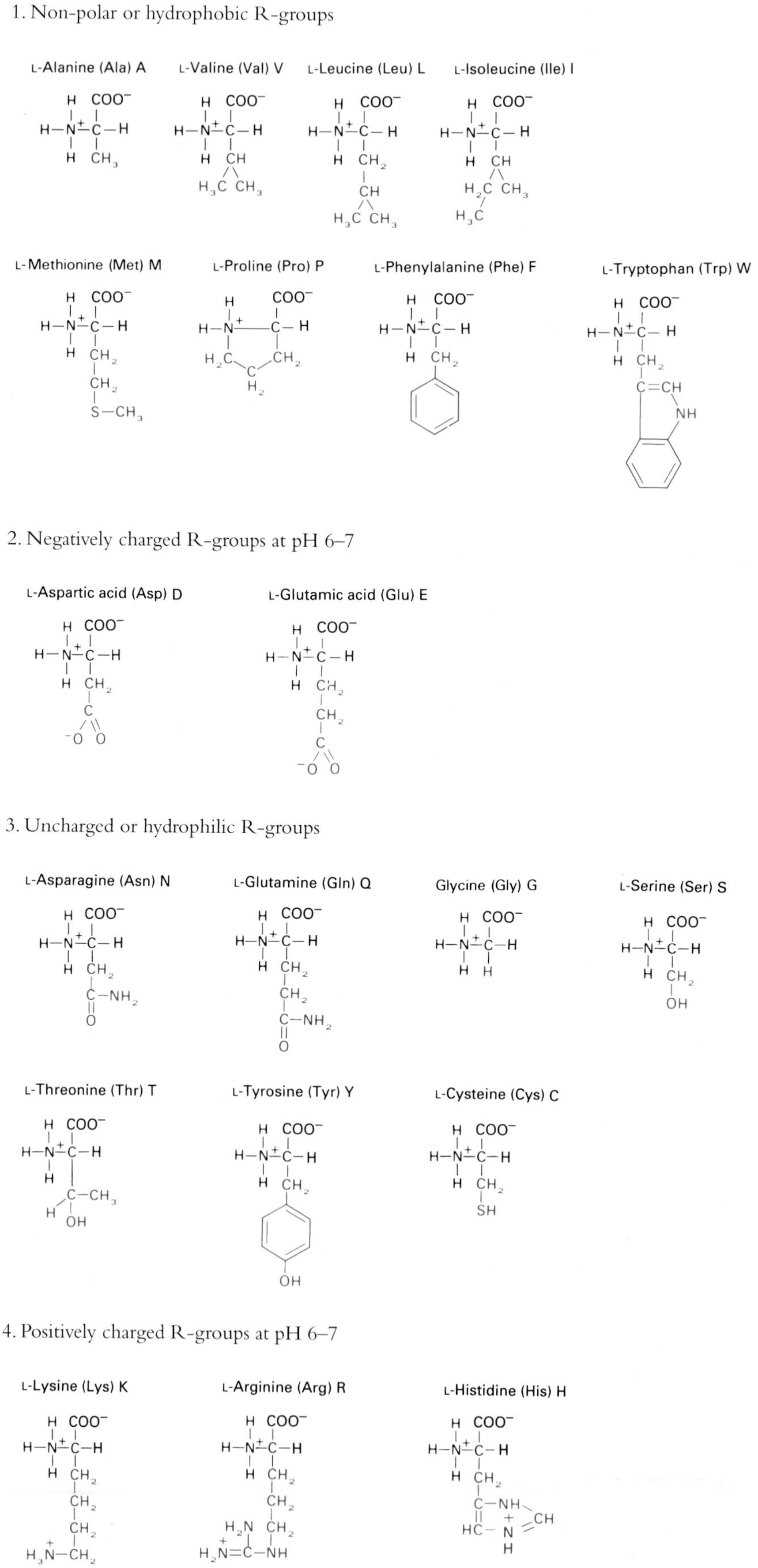

1. Non-polar or hydrophobic R-groups

L-Alanine (Ala) A   L-Valine (Val) V   L-Leucine (Leu) L   L-Isoleucine (Ile) I

L-Methionine (Met) M   L-Proline (Pro) P   L-Phenylalanine (Phe) F   L-Tryptophan (Trp) W

2. Negatively charged R-groups at pH 6–7

L-Aspartic acid (Asp) D   L-Glutamic acid (Glu) E

3. Uncharged or hydrophilic R-groups

L-Asparagine (Asn) N   L-Glutamine (Gln) Q   Glycine (Gly) G   L-Serine (Ser) S

L-Threonine (Thr) T   L-Tyrosine (Tyr) Y   L-Cysteine (Cys) C

4. Positively charged R-groups at pH 6–7

L-Lysine (Lys) K   L-Arginine (Arg) R   L-Histidine (His) H

Fig. 2.2 Structures of the 20 common amino acids grouped according to the nature of their 'R'-group. Note the three- and one-letter notations.

A cystine residue is formed from two cysteines linked through a disulfide bridge (–S–S–) formed from their sulfhydryl (–SH) groups.

The charges on the amino acids indicated in Fig. 2.2 are those that occur at pH 6–7. Acids are defined as proton donors and bases as proton acceptors. It follows that, at pH 6–7, an amino acid in group 2 is present as a free base (an anion) and one in group 4 as a free acid (a cation). The terms 'acidic' and 'basic', as applied to amino acids, should therefore be used with caution because they refer to the protonated forms of group 2 or the unprotonated forms of group 4. A compound such as an amino acid that carries both basic and acidic groups is referred to as amphoteric.

ASYMMETRY IN BIOCHEMISTRY

ASYMMETRY AS APPLIED TO AMINO ACIDS AS AN EXAMPLE

Chirality is derived from the Greek word *cheir* for 'hand' – the left and right hands are mirror images of each other. Such asymmetry in molecular structure is of great importance in biochemistry. A chiral molecule possesses at least one asymmetric centre, such as a carbon atom, to which are joined four groups that are different from each other.

The amino acid alanine can exist in two forms, denoted D-alanine and L-alanine, as shown in Fig. 2.3. The amino acids contained in mammalian proteins are of the L-form. (Sugars are also chiral molecules; D-sugars predominate in mammalian carbohydrates; see p. 110.) In Fig. 2.3, red denotes the oxygen atoms of the carboxyl group, the nitrogen atom of the amino acid group is grey, the carbon atoms are black and the hydrogen atoms are white.

NON-CHIRAL ASYMMETRY

Even if a molecule is not chiral, it can contain identical groups that are sterically distinguishable. A simplified representation of a hypothetical molecule is shown in Fig. 2.4. If A and B are held in space on a surface, then the identical groups X_1 and X_2 can be distinguished. The classic biochemical example is citric acid. Although this molecule has a plane of symmetry, the central carboxyl group and the hydroxyl group can be held in such a way that the two –CH_2COOH groups can be distinguished and the molecule is able

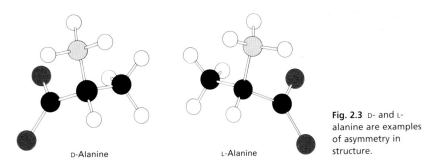

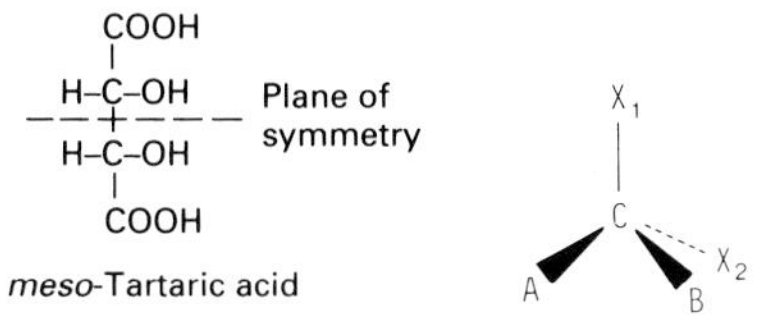

D-Alanine   L-Alanine

Fig. 2.3 D- and L-alanine are examples of asymmetry in structure.

```
      COOH
       |
    H–C–OH    Plane of
    ––+–––    symmetry
    H–C–OH
       |
      COOH
```

meso-Tartaric acid

Fig. 2.4 Example of a *meso* compound (left) and the simple representation of a hypothetical molecule (right).

to interact with an enzyme that has specific binding sites for the different groups in the molecule (see Fig. 9.15, p. 136). Such a molecule is termed 'prochiral' in that it can be made chiral by changing the structure of the group on only one of the central carbon bonds. Note that, if a molecule has a plane of symmetry such that chiral centres on either side of the plane of symmetry exactly compensate, the molecule is termed a *meso* compound (e.g. *meso*-tartaric acid, shown in Fig. 2.4).

R AND *S* CONVENTION

A chiral centre can be denoted *R* or *S*. The method for ascribing the *R* or *S* designation to a centre is as follows:

- List the functional groups in order of their priority assigned by convention. The order for some biochemically important groups is –SH (highest), –OH, –NH_2, –COOH, –CHO, –CH_3, –H (lowest). Then orientate the molecule so that the group of lowest priority points away from the observer.
- If the order of priority (high to low) of the remaining groups is clockwise, the centre is *R*. If the order or priority is anticlockwise, the centre is *S*. Thus the α-carbon of L-alanine has the *S* configuration.

IONIC PROPERTIES OF AMINO ACIDS

ELECTROPHORETIC SEPARATION

As already explained, amino acids have amphoteric properties that allow their separation by electrophoresis at pH 6.0, in which the amino acids move along a medium (paper) under the force of an applied electric field. Such a separation is illustrated in Fig. 2.5. Electrophoresis is commonly carried out on paper but gels can also be used. The amphoteric nature of α-amino acids means that, in the absence

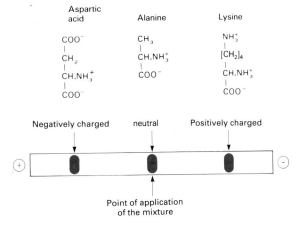

Fig. 2.5 Demonstration of the ionic properties of amino acids by electrophoresis.

of other acids or bases, the carboxyl and amino groups are both fully ionized, giving rise to the term zwitterion (German *Zwitter* = hybrid or hermaphrodite). This is the form that predominates in neutral solution and in crystals, rather than the unionized form.

THE BUFFERING CAPACITY OF AMINO ACIDS

As explained previously, an acid is defined as a proton donor. Acids vary in their tendency to dissociate; stronger acids do so more readily than weaker ones. The strength of an acid is expressed by the term pK_a, which is the pH at which an acid is 50% dissociated. The titration curve of alanine (Fig. 2.6) shows that the –COOH group becomes more dissociated as the pH increases. At pK_1, the change in pH of the solution with increasing additions of NaOH is lowest; in other words, the buffering capacity is greatest.
We have defined a base as a proton acceptor; so, in this case, the proportion of ionized NH_3 decreases as the pH increases and the maximum buffering is at pK_2.

The buffering capacity of histidine

If the R-group of an amino acid is capable of being ionized, then the amino acid will have a third pK. Histidine is very important in this respect because the imidazole group is only weakly basic, having a pK_a of 6.00. It therefore exists as a mixture of the protonated and dissociated forms in solution at the physiological pH of 7.2–7.4. Histidine therefore contributes to the buffering capacity of proteins. The titration curve of histidine is shown in Fig. 2.7.

SEPARATION OF AMINO ACIDS BY ION-EXCHANGE CHROMATOGRAPHY

It is often important to determine the proportion of the different amino acids, either in body fluids such as serum or spinal fluid, or in a protein hydrolysate. For this purpose, a resin bearing either positively charged groups (anion-exchange resin) or negatively charged groups (cation-exchange resin) can be used. Amino acids passed down a column of such a resin bind competitively to the charged groups on the resin.
Figure 2.8 shows the separation of the amino acids present in a peptide hydrolysate on a column of sulfonated

polystyrene (cation-exchange resin). Passage through the column of buffers of increasing pH causes aspartic acid (acidic) to emerge as the first amino acid and arginine (basic) as the last. It is common to detect the amino acids using ninhydrin;

this gives a blue colour after reaction with all α-amino acids (yellow for the amino acid proline), the intensity of colour being related to the amount of the particular amino acid. The whole process can be automated.

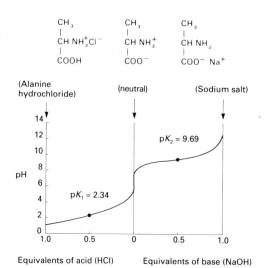

Fig. 2.6 Amino acids possess buffering capacity, as demonstrated by the titration of alanine.

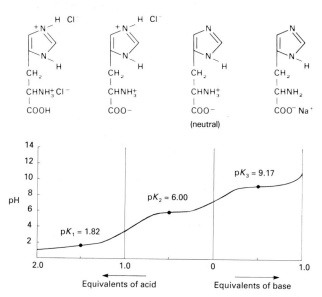

Fig. 2.7 The buffering properties of histidine are of particular physiological importance.

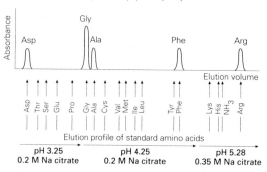

Fig. 2.8 Amino acids can be separated by ion-exchange chromatography and the amount of each determined.

Similar methods can be used for the separation of proteins that carry various net charges.

PEPTIDE STRUCTURE AND THE PEPTIDE BOND

THE PEPTIDE BOND

The peptide bond is formed by the interaction of two amino acids, with the elimination of water between the neighbouring $-NH_2$ and $-COOH$ groups. This is shown in Fig. 2.9. The peptide bond is a rigid structure; this has important implications for the structure of proteins (see p. 56).

Proline can also participate in a peptide bond (Fig. 2.10) but, in contrast to the α-amino acids, there is then no H available for H bonding which, as we will see, is important in the secondary structure of proteins.

NOTATION USED FOR PEPTIDES

The structure of a typical peptide, enkephalin, is shown in Fig. 2.11. In writing the primary structure, one starts with the amino-terminus (also called the N-terminus) and ends with the carboxy-terminus (referred to as the C-terminus). In Fig. 2.11, enkephalin is given in the three-letter code for amino acids. Abbreviated according to the single-letter code it would be written YGGFM. A peptide composed of more than a few amino acid residues is termed a polypeptide. To the extent that such polypeptides are the backbone structures of proteins, there is no formal definition of a transition from polypeptide to protein, but insulin, which has 50 amino acid residues, is commonly regarded as being typical of the smallest protein.

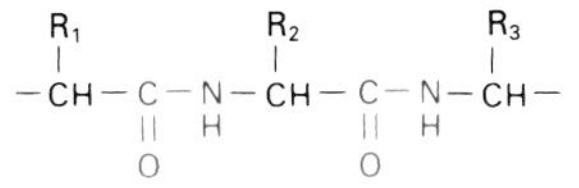

IDENTIFICATION OF PEPTIDE BONDS

The presence of a peptide bond is usually determined by the biuret reaction. Biuret has the formula $NH_2CONHCONH_2$ and is a simple substance possessing a peptide bond. When biuret is treated with $CuSO_4$ in alkaline solution, a purple colour is produced. This is known as the biuret reaction and, as expected, proteins give a strong reaction.

IONIC PROPERTIES OF PEPTIDES

THE NATURE OF THE CHARGED R-GROUPS

The ionizable, dissociable α-amino and α-carboxyl groups of the amino acids are blocked by peptide formation, except for the terminal residues. The ionized state of a protein therefore depends almost entirely on the R-groups; this, in effect, means those on aspartic and glutamic acids, lysine, arginine and histidine. This is illustrated in Fig. 2.12, which shows the structure of a hypothetical peptide containing all these groups. The numbers indicate the pK range of each dissociating group. As indicated above, histidine is very important because its charge can vary over the physiological pH range.

THE ISOELECTRIC POINTS OF PROTEINS

The isoionic point is the pH that results when the protein, freed of all other ions, is dissolved in water. The isoelectric point is the pH at which there is zero migration in an electric field (see below) to either electrode. The isoelectric points of a range of proteins are shown in Table 2.1. On the basis of these values, proteins are described as basic, neutral or acidic, depending on whether their overall charge at physiological pH is positive, approximately zero or negative.

ELECTROPHORESIS OF PROTEINS

Just as amino acids can be separated by electrophoresis so can proteins. Figure 2.13 shows the result of the electrophoresis of human serum proteins on a cellulose strip (paper can also be used) in a buffer at pH 8.6. The separated protein bands are visualized after staining with dye, and a densitometric scan provides an indication of the relative amount of protein in each

Table 2.1 The isoelectric points of some common proteins

Protein	Isoelectric point
Blood proteins	
α_1-Globulin	2.0
Haptoglobin	4.1
Serum albumin	4.7
γ_1-Globulin	5.8
Fibrinogen	5.8
Hemoglobin	7.2
γ_2-Globulin	7.4
Miscellaneous proteins	
Pepsin	1.0
Ovalbumin	4.6
Insulin	5.4
Histones	7.5–11.0
Ribonuclease	9.6
Cytochrome c	9.8
Lysozyme	11.1

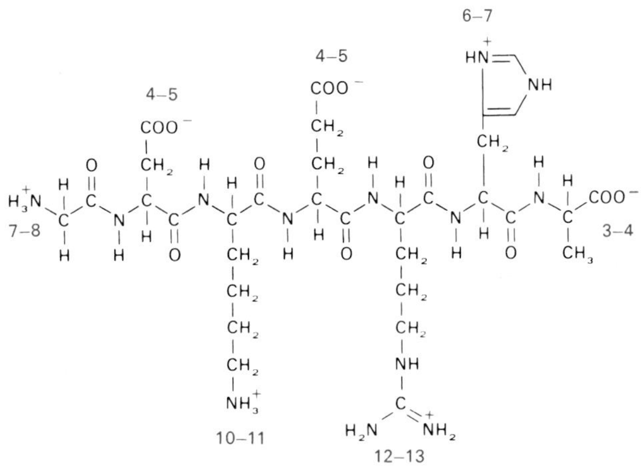

Fig. 2.9 Peptide bonds are formed by the interaction of amino acids.

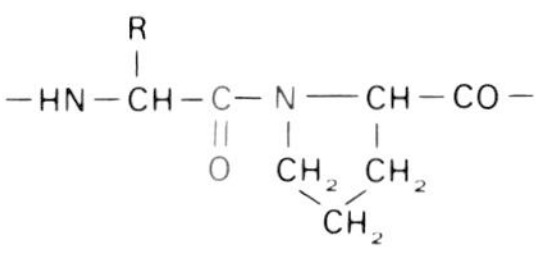

Fig. 2.10 The participation of proline in a peptide bond.

H$_2$N–Tyr–Gly–Gly–Phe–Met–COOH
Enkephalin

Fig. 2.11 The structure of a typical peptide.

glycyl-aspartyl-lysyl-glutamyl-arginyl-histidyl-alanine

Fig. 2.12 Polypeptides possess ionic properties, mainly due to the R-groups on the amino acid residues.

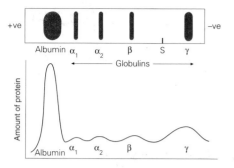

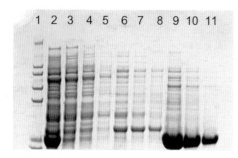

Fig. 2.13 Separation of serum proteins by electrophoresis on cellulose acetate.

Fig. 2.14 An example of the use of SDS PAGE for following the purification of an enzyme from *Pseudomonas aeruginosa* expressed from a plasmid inserted into *E. coli* (see Recombinant DNA p. 49). Lane 1, marker proteins of various M_r down to about 30 K; lane 2, total proteins expressed from the plasmid in the presence of the inducer IPTG; lanes 3–11, the purification of the desired protein by the use of an affinity chromatography column: lane 3, eluent (washing) from the column; lane 4, low salt eluate, first fraction; lane 5, as for lane 4 but later fraction; lanes 6–11, proteins which were eluted from the column by imidazole; lanes 6, 7, 8, eluates from column with 20 mM imidazole; lanes 9, 10, 11, eluates from column with 200 mM imidazole; lane 11, the homogeneity of the desired protein (dimethylarginine dimethylamino hydrolase).

band. 'S' indicates the point of application of the serum before applying the current with the charges shown. Although the mobility of the proteins depends mainly on their relative charge, the size of the proteins also plays a part and this certainly contributes to the position of the large γ-globulin band. Although the serum proteins give the appearance of being separated into discrete bands, it should be remembered that, with the exception of serum albumin, each band contains many different proteins.

POLYACRYLAMIDE GEL ELECTROPHORESIS (PAGE) OF PROTEINS

Polyacrylamide gel can be used instead of cellulose acetate or paper for the separation of native proteins. Such a gel is commonly used in the presence of sodium dodecyl sulfate (SDS). In this case, oligomeric proteins (those composed of several discrete polypeptides) are separated in the form of their subunits.

Figure 2.14 shows the resolution of proteins by SDS-PAGE. The proteins are suspended in a 1% solution of SDS. This detergent disrupts most protein–protein and protein–lipid interactions. Very often, 2-mercaptoethanol is also added, to disrupt disulfide bonds. The electrophoretic mobility of most proteins, but not glycoproteins, depends on their size, as the negative charge contributed by SDS molecules bound to the protein is much larger than the net charge of the protein itself. A pattern of bands appears when the gel is stained with Coomassie Blue.

Agarose can be used in place of polyacrylamide gel for larger proteins or to obtain a different type of separation in the absence of SDS.

Two-dimensional PAGE can also be carried out, using different conditions in each direction: for example, an immobilized pH gradient (pH 4–7) in one direction and an 11–14% polyacrylamide gradient in the other.

NON-COVALENT BONDS IN PROTEINS

The distribution of charged amino acid groups in a polypeptide chain has already been described. The charged groups are important in terms of the folding of the chains because negatively charged groups will repel each other, as will positively charged groups, whereas closely positioned negative and positive charges will attract each other. There are, however, several other important interactions between the R-groups in proteins. These are illustrated in Fig. 2.15.

The ionic interactions already referred to are also known as salt bridges and are illustrated by an interaction between glutamate and arginine. The S–S bonds formed by the oxidation of two sulfhydryl groups are covalent and are particularly likely to be present in proteins when the physiological environment is unfriendly; they enhance the rigidity of the protein. An example is the proteins in the digestive secretions of the pancreas.

The other interactions are described as non-covalent and can be either apolar (i.e. hydrophobic) or polar (i.e. ionic and hydrogen bonding). Hydrophobic interactions result from: (i) van der Waals interactions, which arise from an attraction between atoms due to fluctuating electric dipoles originating from the electronic cloud and positive nucleus; (ii) the hydrophobic effect, which is the tendency of non-polar groups to associate with one another rather than to be in contact with water. Hydrogen bonds arise because, when a hydrogen atom is linked to an oxygen atom, there is a shift of electrons leading to a partial negative charge on the other atom. This produces an electric dipole that can interact with dipoles that exist elsewhere. The most common hydrogen bond is between –N–H and –C=O, as in the α helix and β-pleated sheet (to be described in Chapter 4), but other bonds are possible, as shown in Fig. 2.15.

PURIFICATION OF PROTEINS AND DETERMINATION OF RELATIVE MOLECULAR MASS

PURITY AND HOMOGENEITY

The purification of small molecules has traditionally ended with crystallization and the determination of various physical parameters, such as the melting point, but these procedures are much less applicable to macromolecules such as proteins. Even if proteins are crystallized, they might be contaminated by other proteins, by viruses or by other infective agents such as prions (see p. 60). The objective in the purification of proteins, therefore, is to produce a product that is homogeneous by all known criteria, which usually includes

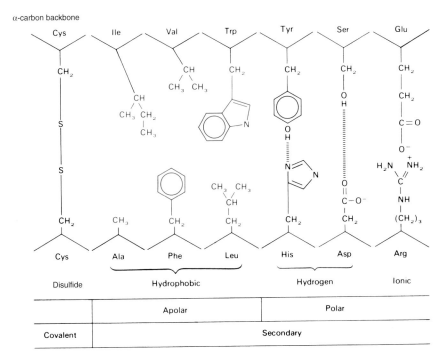

Fig. 2.15 The creation of non-covalent bonds is important in the formation of the tertiary structure of proteins. The various bonds are illustrated.

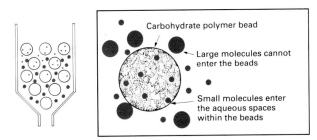

Fig. 2.16 Gel-permeation chromatography can be used for the removal of small molecules from protein solutions and for the separation of proteins according to their size.

attached to the beads in the form of a column. The ligands can be enzyme substrates or antibodies. The proteins are eluted by adding an excess of the ligand or by changing the salt concentration or pH of the elutent. (See p. 78 for immunoaffinity chromatography.)

NOMENCLATURE FOR THE SIZE AND DENSITY OF MACROMOLECULES

Formerly, the size of a molecule was described in terms of its molecular weight, but the term relative molecular mass (abbreviation M_r) is now preferred. Both M_r and molecular weight are ratios and hence it is incorrect to give them units such as daltons (symbol Da). It is thus incorrect to state that 'the M_r or the molecular weight of substance X is 10^5 Da'; the correct usage is '$M_r = 10\,000$'. The dalton is a unit of mass equal to one-twelfth the mass of an atom of carbon-12. Hence, it is correct to say that 'the molecular mass of X is 10^5 Da' or to use expressions such as 'the 16 000-Da peptide'. For entities that do not have a definable M_r, it is correct to state, for example, 'the mass of a ribosome is 10^7 Da'. A kilodalton (symbol kDa) is equal to 1000 Da.

Gel permeation can be used for the determination of the M_r of a protein. Plots of the elution volumes (V_e) of native proteins of known M_r on Sephadex G-75 and G-100 versus log M_r are shown in Fig. 2.17.

LARGE-SCALE SEPARATION OF PROTEINS

The scheme illustrated in Fig. 2.18 shows some of the many methods that are used for the separation of the plasma proteins. Cryoprecipitation depends on the lesser solubility of some proteins in the cold. DEAE (diethylaminoethyl)-, QAE (quaternary aminoethyl)- and SP (sulfopropyl)-Sephadex (or Sepharose) provide separation by ion exchange, as does CM (carboxymethyl)-Sepharose. Although every effort can be taken to produce a product that consists only of the protein of interest, purity cannot be guaranteed. Thus the isolated protein might be contaminated with very small amounts of other substances. Examples of such contamination are: (i) the virus that causes AIDS–HIV (see p. 29) in preparations of factor VIII, which is used in the treatment of people with hemophilia; (ii) the presence of the factor that causes

electrophoresis under various conditions. To achieve this, many different methods are used, based on the characteristic properties of proteins, and in particular their ability to interact specifically with small molecules. The methods used must not impair the structure of the native protein or affect its biological activity. Traditional methods involved the differential solubility of proteins in solutions of ammonium sulfate, but many other methods are now available, such as gel-permeation chromatography, ion-exchange chromatography (similar to that already described for amino acids but using cellulose or Sephadex rather than a resin) and affinity chromatography. Some of these methods are described below.

GEL-PERMEATION CHROMATOGRAPHY

This technique utilizes a matrix based on dextran. This cross-linked polymer of dextran forms a mesh that can be penetrated only by molecules of a certain size (the greater the cross-linking, the smaller the holes of the mesh). The trade name of the dextran is Sephadex; various grades of Sephadex are produced and these differ in the extent of cross-linking. The principle of the method is shown in Fig. 2.16. Large molecules, which penetrate the mesh less readily, have less volume through which to permeate and thus elute more quickly. The matrix is normally packed in a column. The method can be used to separate small molecules, such as salts, from larger molecules, such as proteins, and to separate macromolecules of different sizes. Other materials such as agarose and Sepharose (a proprietary agarose) can be used as the basis of the matrix.

The ability of proteins to bind specifically to other molecules is the basis of affinity chromatography. In this technique ligand molecules that bind to the protein of interest are covalently

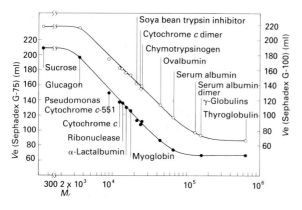

Fig. 2.17 Gel-permeation chromatography can be used to determine the M_r of a protein.

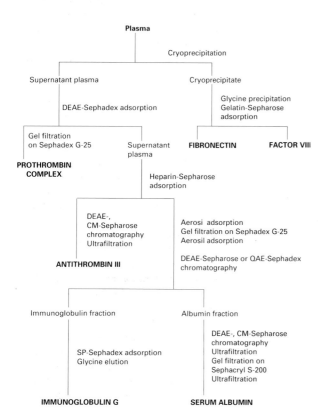

Fig. 2.18 Methods that can be used for the large-scale fractionation of proteins.

Creutzfeldt–Jakob disease (see p. 60) in preparations of human growth hormone; (iii) and the virus that causes hepatitis C in products from blood. Some of these contaminants can be inactivated by heat treatment. In many cases, the alternative of expressing a recombinant DNA for the chosen human protein in a vector such as *E. coli* or yeast (see p. 49) is to be preferred, but care must be taken to eliminate the proteins of the vector from the human protein preparation. Such methods are used for the preparation of erythropoietin, which is used for the treatment of anemia in patients with kidney failure. Serum albumin cannot as yet be obtained in this way.

THE DETERMINATION OF THE AMINO ACID SEQUENCE OF PROTEINS

Proteins have precisely defined amino acid sequences and there are many reasons for wishing to know this sequence for each protein. As shown later (p. 34), it might be possible to achieve this by an indirect method after determining the structure of the gene for the protein and deducing the amino acid sequence from knowledge of the genetic code. Direct methods involve the determination of the N-terminal amino acid followed by Edman degradation. Because this method is limited to about 50 amino acids, it is first necessary

to break larger proteins into smaller polypeptides, either chemically or by the use of proteolytic enzymes (see p. 154). Provided the peptides overlap, it is possible to deduce the sequence of the entire protein. Edman degradation involves the reaction of phenylisothiocyanate with the N-terminal amino acid and its release by mild acid. The procedure is continued in a stepwise, automated manner.

PROTEIN STRUCTURAL HIERARCHIES

The polypeptide chains of proteins fold in various ways, both within chains and with other chains. This folding is essential for the biological activity of proteins and it is this intricate folding that must be preserved during the procedures involved in protein purification. Although it has long been claimed that the manner of folding of the polypeptide chains is determined solely by the amino acid sequence of the chains, it is now accepted that proteins with identical amino acid sequences can exist in differently folded forms, and that such folding can be influenced by the presence of other proteins, known as molecular chaperones (see p. 15).

It is useful to consider protein structure in terms of the four hierarchies shown in Fig. 2.19.

PROTEIN DENATURATION AND RENATURATION

A protein that possesses its own unique biological property is known as a native protein, to distinguish it from a protein that has lost this property and which is described as denatured. A denatured protein has lost its three-dimensional structure, also known as its conformation. Denaturation can be either irreversible or reversible. An example of irreversible denaturation is the application of heat when an egg is boiled; the egg white (albumen) coagulates in an irreversible manner. In fact, this is a common event during cooking that renders proteins more susceptible to the action of proteolytic enzymes when the food is eaten.

Reversible denaturation can be achieved by the careful use of reagents such as urea and mercaptoethanol. Urea destroys the water structure and hence decreases the hydrophobic bonding of the R-groups of the amino acid residues (see Fig. 2.15), resulting in the unfolding and dissociation of the protein molecules. Mercaptoethanol reduces the S–S bonds.

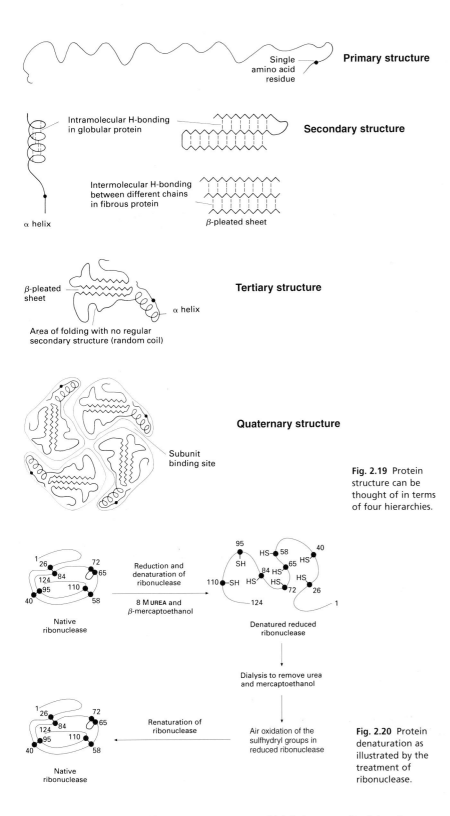

Primary structure

Single amino acid residue

Secondary structure

Intramolecular H-bonding in globular protein

α helix

Intermolecular H-bonding between different chains in fibrous protein

β-pleated sheet

Tertiary structure

β-pleated sheet

α helix

Area of folding with no regular secondary structure (random coil)

Quaternary structure

Subunit binding site

Fig. 2.19 Protein structure can be thought of in terms of four hierarchies.

Native ribonuclease

Reduction and denaturation of ribonuclease

8 M UREA and β-mercaptoethanol

Denatured reduced ribonuclease

Dialysis to remove urea and mercaptoethanol

Renaturation of ribonuclease

Air oxidation of the sulfhydryl groups in reduced ribonuclease

Native ribonuclease

Fig. 2.20 Protein denaturation as illustrated by the treatment of ribonuclease.

It might therefore be possible to renature the protein when the urea and mercaptoethanol are removed. These processes are shown in Fig. 2.20 for ribonuclease.

Renaturation has been taken to indicate that a protein with the 'correct' primary structure will fold spontaneously to give the unique structure required for biological activity. This process is termed 'protein self-

assembly'. It is now realized that there are two means whereby renaturation can be assisted. One involves the enzyme protein disulfide isomerase, an enzyme that plays a role 'correcting' wrongly paired S–S bonds. The other involves molecular chaperones, which have already been referred to. These can be defined as a family of unrelated classes of proteins that mediate the correct assembly of other polypeptides but are not

components of the functional assembled structures. Examples are heat-shock proteins synthesized by cells after their exposure to an abnormally increased temperature.

PEPTIDES, STRUCTURE AND BIOLOGICAL ACTIVITY

EXAMPLES OF SMALL PEPTIDES

There are many naturally-occurring peptides with a wide range of activity, such as hormones, first messengers in neurotransmission, local mediators and antibiotics. These peptides vary in length from the three amino acids of thyrotropin-releasing hormone (TRH) to the 231 amino acids of human gonadotropin. Even the smallest peptides have a very specific activity.

The structures of some typical peptides are shown in Fig. 2.21. The N- and C-termini are often modified. Thus, in TRH, the N-terminus is a cyclized glutamic acid (pyroglutamic acid) and there is an amide at the C-terminus. It is possible that such modifications enhance metabolic stability by protecting the peptides against exopeptidases.

Examples of small peptide hormones produced in the posterior pituitary are oxytocin and vasopressin. The structures of these are shown in Fig. 2.21; again, the C-terminus is an amide. The vasopressins are more correctly named antidiuretic hormone (ADH), because their most important physiological action is to promote reabsorption of water from the distal renal tubule. Oxytocin accelerates birth by stimulating contraction of uterine smooth muscle. These structures illustrate

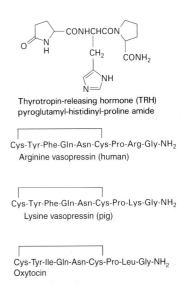

Thyrotropin-releasing hormone (TRH) pyroglutamyl-histidinyl-proline amide

Cys-Tyr-Phe-Gln-Asn-Cys-Pro-Arg-Gly-NH$_2$
Arginine vasopressin (human)

Cys-Tyr-Phe-Gln-Asn-Cys-Pro-Lys-Gly-NH$_2$
Lysine vasopressin (pig)

Cys-Tyr-Ile-Gln-Asn-Cys-Pro-Leu-Gly-NH$_2$
Oxytocin

Fig. 2.21 Structures of some typical peptides.

the specificity of peptides in that small changes of structure are associated with major functional change. Many of the antibiotic peptides are cyclized.

EXAMPLES OF LARGER HORMONES

Somatotropin (growth hormone) and prolactin are protein hormones of the anterior pituitary; lactogen is produced by the placenta. All three hormones are closely related in structure.

Another group of hormones is a family of glycoproteins, which includes thyrotropin, follicle-stimulating hormone (FSH) and chorionic gonadotropin. These compounds all contain numerous N-linked branched carbohydrate chains – hence the name of the group.

Some peptide hormones are first synthesized as larger peptides, which are subsequently split in the tissues into smaller peptides with discrete activities. Such large precursor peptides are called polyproteins. Good examples are the adrenocorticotropin (ACTH) peptides produced from proopiocorticotropin (see p. 33).

THE USE OF THE MASS SPECTROMETER IN PROTEIN STRUCTURE STUDIES

There have been important developments in the approach to protein structure determination in recent years. In particular, techniques in mass spectrometry have been introduced to rapidly identify proteins and to enable the determination of polypeptide amino acid sequence. For identification, the protein is initially digested with trypsin (or similar enzyme) and the peptides formed simultaneously analysed with very high sensitivity by matrix-assisted laser desorption mass spectrometry. The list of peptide masses are then compared *in silico* (i.e. by computer) against the computed masses of all known proteins in the international databases. This technique of peptide fingerprinting usually results in rapid identification of the original protein.

There are also approaches to obtain amino acid sequence information directly from proteins but, more generally, sequence is derived on smaller polypeptides and peptides from a protein by collision-induced dissociation mass spectrometry. In this case the molecular ions of the peptides are collisionally fragmented at their constituent peptide bonds and the sequence deduced from the resulting mass spectrum – a process that also can be carried out automatically by computer. The combination of peptide fingerprinting and sequencing has led to a rapid and sustained expansion in studies of the proteome, in which complex mixtures of proteins are initially separated by two dimensional electrophoresis followed by in-gel digestion and mass spectrometric analysis.

Nucleic acids and protein synthesis

3

The many aspects of the interplay between the nucleic acids of the genomes of organisms and viruses and the expression of their proteins are described. The knowledge of the DNA structure of the genomes of many species enables this endeavour to be pursued at a new level of understanding, legitimately described as the post-genomic era. An understanding of these phenomena underlines their role in the control of metabolism, which is explained in the later chapters of this book. The structure of DNA is explained, as is its compaction into the chromatin of the chromosomes.

There follows an outline of the cell cycle and how it is controlled, together with a description of the multienzyme system involved in the replication of DNA. The activity of restriction enzymes and other enzymes that have actions on DNA are mentioned.

The metabolism of the nucleotides, precursors in the synthesis of the nucleic acids, is described together with the inhibitory action of many drugs and their uses. The Sanger method for the determination of the base sequence of DNA is described. The means whereby DNA is repaired is followed by the mechanism by which mutagenesis is achieved in vitro. The polymerase chain reaction and its uses is explained.

The mechanisms whereby DNA is transcribed into RNA in normal cells and by viruses is described together with the action of reverse transcriptase with particular mention of the virus HIV. The action of many drugs on the replication and transcription of nucleic acids is summarized. The concept and use of RNA interference (RNAi) is introduced.

The many steps involved in the translation of RNA into protein are described. The synthesis of the multichain proteins such as insulin is followed by amino acid activation, transfer RNA and the genetic code. The role of the ribosome, the structure of messenger RNA and the elongation, initiation and termination of polypeptide chains are described. The action of antibiotics on the various steps in protein synthesis is summarized. There follows the concept of split genes, introns, exons and the formation of mature mRNA. Alternative splicing and the generation of antibody diversity are reviewed, followed by the means whereby protein synthesis in both bacteria and animals is controlled. This introduces transcription factors and the general problem of the recognition of sequences in DNA by proteins.

Protein kinesis whereby the newly synthesized proteins are directed to their correct organelle is explained and post-translational modifications are achieved.

The diseases that result when this process is damaged are listed in the case of peroxisomes, the Golgi apparatus and lysosomes. The breakdown of proteins by the lysosomal and ubiquitin systems is explained.

There follows a description of recombinant DNA and its applications, particularly with respect to antenatal diagnosis. The chapter ends with an explanation of the means of achieving transgenesis and knock-out animals, and of reverse genetics and the effect of trinucleotide repeats in human disease. There is a glossary of some useful terms.

INTRODUCTION: REPLICATION, TRANSCRIPTION AND TRANSLATION

Before embarking on the more detailed aspects of the biosynthesis of nucleic acids and proteins, it is as well to be clear about the overall characteristics of the scheme that is shown in Fig. 3.1. 'Replication' refers to the biosynthesis of either DNA or RNA, where the parental nucleic acid serves as a template to direct the structure of the product. 'Transcription' means the change in the nature of the nucleic acid from DNA to RNA, and 'reverse transcription' means the reverse process. When DNA is transcribed into RNA, three different kinds of RNA can be identified: messenger RNA (mRNA), transfer RNA (tRNA) and ribosomal RNA (rRNA). The dashed lines indicate the processes that are confined to viruses and indicate that the genome of a virus can be either DNA or RNA. The viral RNA can either be replicated directly or first transcribed back into DNA. 'Translation' means the change from RNA to polypeptide; the RNA, in this case mRNA, serving as a template that directs the primary structure of the polypeptide. The polypeptide is often then modified by hydroxylation, phosphorylation or glycosylation of the R groups of selected amino acid residues. This process is known as post-translational modification.

The so-called central dogma of Crick was that the information concerning the structure of polypeptides had to pass from nucleic acid to polypeptide and could not flow from polypeptide to nucleic acid or to another polypeptide. Although there have been various discoveries since the dogma was first pronounced in 1958, the dogma has held and should always be kept in mind.

NUCLEIC ACID STRUCTURE AND SYNTHESIS

GENERAL ASPECTS OF STRUCTURE

Nucleic acids are polymers

There are two types of nucleic acid: deoxyribonucleic acid (DNA) and ribonucleic acid (RNA). Nucleic acids are polymers, the monomeric unit being a nucleotide, so that all nucleic acids are polynucleotides. A nucleotide has three components:

phosphate–5′–sugar–1′–N–base

In DNA the sugar is deoxyribose, in RNA it is ribose. (The 2′-hydroxyl present in RNA makes it susceptible to alkaline hydrolysis, whereas DNA is resistant. However, both DNA and RNA are hydrolysed by acid.) The nucleotides are linked in the polynucleotides through the formation of a phosphodiester bond. The basic structure of a polynucleotide is, therefore, as shown in Fig. 3.2.

The polynucleotide chain has polarity, that is, it is not the same in each direction. By convention, the order of the nucleotides containing the different bases is read from the 5′ end to the 3′ end. Chains of opposite polarity are said to be antiparallel.

Figure 3.3 shows part of a chain of RNA; in DNA the 2′-OH is replaced by H. The carbon atoms within the bases are numbered 1, 2, 3, etc. and those in deoxyribose and ribose 1′, 2′, 3′, etc.

Components

There are typically only four different bases in either DNA or RNA. The only

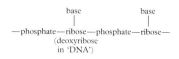

Fig. 3.2 The structure of a polynucleotide. It has three components: phosphate, ribose and a base.

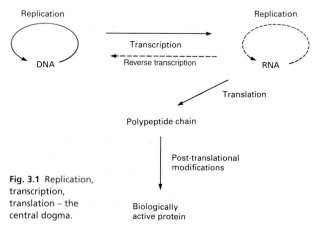

Fig. 3.1 Replication, transcription, translation – the central dogma.

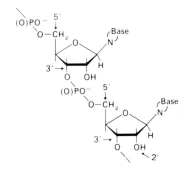

Fig. 3.3 The linkage of the nucleotide in RNA. In DNA the 2′-OH is replaced by H.

Pyrimidine bases

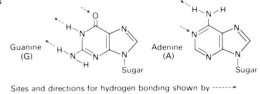

Cytosine
(C)

Uracil
(U)

(methyl-U
= thymine (T))

Sugar

Purine bases

Guanine
(G)

Adenine
(A)

Sugar

Sugar

Sites and directions for hydrogen bonding shown by ------►

Fig. 3.4 Structure of the pyrimidine and purine bases. The site of attachment of the sugar (ribose in RNA, deoxyribose in DNA) is indicated.

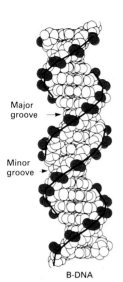

Major groove

Minor groove

B-DNA

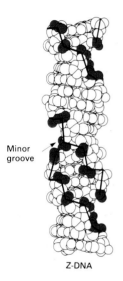

Minor groove

Z-DNA

Table 3.1 Nomenclature of the bases and the nucleosides and nucleotides derived from them

Base	Nucleoside*	Nucleotide†
Purines		
Adenine	Adenosine (A)	Adenylic acid (AMP)
Guanine	Guanosine (G)	Guanylic acid (GMP)
Hypoxanthine	Inosine (I)	Inosinic acid (IMP)
Pyrimidines		
Cytosine	Cytidine (C)	Cytidylic acid (CMP)
Uracil (in RNA)	Uridine (U)	Uridylic acid (UMP)
Thymine (= 5-methyluracil) in DNA	Thymidine (T)	Thymidylic acid (TMP)

*In polymers with repeating units, the letters indicate nucleotides, e.g. poly(A) and poly(dT).
†When the sugar is deoxyribose, the nucleoside or nucleotide is abbreviated dT, dAMP, etc. dNTP signifies unspecified deoxynucleoside triphosphate.

difference between them is that DNA contains thymine whereas RNA contains uracil. The names and structures of the bases are shown in Fig. 3.4. In tRNA, inosine is also present. Inosine is the nucleoside of hypoxanthine, which is deaminated adenine. tRNA also contains other so-called unusual bases such as pseudouridine, ribothymidine and dihydrouridine.

Whereas a nucleotide has three components, a nucleoside has two components:

–sugar–1′–N–base

It follows that a nucleotide with three phosphate groups attached to a nucleoside at the 5′ position of the sugar is called a nucleoside triphosphate; thus ATP stands for adenosine triphosphate:

P–P–P–5′–ribose–1–adenine

The names adenosine diphosphate (ADP) and adenosine monophosphate (AMP) and related terms for other bases are similarly obtained. These are listed in Table 3.1.

Nucleic acids are characterized by the order in which the four different nucleotides occur in the polynucleotide chain. As already mentioned, the base sequence is specified in the direction 5′ to 3′; hence, pApCpGpApT specifies that the sequence in the polynucleotide starts with A at the 5′ end and has T at the 3′ end. The 'p' in the sequence above indicates the presence of one phosphate group; the capital letter indicates the nucleotide base.

CONFORMATION OF THE DNA DOUBLE HELIX

DNA exists as a double helix. The two strands run in opposite directions (antiparallel) but can vary in conformation – a feature known as structural polymorphism. There are two right-handed double-helical DNA conformations: A-DNA and B-DNA (the chains turn to the right as they move upwards). B-DNA is characterized by a regular repeat of a minor groove and major groove as shown in Fig. 3.5. The phosphate groups are shown in red. Another quite different

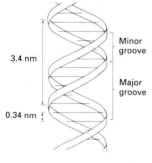

3.4 nm

0.34 nm

Minor groove

Major groove

Fig. 3.5 The conformation of the DNA double helix. When the relative humidity is reduced, B-DNA undergoes a reversible conformational change to A-DNA.

form of DNA is Z-DNA, which has a left-handed helix. The irregularity of the Z-DNA backbone is illustrated by the heavy line that connects the phosphate groups. There is speculation that the conformation of DNA might change in vivo and that this could be important in gene expression. Thus, transcription of

Table 3.2 The sizes of DNA molecules from various sources		
Source	Number of base pairs	Length (μm)
Viruses		
Polyoma SV40	5.1×10^3	1.7
Bacteriophage T2	1.66×10^5	55
Bacteria		
Escherichia coli	4.7×10^6	1360
Human	2.9×10^9	990 000

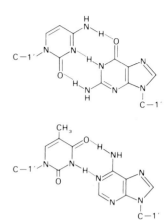

Fig. 3.7 Base pairing. The base pair C...G is shown above, T:A is below.

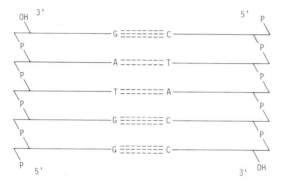

Fig. 3.6 Hydrogen bonding between the antiparallel strands of DNA.

SECONDARY STRUCTURE OF DNA

DNA molecules are either linear or circular; human chromosomes are linear whereas many viral and bacterial chromosomes are circular. When DNA molecules with both ends anchored are twisted about their long axis, the strain is relieved by the development of long-range bends and twists called supercoils or superhelices. (Try twisting a double-stranded electric cord.) Supercoiling is biologically important because it can influence gene expresssion. The degree of supercoiling can be regulated by enzymes called topoisomerases. Type I enzymes nick one strand whereas type II enzymes nick both strands and rejoin the ends. These enzymes also relieve the supercoiling that occurs when DNA is unwound before replication (see p. 24).

THE STRUCTURE OF CHROMATIN

General principles

Chromatin is the DNA–protein complex of an entangled mass of fibres in which, in the non-dividing cell, the chromosomes are segregated. The DNA molecule of a

DNA (see p. 28) probably occurs at the junction of B- and Z-DNA where unfolding takes place.

DENATURATION AND HYBRIDIZATION

The size of DNA

The size of the DNA within a cell differs markedly according to the source, as shown in Table 3.2. RNA is usually a much smaller molecule than DNA.

Melting and annealing

Unlike DNA, RNA is usually single stranded but is characterized by the presence of many intrachain hydrogen bonds. A typical example is the clover-leaf structure of tRNA, which is explained on p. 35.

The two chains in double-stranded DNA are linked by hydrogen bonds between pairs of purine and pyrimidine bases as shown in Fig. 3.6. The proportion of the different bases in DNA is such that A = T and G = C. This is in accord with A hydrogen-bonding with T, and G hydrogen-bonding with C. This is known as base pairing (see Fig. 3.7). It should be noted that the link between G and C is stronger than the link between A and T. The antiparallel strands in DNA linked by base pairs (bp) are said to be complementary strands.

Whereas denaturation of a protein implies the loss of tertiary structure, denaturation of double-stranded DNA involves the separation of the two complementary strands. Denaturation is usually effected experimentally by heating, the temperature at which 50% of the two strands are separated being termed the melting temperature (T_m). The reverse phenomenon, whereby the two strands reassociate, is termed annealing; this is illustrated in Fig. 3.8. Instead of heating, denaturation of DNA can be achieved by raising the pH to about 12 (0.5 M NaOH).

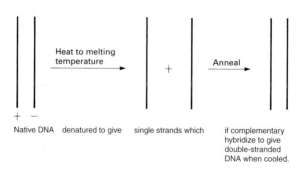

Native DNA   denatured to give   single strands which   if complementary hybridize to give double-stranded DNA when cooled.

Fig. 3.8 Denaturation and annealing of DNA.

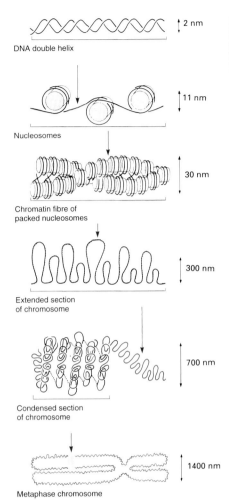

Fig. 3.9 A schematic view of the structure of chromosomes.

DNA double helix · 2 nm

Nucleosomes · 11 nm

Chromatin fibre of packed nucleosomes · 30 nm

Extended section of chromosome · 300 nm

Condensed section of chromosome · 700 nm

Metaphase chromosome · 1400 nm

Table 3.3 Types of histones

Histone type	Lys/Arg ratio	Number of amino acid residues	M_r ($\times 10^{-3}$)	
H1	20.0	215	21.0	
H2A	1.25	129	14.5	
H2B	2.5	125	13.8	Components of nucleosomes
H3	0.72	135	15.3	
H4	0.79	102	11.3	

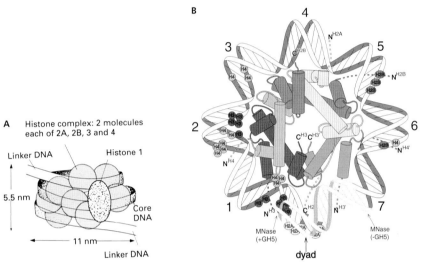

Fig. 3.10 The structure of nucleosomes. (A) Sketch of the arrangement of the histones encircled by DNA in two turns. (B) The structure of the nucleosome core at a resolution of 2.8 Å; half of the structure is shown. One turn (73 bp) of the DNA superhelix is visible and the view is down the superhelix axis. The different histones are indicated by different shades of red; helical regions in the proteins are represented by cylinders. The centre of the nucleosome (the dyad position) is indicated, and it terminates at site 7.

chromosome of a higher organism would stretch over many centimetres if laid out straight and so must be highly folded to form the compact structure (a process known as compaction) found in the nucleus. The DNA must also be organized into functional units that permit the expression of genes and their replication. A schematic view of the different levels of organization in the structure of a chromosome is shown in Fig. 3.9.

The structure of nucleosomes

A characteristic feature of the nucleus of eukaryotic cells, unlike prokaryotic cells, is the association of small basic proteins with the DNA. These are called histones. Table 3.3 shows some of the characteristics of the histones. Four of the five types of histones group in pairs to form a particle around which the DNA is wrapped. The product is known as a nucleosome. The nucleosomes, which occur about every 200 bp, implying that an average cell

nucleus contains 25 million, form a filament that can coil into a helical solenoid structure. Figure 3.10A shows in diagrammatic form the arrangement of the histones encircled by 146 bp of DNA in two turns. At the point of entry and leaving, the DNA is sealed by another histone, H1. Figure 3.10B shows the structure of a reconstituted nucleosome determined by X-ray diffraction. The DNA contacts the histone octamer at 14 main points, most of which have quite different structures, so that the DNA does not follow a regular path. Each histone consists of a structured, three-helix domain, as well as two unstructured tails that extend beyond the DNA. These might play an important role in making contact with adjacent nucleosomes and are probably the site where the histones are modified by acetyltransferases, which play a role in the regulation of transcription. The DNA on the outside of the octamers has been likened to a piece of Velcro, which could

be displaced a little at a time as the enzyme reactions involved in DNA replication proceed. Transcription of a gene is highest when the associated histones are highly acetylated. Histone deacetylation causes chromatin to assume a more condensed transcriptionally inactive form (see p. 28).

BIOLOGICAL ACTIVITY AND REPLICATION OF DNA

Methods of demonstrating activity

The biological activity of DNA was first demonstrated in 1944 by Avery, MacLeod and McCarty, who showed that the active principle in their experiments with extracts of strains of pneumococci (first reported by Griffith in 1928) was DNA. The results of the experiments are illustrated in Fig. 3.11. Two strains of pneumococci were used: (1) a pathogenic wild strain, known as smooth or S-strain because of the kind of colony it forms and the fact that it contains capsular

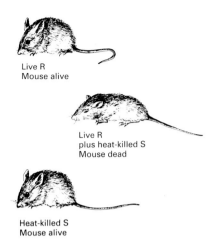

Fig. 3.11 Demonstration of the biological activity of DNA.

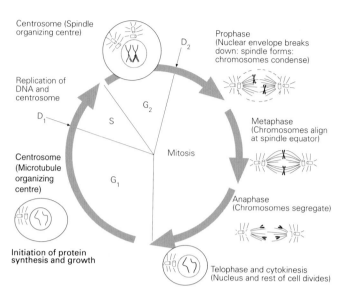

Fig. 3.12 The cell cycle.

polysaccharide; and (2) a non-pathogenic mutant rough or R-strain, which did not possess capsular polysaccharide because it lacked an essential enzyme. An extract of heat-killed S-strain had no effect when injected into a mouse but, when it was injected together with R-strain pneumococci, the mouse died. Moreover, the blood of the dead mouse was shown to contain live S-strain pneumococci. Thus the heat-killed extract from S-strain had transformed live R-strain (non-pathogenic) into live S-strain (pathogenic).

Since 1944, many experiments have demonstrated the biological role of DNA and even of RNA. The most sophisticated of these are described in the section on recombinant DNA (see p. 49). Other methods have involved the use of bacterial (bacteriophage, phage) and plant viruses. Phage DNA can be shown to infect a suitable host cell and cause it to lyse as a result of phage replication. In the tobacco mosaic plant virus the genome is RNA, which is itself infective. The primary structure of the coat protein of the resulting virus depends crucially on the structure of the infecting nucleic acid.

The cell cycle

All living cells either are undergoing a programme of cell division or are planning to die, a process now described as apoptosis (see Chapter 16). In eukaryotic cells we can distinguish two phases during the cell division cycle (shown in Fig. 3.12): (1) the interphase, during which the cell grows; and (2) mitosis, during which the nucleus and then the rest of the cell divides. In terms of the time to pass through the various phases, mitosis takes up about 40% of the total time in the cells of early

embryos and less than 10% in most other cells. Interphase, shown on the left-hand side of Fig. 3.12, can be divided into three parts. In S phase, the chromosomes replicate and DNA synthesis (S) occurs. Cell mass increases continuously throughout the cycle whereas the DNA content increases during S phase and falls dramatically thereafter, so that the DNA content of the non-dividing cell is constant. S phase is preceded by a gap, G_1, and is followed by another gap, G_2. The cycle contains two decision-making points: at D_1 (start) the cell decides whether to replicate its DNA, and at D_2 whether to initiate mitosis. The protein Cdc2 has been identified as the main regulator of passage through both points. At D_1 a quiescent cell is said to have entered G_0. The adult cells, from which the nucleus in the cloned sheep Dolly was obtained, were starved and in G_0. A family of proteins known as the cyclins, which periodically rise and fall in concentration in step with the eukaryotic cell cycle, activate crucial protein kinases (see p. 91) by forming complexes and thereby help to control progression from one stage of the cell cycle to the next. Mutations in the 'machinery' that controls the cell cycle feature prominently in many cancers (see Oncogenes and cancer, p. 221). The work with Dolly showed that in a differentiated cell the nucleus retains its DNA intact. This confirmed a previous finding that specialized cells in the body are genetically equivalent and that they differ only in the genes they express and not the genes they contain. The specialized cells can be switched back to an embryonic state from which they can be

made to form a whole range of different cell types. Such a switch might occur when cells become cancerous e.g. hepatoma cells in the liver express α-fetoprotein, which is normally present only in the embryo (see p. 69).

Semiconservative replication in vivo

DNA is replicated in the cell by a process that ensures that one of the parent strands is present in the daughter molecules, so-called semiconservative replication. The experiments that demonstrated this were done by Meselson and Stahl and are illustrated in Fig. 3.13. These workers grew E. coli in the presence of ^{15}N, the heavy isotope of nitrogen. They determined the density of the resulting DNA and showed that after one generation it was intermediate between the density of light DNA (containing ^{14}N) and heavy DNA (containing ^{15}N). The copying of a DNA template strand into a complementary strand is a common feature in DNA replication.

Replication of double-stranded DNA

In the living cell, the most common mechanism of DNA replication is for it to proceed simultaneously in both directions along the two strands of DNA. In the simplest case of E. coli, unwinding and replication of the double-stranded circular DNA leads to the production of a structure that resembles a circle with an inner loop, as shown in Fig. 3.14. In this case, replication is from a single initiation point.

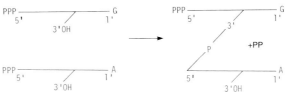

Fig. 3.15 DNA polymerases synthesize polynucleotides in the direction 5'→3'.

The horizontal line indicates the presence of deoxyribose and the numbers the identity of the carbon atoms of the sugar.

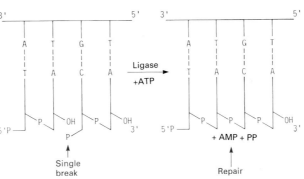

Fig. 3.16 Polynucleotide is synthesized on a DNA template to produce antiparallel chains.

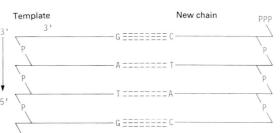

Fig. 3.17 Fragments of DNA are sealed by DNA ligase.

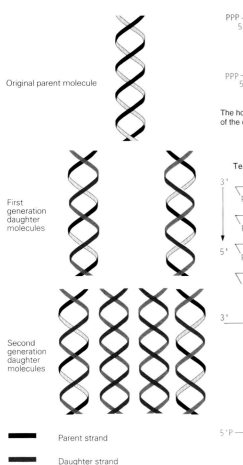

Fig. 3.13 The Meselson–Stahl experiment to demonstrate that DNA replication in vivo is by a semiconservative process.

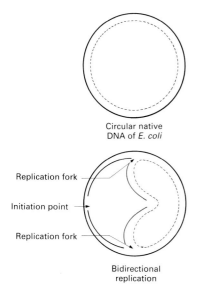

Fig. 3.14 The replication of double-stranded DNA in *Escherichia coli*.

Enzymes involved in replication

DNA is synthesized by enzymes called DNA polymerases, all of which utilize deoxynucleoside triphosphates as substrates; the polynucleotide is formed in the direction 5'→3'. The essential features are illustrated in Fig. 3.15. A DNA template is used to direct the order of bases in the newly synthesized polynucleotide such that it is complementary to the template DNA, as shown in Fig. 3.16.

There are three types of DNA polymerase in *E. coli*. It will be shown that, although DNA polymerase III plays the major role in synthesis, DNA polymerase I is also important. Fragments of DNA bound by a continuous template are sealed by an enzyme called DNA ligase (see Fig. 3.17). This enzyme plays a role both in the synthesis of DNA in vivo and in the repair of single breaks in DNA. In animal cells, a covalent enzyme–AMP complex is formed as an intermediate. In bacteria, ATP is replaced by NAD⁺.

Replication of double-stranded DNA

To explain the apparent growth of both strands of DNA in the same direction when the enzymes synthesize new strands in only one direction, namely 5'→3', it was postulated that one of the strands was first synthesized in fragments; the mechanism is shown in Fig. 3.18. When DNA was examined shortly after the start of synthesis, small fragments were found; these were called Okazaki fragments, after the originator.

The role of RNA in DNA biosynthesis

It came as a surprise that DNA synthesis also required the cell to be synthesizing RNA. A specific enzyme, primase, is involved, as shown in Fig. 3.19. All DNA synthesis is initiated by the synthesis of a short chain of RNA, again in the direction 5'→3', using nucleoside triphosphates (NTPs) as substrate. The enzyme is selective with respect to the site for the initiation of synthesis. On the leading strand, only one primer is synthesized. On the lagging strand, many initiation sites are involved as the two strands of the parental DNA separate. The primer RNA is removed by DNA polymerase I and the gaps are filled by the same enzyme. The fragments are sealed by DNA ligase. This mechanism leads to problems in the replication of the ends of chromosomes,

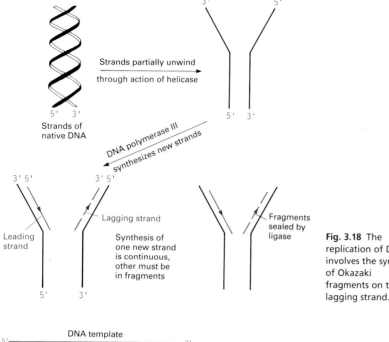

Strands partially unwind through action of helicase

Strands of native DNA

DNA polymerase III synthesizes new strands

Leading strand

Lagging strand

Synthesis of one new strand is continuous, other must be in fragments

Fragments sealed by ligase

Fig. 3.18 The replication of DNA involves the synthesis of Okazaki fragments on the lagging strand.

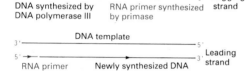

DNA template

DNA synthesized by DNA polymerase III

RNA primer synthesized by primase

Lagging strand

DNA template

RNA primer

Newly synthesized DNA

Leading strand

Fig. 3.19 DNA replication also involves the synthesis of RNA.

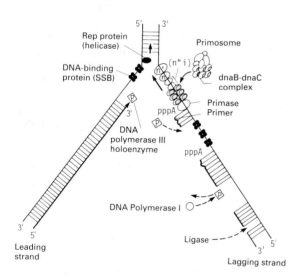

Rep protein (helicase)

DNA-binding protein (SSB)

Primosome

(n''i)

dnaB-dnaC complex

Primase Primer

pppA

DNA polymerase III holoenzyme

pppA

DNA Polymerase I

Ligase

Leading strand

Lagging strand

Fig. 3.20 DNA replication in vivo depends on the activity of many proteins participating in a multienzyme system.

will be removed by DNA polymerase I. New DNA is synthesized by DNA polymerase III holoenzyme, consisting of eight polypeptide chains. The DNA ahead of the polymerase on the leading strand is unwound by helicase (the Rep protein). On the lagging strand the gaps between the fragments of DNA are filled by DNA polymerase I and the fragments joined by DNA ligase.

At least four DNA polymerases have been identified in eukaryotes. These are designated by Greek letters: α and δ are involved in the replication of nuclear DNA, β with editing and repair, and γ with the replication of mitochondrial DNA. If the genome of a virus is composed of DNA then replication proceeds in a similar way to that described for the normal cell. Viruses have the ability to take over and utilize the normal metabolism of the cell so that, in the case of lytic phages, for example, infection causes the entire DNA replication activity to be switched to the replication of phage DNA.

OTHER ENZYMES WITH DNA SYNTHETIC ACTIVITY

Terminal transferase

Terminal transferase enzyme from calf thymus catalyses the addition of homopolymers to the 3′ terminus of deoxypolynucleotide chains as shown for the addition of poly(dT) in Fig. 3.21. Poly(dA), poly(dC) and poly(dG) can also be added. This enzyme is particularly useful in the formation of recombinant DNA, as will be described later. Different fragments of DNA can be linked after the addition of tails that are complementary to each other, e.g. poly(dA) and poly(dT).

Reverse transcriptase

This enzyme catalyses the synthesis of DNA on a single-stranded RNA chain. The physiological role of this enzyme in the retroviruses will be described later but it has been extremely important for the cloning of DNA. Again, synthesis is initiated by an RNA primer, tRNA being used for this purpose. As shown in Fig. 3.21, a hybrid double chain of RNA and DNA is formed. The enzyme is also able to remove the RNA strand. As will be shown, this enzyme is useful in recombinant DNA technology, particularly in respect to the synthesis of complementary DNA (cDNA) in which a copy of mRNA is synthesized.

known as telomeres. The resolution of the problem by telomerase is described in Chapter 16.

The multienzyme system for DNA synthesis

The enzymes and proteins operating at the fork in the bidirectional replication of DNA in *E. coli* are illustrated in Fig. 3.20. At least 15 replication proteins (comprising

over 30 polypeptides) have been characterized. The dnaA protein binds to DNA to be joined by a complex of the dnaB and dnaC proteins. dnaB is a helicase, which catalyses the ATP-driven unwinding of the double helix. The unwound portion of the DNA is then stabilized by single-stranded binding protein (SSB). An RNA primer is formed by primase in a multisubunit assembly called the primosome. At the end of replication this

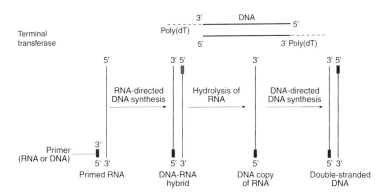

Fig. 3.21 Two enzymes with DNA synthetic activity. Above, terminal transferase usefully adds tails to DNA. Below, reverse transcriptase transcribes the base sequence of RNA into DNA.

ENZYMES THAT DEGRADE DNA

Restriction enzymes: action and nomenclature and S₁ nuclease

Restriction enzymes are the means whereby a host bacterium protects itself from foreign DNA; an infecting phage is said to be restricted by the host. These enzymes recognize a particular target sequence in duplex DNA and are, therefore, essential tools in both the determination of the primary structure of DNA and in recombinant DNA technology, as will be shown later. The most useful enzymes are known as type II, of which several hundred have now been characterized, having been isolated from a wide variety of bacteria. The nomenclature used for these enzymes is as follows: the species name of the host organism is identified by the first letter of the genus name and the first two letters of the specific epithet to a three-letter abbreviation. Thus *Escherichia coli = Eco* and *Haemophilus influenzae = Hin*. Strain or type identification is given by a further letter, hence *Hind*. Because of the symmetry of the recognition sequence, the restriction enzyme might generate fragments with mutually cohesive termini as shown in Fig. 3.22A. Other enzymes generate fragments with blunt ends.

S₁ nuclease degrades any non-base-paired region in double-stranded DNA. It is particularly useful, therefore, for the removal of nucleotides at the ends of sealed chains, as shown in Fig. 3.22B.

METABOLISM OF NUCLEOTIDES

General principles

As we have seen, deoxynucleoside triphosphates (dNTPs) and nucleoside triphosphates (NTPs) are the substrates for the synthesis of DNA and RNA, and

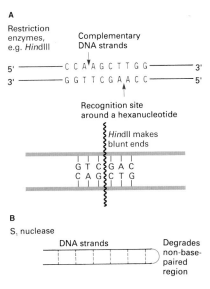

Fig. 3.22 Two types of enzyme break DNA strands. (A) Restriction enzymes that cut DNA at specific sites. These can generate either fragments with mutually cohesive termini (top) or fragments with blunt ends (bottom). (B) S₁ nuclease removes DNA strands that are not base paired.

hence any change in the availability of these substrates affects the synthesis of DNA and RNA. The metabolic pathways for the metabolism of the nucleotides are shown in Fig. 3.23.

CLINICAL IMPLICATIONS IN NUCLEOTIDE METABOLISM

Action of drugs

Various drugs that interfere with the formation of nucleotides have been used for different purposes, antibacterials, cancer chemotherapy and antimalarials, as well as the alleviation of gout. The points of attack of some of these drugs are shown in Fig. 3.23. The folate coenzymes (see p. 105) are involved at several points and can be inhibited by folate antagonists such

as fluorouracil. In the conversion of dUMP to dTMP, the methyl donor is N^5,N^{10}-methylenetetrahydrofolate; this is regenerated by dihydrofolate reductase, which is inhibited by aminopterin, methotrexate and proguanil (the last was formerly used as an antimalarial). The free purine bases formed by the degradation of nucleic acids and nucleotides are converted to purine nucleotides by a salvage pathway.

Gout

Gout, which is characterized by elevated levels of uric acid in the blood, can be alleviated by the drug allopurinol, the action of which is shown in Fig. 3.23. This results in a reduction in the formation of uric acid and an increase in the excretion of the more soluble xanthine and hypoxanthine.

DETERMINATION OF THE BASE SEQUENCE OF DNA

The Sanger method

Various methods have been used for the determination of the base sequence of DNA, the most common being that devised by Sanger and his colleagues; this is illustrated in Fig. 3.24. The 2′,3′-dideoxynucleotides of each of the four bases are prepared. These molecules are incorporated into DNA by *E. coli* DNA polymerase, but, once incorporated, the dideoxynucleotide (ddNTP) cannot form a phosphodiester bond with the next incoming dNTP and so the growth of the chain stops. A sequencing reaction consists of a DNA strand to be sequenced; a short, labelled piece of DNA (the primer) that is complementary to the end of that strand; a carefully controlled ratio of one particular ddNTP with its normal dNTP and the three other dNTPs. If the correct ratio of ddNTP to dNTP is chosen, a series of labelled strands will result, the lengths of which depend on the location of a particular base relative to the end of the DNA. A DNA strand to be sequenced, along with labelled primer, is split into four DNA polymerase reactions, each containing one of the four ddNTPs. The resultant labelled fragments are separated by size on a gel by electrophoresis.

The structure of the human genome and fingerprinting

The automation of the described Sanger method permitted the completion, in

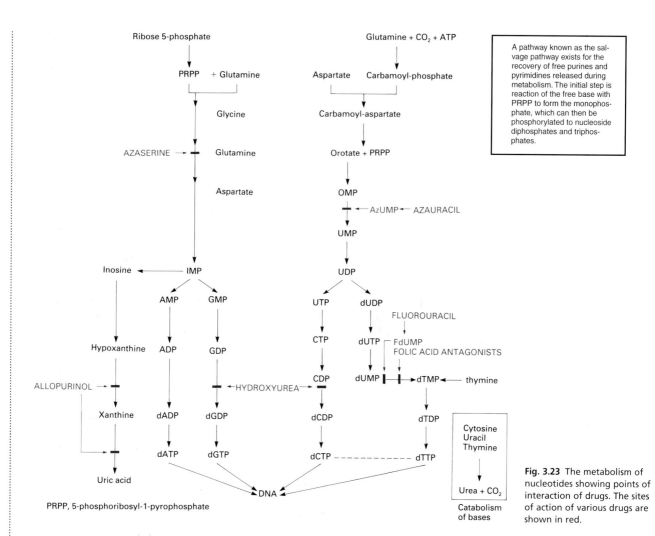

Fig. 3.23 The metabolism of nucleotides showing points of interaction of drugs. The sites of action of various drugs are shown in red.

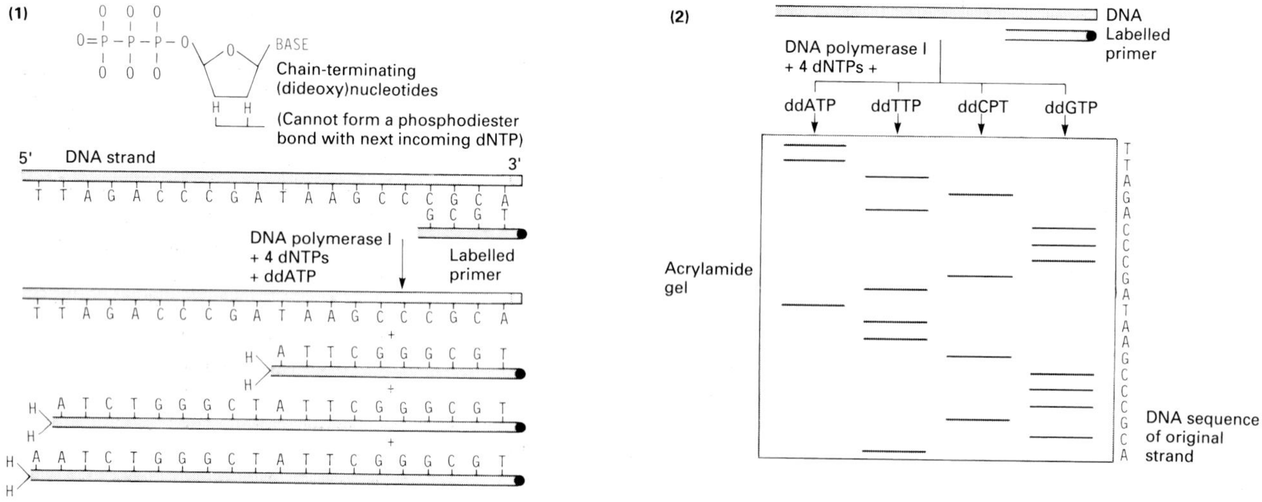

A pathway known as the salvage pathway exists for the recovery of free purines and pyrimidines released during metabolism. The initial step is reaction of the free base with PRPP to form the monophosphate, which can then be phosphorylated to nucleoside diphosphates and triphosphates.

PRPP, 5-phosphoribosyl-1-pyrophosphate

Fig. 3.24 Determination of the base sequence of DNA by the Sanger dideoxynucleotide method.

2003, of the base sequence of the entire human genome. This has greatly enhanced our ability to search for human genes and to detect those responsible for many diseases. A surprise has been the relatively small number of human genes so far

detected – fewer than 35 000. These occupy only about 5% of the DNA of the chromosomes. About half of the genes in the fruit fly are related to proteins found in the human genome, which emphasizes the value of determining the genome of other

species (see p. 218). As with other eukaryotic genomes, that of the human contains many repetitive sequences, which show two patterns of distribution in the chromosomes. Satellite DNAs are clustered in discrete areas such as the centromeres, whereas other types – such as the *Alu* class – are dispersed throughout the genome; this class constitutes 13% of the total DNA. There is considerable variability of the number of these sequences at each locus (variable number of tandem repeats, VNTR). As individuals usually inherit a different variant from their mother and from their father, the overall pattern for each person is distinct, which means that the band pattern on electrophoresis of the DNA (the fingerprint) can be used to identify an individual uniquely.

IN VITRO MUTAGENESIS

This is defined as the process of engineering specific changes in a DNA sequence in vitro to determine the effect on the function of that sequence. The DNA is first cloned so that a sufficient amount of homogeneous DNA is available (this will be described later, see p. 50). Three types of alteration can be made: deletions, insertions and replacements. Deletions can be effected by the use of restriction enzymes. Insertions are effected by the ligation of oligonucleotide linkers into restriction sites after cutting with the appropriate restriction enzyme. Replacements, which involve the alteration of a sequence at a specific point, can be achieved by making a small deletion at a restriction site and inserting into the gap an oligonucleotide linker of the same size but of different sequence. This process has been termed 'protein engineering'. In the procedure illustrated in Fig. 3.25, the gene is first cloned into a single-stranded vector, such as phage M13. A polynucleotide of about 20 nucleotides long is synthesized, which is complementary in sequence to the cloned gene at the site of the desired mutation but contains a few deliberate mistakes. The correctly matched base pairs on either side of the mistakes enable the polynucleotide to anneal to the plasmid. DNA polymerases are used to complete the circle and the product is introduced into bacteria.

DNA REPAIR

Cells have a large repertoire of repair kits to deal with damage by various external agents and to safeguard DNA against their consequences. Ultraviolet (UV) radiation can cause the formation of so-called pyrimidine dimers; this structure is illustrated in Fig. 3.26. These pyrimidine dimers can be removed by DNA photolyases or by a process known as

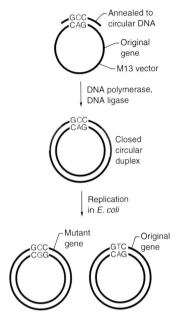

Fig. 3.25 The use of a mismatched synthetic oligonucleotide primer to introduce mutations into a gene cloned into a single-strand vector.

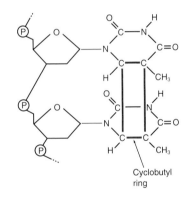

Fig. 3.26 The cyclobutylthymine dimer. The 1.6-Å long covalent bonds joining the thymine rings (red) are much shorter than the normal 3.4 Å spacing between stacked rings in B-DNA, thereby locally distorting the DNA.

nucleotide excision repair (NER), which has more relevance to humans. In the rare inherited disease xeroderma pigmentosum, the skin cells are unable to repair UV-induced DNA lesions. Individuals suffering from this autosomal recessive condition are extremely sensitive to sunlight. Cultured skin fibroblasts from such individuals are defective in the NER of pyrimidine dimers (see also tumour suppressor genes in Chapter 16). Another way of eliminating modified bases is by base excision; this involves DNA glycosylases, which cleave the glycosidic bond leaving a deoxyribose residue in the DNA backbone.

In both NER repair and base excision, endonucleases usually extend the removal beyond the defect, which is subsequently filled in by the action of polymerase I and the gap sealed by ligase.

THE POLYMERASE CHAIN REACTION (PCR)

Principles

With a knowledge of the sequence of bases that flank the region of the DNA to be amplified, oligonucleotides complementary to these sequences are prepared. The DNA containing the sequences to be amplified is heat denatured, as illustrated in Fig. 3.27, step 1, and annealed to the primers, step 2. Polymerase chain extension is carried out from the primer termini (step 3). Subsequent cycles of denaturation, annealing and primer extension are then carried out. By using a thermostable DNA polymerase (*Taq*), which is not destroyed at the temperature of the heat denaturation, the addition of fresh enzyme at each cycle is avoided. Apparatus is available to automate the recycling process. The use of additional primers around the bases of interest increases the sensitivity of the process; this is known as Nested PCR. Trace amounts of RNA can be analysed in the same way by first transcribing it into DNA by reverse transcriptase.

Uses of the PCR

By means of the PCR a 10 to 100 000-fold amplification of the DNA stretch required can be obtained. The method now has a very wide application and amounts of DNA as small as the DNA content of a single cell can be replicated. PCR is, therefore, used for the detection of DNA in blood and semen in criminal investigations, including suspected rape. Human DNA contains blocks of nucleotides that have been repeated in tandem fashion and are to be found in the non-coding regions of the genome. It is the number of times these blocks are repeated that produces the variation between individuals. These hypervariable regions are termed minisatellites. Fragments of DNA containing the minisatellites can be detected after separation by electrophoresis using probes. With PCR, very short repeating units are selected (short tandem repeats, STR). PCR is also used for the identification of virus infections and for the mutations in genes as described on p. 51.

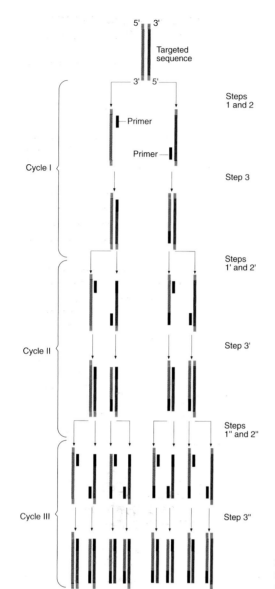

5' 3'

Targeted sequence

3' 5'

Steps 1 and 2

Primer

Primer

Cycle I

Step 3

Steps 1' and 2'

Cycle II

Step 3'

Steps 1" and 2"

Cycle III

Step 3"

Fig. 3.27 The polymerase chain reaction permits amplification of the amount of chosen stretches of DNA.

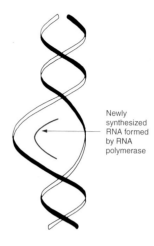

Newly synthesized RNA formed by RNA polymerase

Fig. 3.28 The transcription of DNA to produce RNA involves the separation of the strands of DNA and DNA-dependent RNA polymerase.

rRNA. RNA polymerase II is located in the nucleoplasm and synthesizes the precursors of mRNA. RNA polymerase III is located in the nucleoplasm and synthesizes the precursors of 5S rRNA, the tRNAs and a variety of small nuclear and cytoplasmic RNAs. The control of the transcription of structural genes is exercised through RNA polymerase II, so this enzyme will feature again in a later section (p. 41).

The antibiotic actinomycin D inhibits transcription by binding to the DNA template, whereas rifampicin causes such inhibition by binding to RNA polymerase.

In viruses

When the genome of a virus consists of double-stranded DNA, transcription will proceed as described for normal cells, usually using the host's RNA polymerase in the nucleus. An exception is the case of vaccinia virus, which causes cowpox. In this case, replication takes place in the cytoplasm and the virion particles carry their own RNA polymerase. If the viral DNA is single-stranded, its replication involves a double-stranded replicative form, the viral DNA being synthesized by the asymmetric synthesis of just one of the two strands.

In some cases, the genome of the virus is RNA, which occurs in two different forms. If the RNA serves as mRNA, it is denoted as (+). An example is poliomyelitis virus. The way in which this virus replicates many (+) strands is shown in Fig. 3.29. The polymerase involved is a multisubunit protein of four subunits, only one of which is virus specific, the other subunits being provided by the host cell. If the viral RNA

THE MECHANISM OF TRANSCRIPTION

In normal cells

The synthesis of RNA utilizing a DNA template is effected by DNA-dependent RNA polymerases, which use nucleoside triphosphates as substrates and effect the synthesis of chains in the direction $5' \rightarrow 3'$, reminiscent of the action of DNA polymerases. Only one strand of the DNA double helix is used as the template. Because the double-stranded DNA is conserved, the synthesis is described as conservative, but as only one strand is produced it is said to be asymmetric. The strand of DNA that is used as the template is known as the template or antisense strand; the other strand is known

as the coding or sense strand. (The base sequence of the synthesized RNA will be the same as that of the coding strand except for the substitution of uracil for thymine.) RNA polymerases are large and complex multisubunit enzymes that have the ability to select the site at which synthesis is initiated on the DNA template. Unlike DNA polymerases, they do not require a primer. The two strands of DNA separate at the site of synthesis, as shown in Fig. 3.28.

The nuclei of eukaryotic cells contain three distinct types of RNA polymerases, which differ in the RNAs that they synthesize. RNA polymerase I is located in the nucleoli, where the ribosomal genes are located, and synthesizes the precursors of most of the ribosomal RNAs (rRNAs), but not that for 5S

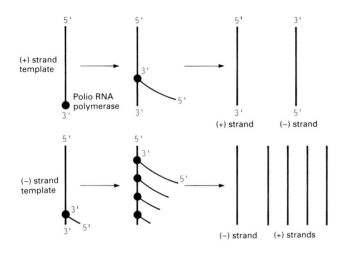

Fig. 3.29 An example of the replication of an RNA virus: poliomyelitis.

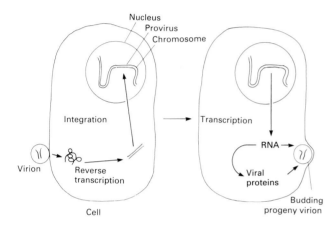

Fig. 3.30 Incorporation of the information in the RNA of a retrovirus into the DNA of the host.

is (−), the host cell cannot replicate it and the virion has to carry a replica to cause the formation of (+) strands, which serve as mRNA. Examples of such viruses are influenza, measles and rabies viruses.

REVERSE TRANSCRIPTION

General principles

Cancer-causing viruses, also called oncogenic viruses, can have as their genome either DNA or RNA. Examples of such DNA viruses are polyoma virus, Simian virus SV40 and Epstein–Barr virus (EBV). The RNA viruses are known as retroviruses; they are the only cancer-producing RNA viruses and used to be called oncorna (oncogenic RNA) viruses. They act either by introducing an oncogene into the host DNA, which leads to the synthesis of altered proteins, or by causing the production of excessive amounts of normal proteins that play a key role in growth regulation (see also p. 221). The normal cells are said to be transformed to neoplastic cells, which not

only grow faster than normal but are also immortal. Normal cells contain genes that might be mutated (often by only one base change) to become cancer producing; such genes are called protooncogenes and, unlike oncogenes, they contain introns (see p. 39). It is probable that viral oncogenes were derived from protooncogenes. It came as a surprise that the synthesis of DNA was essential for the propagation of oncorna viruses. It was then discovered that the structure of their RNA was integrated into the host genome and that an RNA-directed DNA polymerase, known as reverse transcriptase, was involved. The idea that information from RNA could be channelled back to DNA appeared to some experts as a contradiction of the central dogma of Crick (see p. 18) concerning information transfer, but it is not really so. The mechanism of action of reverse transcriptase is illustrated in Fig. 3.21. The way in which the base sequence of the viral RNA is copied into the host chromosome to become a provirus is illustrated in Fig. 3.30.

CLINICAL IMPLICATIONS – HUMAN IMMUNODEFICIENCY VIRUS (HIV)

The structure of human immunodeficiency virus (HIV-1), the retrovirus that is the causative agent for acquired immunodeficiency syndrome (AIDS), is shown in Fig. 3.31. The HIV virion is about 100 nm in diameter. The distribution of the various proteins is shown. HIV enters T4 lymphocytes by the interaction of gp120 with a plasma membrane receptor CD4, although a further chemokine receptor, called CCR5, is required for the entry of the virus in the early stages of infection. The viral core enters the cytosol of the host cells. This results in destruction of T4 lymphocytes, which are vital contributors to the immune response. The primary structure of gp120 undergoes rapid mutation, a fact that makes the preparation of an effective vaccine difficult. The primary translation product of the provirion is a polyprotein, which requires to be split by a protease. Several drugs are aimed at the inhibition of this protease (see Antiviral drugs, below). Another human retrovirus is human T-cell lymphotrophic virus (HTLV), which causes a form of leukemia (see Chapter 16).

CLINICAL IMPLICATIONS – ACTION OF ANTIBIOTICS AND ANTIMETABOLITES ON REPLICATION AND TRANSCRIPTION

General principles

The processes of replication and transcription are obviously potentially important sites for the action of drugs, either to protect eukaryotic cells from the action of bacteria and viruses or to inhibit the growth of neoplastic cells. Sometimes it is necessary to protect animal cells from the action of other eukaryotic cells such as fungi (e.g. yeasts), protozoa and amoebae, but this presents problems because they share a common metabolism with higher eukaryotes. In principle, it is easier to inhibit differentially the growth of bacteria. An example is the action of rifampicin, which inhibits bacterial DNA replication by interaction with RNA polymerase but has little effect on replication by eukaryotes. Drugs that are used in the chemotherapy of cancer are rather non-specific in that they are designed to inhibit the activity of all rapidly dividing cells, including the mucosal cells of the intestine and the hair follicles. The toxicity of such drugs can be limited to some extent by using a cocktail of various drugs in which

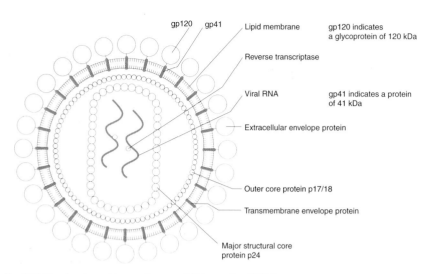

Fig. 3.31 The structure of human immunodeficiency virus (HIV-1).

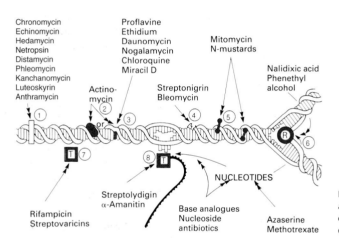

Fig. 3.32 The site of action of chemotherapeutic drugs.

Antiviral drugs

Because the viruses enter into such a close integration with the replication of the host nucleic acids, it has been difficult to devise drugs that interfere specifically with the replication of the virus (i.e. are not toxic to the host), although some progress has been made. Thus aciclovir (acycloguanosine) is a guanine derivative that is phosphorylated in herpes virus-infected cells much faster than in uninfected cells due to the action of a herpes-specific thymidine kinase. The product, acycloguanosine triphosphate, inhibits herpes virus DNA polymerase more effectively than the host cell DNA polymerase. AZT (zidovudine) (3′-azido-3′-deoxythymidine) undergoes phosphorylation in human T cells to a nucleoside 5′-triphosphate, which competes with TTP and serves as a chain-terminating inhibitor of HIV reverse transcriptase. The structures of aciclovir and AZT are shown in Fig. 3.33. The HIV protease encoded by the viral *pol* gene belongs to the aspartyl family of proteases. The structure of the HIV protease revealed by X-ray crystallography has facilitated the design of non-peptide inhibitors. To reduce the development of resistance, the drugs are given as a triple therapy, each drug having a different site of inhibition. Although the drugs do not cure the patient of the HIV infection, they markedly reduce the viral load and substantially prolong life.

Antisense RNA and RNA interference (RNAi)

Antisense RNA is defined as a short RNA transcript that lacks coding capacity but has a high degree of complementarity to another RNA that enables the two to hybridize. Such an antisense RNA can act as a repressor of the normal function or expression of the targeted RNA. Thus, antisense RNA has been transferred to cells to inhibit the synthesis of a specific

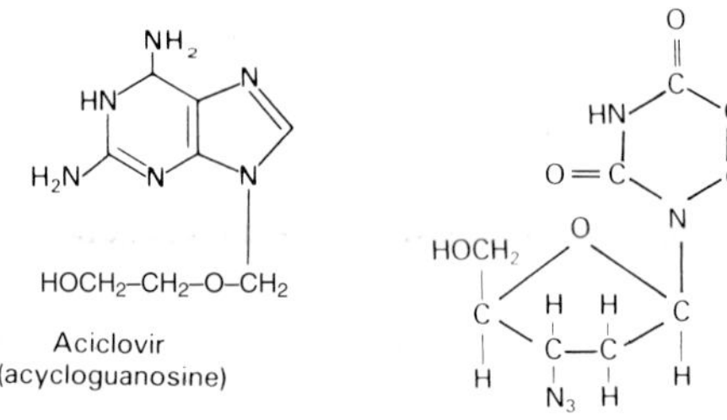

each is present at a low concentration. Inhibitors of steps in the biosynthesis of DNA precursors have already been described (see p. 26).

Drugs that interact with DNA to inhibit replication or transcription

These inhibitors act in various ways, as indicated in Fig. 3.32.

1. Drugs that bind non-covalently to DNA by unknown mechanisms and prevent replication.
2. Actinomycin D binds to DNA without distortion of the helix structure to prevent transcription; doxorubicin (Adriamycin); chronomycin A and distamycin act in a similar manner.
3. Substances that bind to DNA with distortion of the helix structure.
4. Drugs that break the strands of DNA.
5. The nitrogen mustards and mitomycin C are typical alkylating agents and cause cross-linking of the DNA strands; chlorambucil, cyclophosphamide and

busulfan (Myeleran) act in a similar manner.
6. Substances that prevent replication by binding at the fork.
7. As mentioned above, rifampicin inhibits RNA polymerase.
8. α-Amanitin from mushrooms inhibits eukaryotic polymerase II; the platinum drugs (cisplatin and carboplatin) induce both inter- and intrastrand cross-links; hexamethylmelamine and dacarbazine (DTIC) both methylate DNA.

Fig. 3.33 The structure of two antiviral drugs: aciclovir and AZT.

Aciclovir (acycloguanosine)

AZT (zidovudine) (Retrovir) (3'-azido-3'-deoxythymidine)

protein. Antisense RNA has been largely superseded by RNAi, which silences a target gene through the specific destruction of that gene's mRNA. Double-stranded RNA (dsRNA) is central to the technique. When dsRNA with identical sequences to a specific mRNA is introduced into cells, the mRNA is recognized and degraded by a multiprotein body called the RNA-induced silencing complex. The destruction of the target mRNA leads to a drop in the levels of the encoded protein and thus inhibition of the target gene. In worms and flies, dsRNA of hundreds of nucleotides can be used but in mammalian cells long dsRNA induces an antiviral response. Instead, small interfering RNAs (siRNAs) about 21 nucleotides long are efficiently used by the RNA-induced silencing complex. siRNA can either be synthesized and introduced into the cells or can be made directly in the cells through the expression of short hairpin RNAs (shRNAs). Such shRNA can be used to induce RNAi in transgenic mice (see p. 51), so the technique can be used to investigate gene function in whole animals.

BIOSYNTHESIS OF PROTEINS: TRANSLATION

GENERAL PRINCIPLES

Bodily requirements

The body requires a net increase in the amount of protein to provide for growth, the replacement of cells after their death (e.g. in the brush border of the intestine) and the production of milk proteins during lactation. Such an increase can result from an increase in the rate of synthesis or a decrease in the rate of breakdown. Adult man synthesizes about 400 g of protein every day.

Metabolic turnover

When isotopically labelled amino acids were administered to rats, it came as a surprise to find that most of the body proteins were being constantly synthesized and degraded to free amino acids (see Fig. 3.34). This led to the general concept of the dynamic state of body constituents. It was subsequently shown that the various proteins were turned over at different rates and that the rate of turnover depended on various pathological conditions. In general terms, the protein synthetic machinery of the body is always operating at full

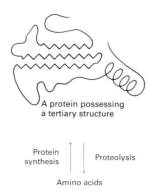

Protein synthesis | Proteolysis

Amino acids

Fig. 3.34 The synthesis of protein from free amino acids.

capacity, so that if more of a particular protein is required then the rate of synthesis of other proteins must be reduced. The rate of turnover of a protein is usually expressed in terms of its biological half-life. The most stable protein in the body is collagen, which is also the most abundant. Even so, the collagen in some tissues turns over faster than the average in other tissues. The brain proteins are also thought to have a low rate of turnover, although there is now some doubt as to the validity of this view.

Intermediates in protein synthesis

Because proteolytic enzymes can degrade proteins to polypeptides, it seemed possible that these might be the substrates for protein synthesis. Indeed, in view of the similarity of the domains within the different proteins – even those possessing different functions – the possibility that the primary structures of proteins might be modified by the exchange of amino acids within existing polypeptide chains was considered. It is now apparent that in virtually all cases the polypeptide backbone of all proteins is synthesized from free amino acids.

Specialization between organs

Although, as we have seen, the DNA in all cells of the body has the potential to provide the genetic information for the synthesis of all bodily proteins, the various tissues and organs specialize in respect of the proteins they synthesize (Fig. 3.35). Thus, some cells synthesize only a single protein, such as the synthesis of hemoglobin by the reticulocytes. Other cells synthesize a broad range of proteins; for example, the hepatocytes in the liver synthesize all the serum proteins except for the γ-globulins. This means that there must

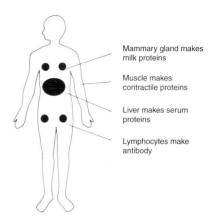

Mammary gland makes milk proteins

Muscle makes contractile proteins

Liver makes serum proteins

Lymphocytes make antibody

Fig. 3.35 The various organs of the body synthesize different proteins through the differential expression of their common DNA.

be methods for the control of differential protein synthesis. That such controls are potentially reversible is shown by the fact that DNA taken from adult (i.e. differentiated) cells can be used for the generation of an embryo, the so-called cloning experiment in sheep. Sometimes tumours possess the ability to synthesize proteins other than those expected of their cell of origin e.g. the synthesis of α-fetoprotein (typical of the embryo) by hepatoma cells; this phenomenon is known as ectopic protein synthesis.

ASSEMBLY OF AMINO ACIDS ON A TEMPLATE

Evidence in support of the template hypothesis

Before the method whereby proteins were synthesized in vivo was known, it was postulated that the amino acids would be linked together under the direction of specific enzymes. Although this was subsequently found to be true for the synthesis of many biologically active peptides derived from microorganisms, it is not so for the synthesis of proteins. In microorganisms, the biosynthetic systems that catalyse the formation of biologically active peptides, especially those that have antibacterial activity, consist of interacting multienzymes that are often very large (with an M_r up to 1 700 000). The respective genes of repeating modules each encode the incorporation of one amino acid residue. ATP is used as an energy source. In view of their size, the enzymic synthesis of proteins would demand an enormous range of specific enzymes. The concept of assembly of the amino acids on a template was contemplated even before

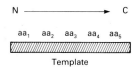

Fig. 3.36 The amino acids (aa) are temporally assembled on a template, in an order starting from the N-terminus of the polypeptide.

Glycine (Gly, G)	Proline (Pro, P)	Asparagine (Asp, N)
Valine (Val, V)	Tryptophan (Trp, W)	Lysine (Lys, K)
Alanine (Ala, A)	Tyrosine (Tyr, Y)	Arginine (Arg, R)
Leucine (Leu, L)	Phenylalanine (Phe, F)	Histidine (His, H)
Isoleucine (Ile, I)	Glutamic acid (Glu, E)	Methionine (Met, M)
Serine (Ser, S)	Glutamine (Gln, Q)	Cysteine (Cys, C)
Threonine (Thr, T)	Aspartic acid (Asp, D)	

the nature of the template was known; it was subsequently shown to be RNA. Studies on the synthesis of hemoglobin showed that the participating amino acids are assembled from the amino-terminus (N-terminus), as shown in Fig. 3.36.

The nature of participating amino acids and achievement of tertiary structure

Although proteins contain a wide variety of different amino acids, only 20 participate in the assembly on the template; these are listed in Table 3.4. Some of the amino acid residues are subsequently modified after incorporation into the polypeptide chains. This process is known as post-translational modification. Among the amino acids incorporated are glutamine and asparagine but other amino acids that commonly occur in proteins, such as hydroxyproline and hydroxylysine, and phosphoserine, phosphothreonine and phosphotyrosine, are not included. In such cases the parent amino acids undergo hydroxylation or phosphorylation after their incorporation into the polypeptide chain. Cystine is formed from two cysteine residues. Whereas molecular chaperones can influence the tertiary structure of a protein (see pp. 14 and 15) this section, on protein synthesis, will be concerned primarily with the biosynthesis of polypeptides with the correct primary structure.

Synthesis of multichain proteins

As we have seen, some proteins comprise several different polypeptide chains. The association of such chains might be by means of weak non-covalent bonds, as with hemoglobin (see Fig. 3.37), in which case the chains associate spontaneously and no novel mechanism is required. In other cases, association might be promoted by the presence of another protein, known as a molecular chaperone. An example is that of the immunoglobulins, where Ig-binding protein, present within the rough endoplasmic reticulum of the plasma cells,

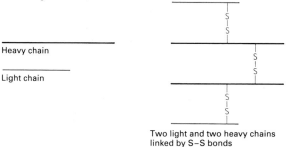

Fig. 3.37 The biosynthesis of multichain proteins. The separate chains usually associate spontaneously.

assists in combining the heavy and light chains. Proteins that are destined to be exported from a cell are usually synthesized in a precursor form with an additional peptide at the N-terminus. Such proteins (e.g. serum albumin) are known as proproteins and the peptide as a propeptide. The propeptide is removed by an enzyme called furin, a member of a superfamily of PC proteases, during the passage of the protein through the Golgi apparatus to give rise to the mature protein. Many propeptides, including those in the blood coagulation cascade and numerous viral proteins, are linked to the mature protein through two adjacent basic amino acids (see, for example, proopiomelanocortin, p. 33). The biosynthesis of collagen, which has multiple chains, also involves the synthesis of a precursor protein, procollagen, which has N- and C-terminal-extension peptides that serve to align the association of the chains. The structure and biosynthesis of collagen is described in Chapter 5 (p. 72).

The synthesis of insulin calls for particular consideration.

The biosynthesis of insulin

Insulin is closely related structurally to relaxin and insulin-like growth factors-1 and -2 (somatomedins), which are synthesized in the liver and certain target tissues under the control of growth hormone (somatotropin), which is secreted by the anterior pituitary. Insulin consists of two chains, shown in Fig. 3.38 in red. It is synthesized as a precursor, proinsulin, in which the two chains are linked by a connecting peptide, amino acid residues 31–63. Proinsulin, which has only 5% of the biological activity of insulin, is converted to insulin within the Golgi apparatus. In the conversion, the proteases PC2 and PC3 each cleave on the carboxyl side of a pair of basic amino acids KR (63 and 1) and RR (33 and 32). A carboxypeptidase-B-like protease (carboxypeptidase H) then acts to remove the remaining RR to form insulin. The connecting peptide without the terminal RR is known as the C-peptide. (Although this peptide has no insulin-like action, it is thought to serve various functions.)

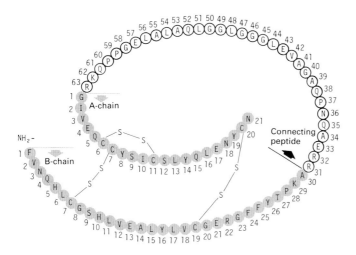

Fig. 3.38 The conversion of pig proinsulin to insulin.

Proinsulin, like most secreted proteins (as will be explained, see p. 45), is synthesized as a precursor with an extra N-terminal peptide (the signal peptide), the complete molecule being known as preproinsulin; however, the additional prepeptide is removed before the synthesis of proinsulin is completed so that preproinsulin under in vivo conditions does not exist in its entirety.

The synthesis of polyproteins

As mentioned in Chapter 2 (p. 16), in the case of some peptide hormones the active peptide is split from a larger protein. When the precursor protein gives rise to more than one mature protein it is known as a polyprotein. The cleavage pattern of a particular polyprotein can vary in different tissues; thus the same gene product can yield different sets of polypeptide hormones. An example of this is proopiomelanocortin, which is the precursor of adrenocorticotropic hormone (ACTH) and other hormones, as depicted

in Fig. 3.39. The initial translation product in the pituitary contains a signal peptide at the N-terminus, which is removed to give proopiomelanocortin, with an M_r of 31 000. The dark vertical bars represent proteolytic cleavage sites for specific enzymes, which comprise a family of proteases named Kex2, PC2 and PC3. The cleavage sites are Arg–Lys, Lys–Arg or Lys–Lys. In the corticotropic cell of the anterior pituitary, enzymes are present that cleave at sites 3 and 5, releasing the major products ACTH and β-lipotropin into the general circulation. In the pars intermedia, especially in sub-human vertebrates, these products are further cleaved at major sites 4, 6 and 7 to release α-MSH (melanocyte-stimulating hormone), CLIP (corticotropin-like intermediate lobe peptide), γ-lipotropin and β-endorphin into the general circulation. Some β-lipotropin might be further degraded to form β-endorphin. This contains a pentapeptide, enkephalin, which can be released by hydrolysis at 8. β-Endorphin has morphine-like properties (*endogenous*

morphine) in that it and enkephalin bind to opiate receptors in nervous tissue. β-Lipotropin was once thought, erroneously, to mobilize fatty acids from adipose tissue.

Although, as indicated, β-endorphin can give rise to Met-enkephalin, it was subsequently shown that the enkephalins in the adrenals and brain arise from proenkephalins, which contain multiple copies (often six) of the enkephalins sandwiched between pairs of basic amino acid residues.

STEPS IN THE SYNTHESIS OF PROTEINS FROM FREE AMINO ACIDS

Amino acid activation

The first step in protein synthesis involves the activation of the amino acids. Because polypeptides are polymers, energy must be utilized in their formation. Hence an activated amino acid was sought. It was soon shown that the activation took place on the carboxyl group of the amino acid by a reaction involving ATP to yield an amino acid adenylate and pyrophosphate, as shown in Fig. 3.40. There is a specific enzyme for the activation of each of the 20 different amino acids.

Attachment of amino acid to transfer RNA

The second step involves the transfer of the activated amino acid to transfer RNA (tRNA) (see Fig. 3.41). In this transfer the same enzymes are involved as those that catalyse the first step. There is at least one specific tRNA for each of the 20 amino acids but all have the same three nucleotides at the 3'-terminus, namely CCA, to which the amino acid residue is attached. The link is by means of an ester bond, which facilitates the subsequent utilization of the amino acid in the formation of a peptide bond.

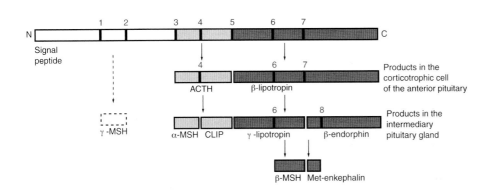

Fig. 3.39 Peptide hormones often result from the fragmentation of a larger precursor protein. The break-up of preproopiomelanocortin.

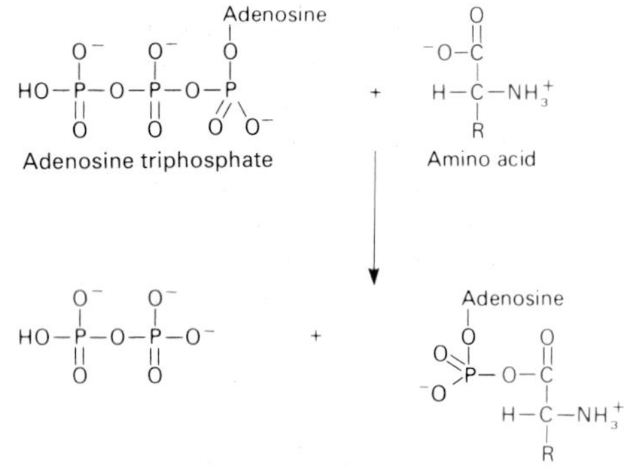

Adenosine

$$HO-P-O-P-O-P \quad + \quad H-C-NH_3^+$$

Adenosine triphosphate

Amino acid

$$HO-P-O-P-O^- \quad + \quad$$

Adenosine

H-C-NH₃⁺

Fig. 3.40 Step 1. The activation of amino acids.

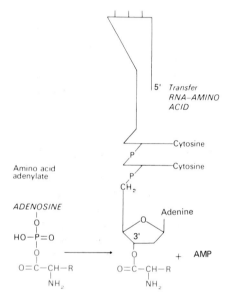

5' *Transfer RNA–AMINO ACID*

Cytosine

Cytosine

CH_2

Amino acid adenylate

ADENOSINE

$HO-P=O$

Adenine

3'

+ AMP

$$O=C-CH-R \quad\quad O=C-CH-R$$
$$NH_2 \quad\quad\quad NH_2$$

Fig. 3.41 Step 2. The transfer of the activated amino acid to transfer RNA (tRNA).

THE GENETIC CODE

Role of the 64 codons

Theoretical considerations led to the prediction that the code for the translation of the sequence of four different nucleotides – the base sequence – in mRNA into the order of the 20 amino acids in a polypeptide would be at least a triplet of bases, called a codon. This prediction was later supported by genetic experiments involving missense mutations. The code shown in Fig. 3.42 has 61 triplets coding for the amino acids. Three triplets indicate the termination (marked Term★) of a polypeptide chain (so-called nonsense codons because they do not code for an amino acid). Two other triplets are used for initiation (marked Init.†) as well as for Met and Val, respectively, although the triplet for Val is seldom used for this purpose. The genetic code is generally found to be universal in that it appears to be valid for all living cells whether eukaryotic or prokaryotic. The code for mitochondria differs in some respects from that indicated. Thus, in humans, UGA is used for Trp rather than Term, AUA for Met rather than Ile, and AGA for Term rather than Arg.

The genetic code in vivo

The genetic code was determined mainly using cell-free systems. Its reality can be checked in two ways. First, whether it accounts for single amino acid changes (missense mutations) in a protein, such as occurs for hemoglobin in sickle-cell disease, on the basis that it is a single-point mutation. As shown in Fig. 3.43 it passes this test. The change from glutamic acid to valine in position 6 of the β chain arises as a result of a change of A for U in either of the possible codons for the two amino acids. The second check is whether the known structure of an mRNA accords with the structure of the corresponding polypeptide. The polypeptide and mRNA are found to be collinear, the mRNA being read from 5'→3'. From such considerations it is right to conclude that the genetic code holds for the living cell.

Initiation and reading frames

Recognition of the initiator codon determines the reading frame, i.e. which bases will form the triplets for successive codons. As shown in Fig. 3.44, the sequence of bases starts with AUG. As AUG also codes for methionine, all proteins start with this amino acid residue but, as there are many AUG codons in a given mRNA, special means have to be in place to designate the AUG codon that signifies initiation. The mRNA shown in Fig. 3.44 ends with UAG – one of the three codons used for termination. In the mRNA for any particular protein several codons might be used for a particular amino acid, such as glycine, as indicated. Thus there is degeneracy within a particular mRNA.

STRUCTURE OF TRANSFER RNA

Secondary structure and location of anticodons

In the early studies there was much speculation as to the way in which any particular amino acid would become associated with its codon on the mRNA. Crick predicted that it would be through the medium of a small adaptor RNA, which would bear an anticodon. The discovery of transfer RNA (tRNA, originally called soluble RNA because it was not associated with any particles in a disrupted cell) supported this hypothesis and it was subsequently shown that tRNA

Second base of codon:						
	U	C	A	G		
U	UUU ⎤ Phe UUC ⎦ UUA ⎤ Leu UUG ⎦	UCU ⎤ UCC ⎥ Ser UCA ⎥ UCG ⎦	UAU ⎤ Tyr UAC ⎦ UAA ⎤ Term★ UAG ⎦	UGU ⎤ Cys UGC ⎦ UGA Term★ UGG Trp	U C A G	
C	CUU ⎤ CUC ⎥ Leu CUA ⎥ CUG ⎦	CCU ⎤ CCC ⎥ Pro CCA ⎥ CCG ⎦	CAU ⎤ His CAC ⎦ CAA ⎤ Gln GAG ⎦	CGU ⎤ CGC ⎥ Arg CGA ⎥ CGG ⎦	U C A G	
A	AUU ⎤ AUC ⎥ Ile AUA ⎦ AUG Met+Init.†	ACU ⎤ ACC ⎥ Thr ACA ⎥ ACG ⎦	AAU ⎤ Asn AAC ⎦ AAA ⎤ Lys AAG ⎦	AGU ⎤ Ser AGC ⎦ AGA ⎤ Arg AGG ⎦	U C A G	
G	GUU ⎤ GUC ⎥ Val GUA ⎦ GUG Val+Init.†	GCU ⎤ GCC ⎥ Ala GCA ⎥ GCG ⎦	GAU ⎤ Asp GAC ⎦ GAA ⎤ Glu GAG ⎦	GGU ⎤ GGC ⎥ Gly GGA ⎥ GGG ⎦	U C A G	

(First base of codon / Third base of codon)

Fig. 3.42 The genetic code. Init. and Term indicate initiation and termination, respectively.

	HbA Glu	HbS Val
Possible ⎫ codons ⎬	GAA GAG	GUA GUG

Fig. 3.43 The mRNA for sickle-cell hemoglobin.

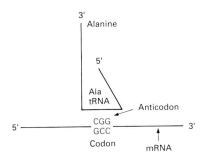

NH₂ term

Met Pro Ser Ala Gly Gly
AUGCCGUCGGCGGGCGGUUAG

5'   3'

COOH term

Fig. 3.44 Utilization of the codons in mRNA.

Fig. 3.45 Coupling of the anticodon on tRNA to the complementary codon on mRNA.

bearing an amino acid has the unique property of locating itself at the correct codon. The structure of the anticodon, indicated by CGG (3'→5') in Fig. 3.45, can be predicted, with certain reservations as will be explained, from our knowledge of base pairing (A–U, G–C).

Structure of alanine tRNA

A common feature of all tRNAs is that they contain many intramolecular base pairs and also many modified bases (e.g. methylguanosine, MeG). The significance of these modified bases is not known with any certainty.

Having determined the primary structure of alanine tRNA, Holley studied the way in which the maximum number of intramolecular base pairs could be formed. Fig. 3.46 shows that all the bases except those shown in the loops could be so base paired, producing a structure in the form of a clover leaf. The primary structure of all the other tRNAs studied conforms

with the clover leaf, as do the few tertiary structures determined by X-ray crystallography. As expected, a triplet of unpaired bases is present that could serve as an anticodon. These are in the so-called anticodon loop. I stands for inosine, which is deaminated adenosine (A), and would normally pair as A.

The wobble hypothesis

From the genetic code, 61 different tRNAs might be expected to exist (one for each sense codon). However, because one anticodon can pair with more than one codon, there are probably no more than 40 different tRNAs. Crick predicted that, whereas there would be G–C, A–U pairing at the first two codon bases, the pairing at the third base might be more imprecise. This was called the wobble hypothesis, for which there is now ample support. Thus, in the third position, I can pair with U, C or A. This is shown in Fig. 3.47 and explains why there are only two different tRNAs for alanine, which has four codons.

THE ROLE OF THE RIBOSOME

Ribosome structure

The biosynthesis of polypeptides involves the participation of particles, i.e. it is not effected in a soluble system. These particles

5' Codons   3' GCU   GCC   GCA   GCG
3' Anticodons 5' CGI   CGI   CGI   CGC

Fig. 3.47 The base pairing of the two tRNAs for alanine with the four codons for alanine.

are called ribosomes. They contain proteins, RNA and magnesium ions (Mg^{2+}). The ribosomes from prokaryotes and eukaryotes are similar in structure even though the ratio of protein to RNA differs and there are subtle differences in their biological activity. Ribosomes from different sources are characterized by their sedimentation coefficients (expressed in Svedberg units, S), as shown in Table 3.5. A ribosome consists of two subunits, one being about twice the size of the other, hence the names large and small subunit. Again, the subunits are characterized by their S values; those from prokaryotes are named 50S (large) and 30S (small) and those from eukaryotes 60S and 40S. The ribosomes from mitochondria are smaller than those in the rest of the eukaryotic cell (they are sometimes known as mitoribosomes to differentiate them from cytoribosomes) and resemble prokaryotic ribosomes. Mitoribosomes vary in size according to their source.

Characteristics of ribosomal RNA

The size of the RNA within the different ribosomal subunits, ribosomal RNA (rRNA), differs, as does the number of different rRNAs. As shown in Table 3.6, the 50S subunit from prokaryotes contains two kinds of RNA, 23S and 5S, whereas

Table 3.5 Sedimentation coefficients (in Svedberg units, S) of ribosomes and their subunits

	Intact ribosome	Large subunit	Small subunit
Prokaryotes	70S	50S	30S
Eukaryotes	80S	60S	40S

Table 3.6 Characteristics of the RNA within the ribosomal subunits

Ribosomal subunit	S of RNA	M_r
50S	23S	0.98×10^6
	5S	4×10^4
30S	16S	0.9×10^6
60S	28S	1.7×10^6
	5.8S	5.1×10^4
	5S	3.9×10^4
40S	18S	0.7×10^6

M_r, relative molecular mass; S, Svedberg unit.

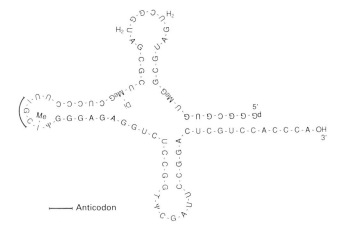

Fig. 3.46 The secondary structure of alanine tRNA showing the anticodon loop.

Anticodon

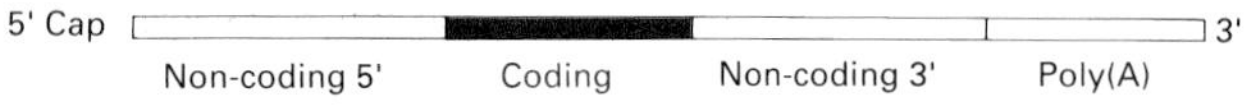

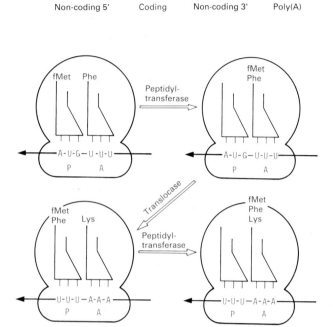

5' Cap | Non-coding 5' | Coding | Non-coding 3' | Poly(A) | 3'

Fig. 3.48 The structure of mRNA from eukaryotes.

Fig. 3.49 The ribosome and chain elongation.

the 30S subunit contains only one kind of RNA, 16S. A similar situation is found for eukaryotes except that the 60S subunit contains three kinds of RNA.

Messenger RNA and its structure

rRNA is not the template on which the amino acids are assembled. The template consists of another type of RNA, messenger RNA (mRNA), which becomes associated with the ribosomes to form polyribosomes. Figure 3.48 shows the structural characteristics of a typical mRNA. At the 5′ end (described as upstream), there is a region that does not code for amino acids (the so-called 5′ non-coding region). In bacteria there is evidence that the base sequence of this region is complementary to the 3′ end of the 16S RNA, and hence it is postulated that the region has a role in the association of mRNA with the 30S ribosomal subunit (this sequence is sometimes called the Shine–Dalgarno sequence after those who originally identified it). In many eukaryote mRNAs there is a cap at the 5′ end consisting of 7-methylguanosine which is attached by a triphosphate bridge. The 3′ end usually possesses a tail of A, the poly(A) tail, which does not code for amino acids.

The editing of mRNA

One or more bases in mRNA might be modified in vivo, a process known as RNA editing. Most of the known cases concern

mitochondria but in the mRNA for apolipoprotein B-100 (see p. 164) a cytidine is deaminated to a uridine. Thus, the codon for glutamine (CAA) (see Fig. 3.42) becomes a stop codon (UAA) and a shortened form of protein (apo B-48) results. The site-specific deamination is effected by an enzyme complex containing a protein, apobec-1, which is homologous with an enzyme, activation induced deaminase, which deaminates C in a specific sequence of DNA in lymphocyte B cells and is important in the generation of gene diversification in adaptive and innate immunity.

Chain elongation

Chain elongation involves a shuttle movement of tRNA between two sites on the ribosome, labelled sites P (peptidyl) and A (aminoacyl) in Fig. 3.49. The aminoacyl tRNA normally enters the A site whereas the nascent peptide attached to tRNA is attached to the P site. When the two tRNAs are assembled on the ribosome, a peptide bond is formed by a nucleophilic attack by the α-amino group of the amino acid attached to the incoming tRNA at site A on the carboxyl group of the nascent chain already attached at site P to the tRNA. (The significance of fMet will be explained below.) The tRNA is then released from site P of the ribosome. The formation of the new peptide bond is catalysed by the enzyme peptidyltransferase. The tRNA bearing the

newly extended peptide is then moved from the A site to the P site, a process known as translocation. This is catalysed by the enzyme translocase. After peptide bond formation the tRNA moves to the E site before finally leaving the ribosome.

Chain initiation

As already explained, the aminoacyl tRNA normally enters the A site, so the task of chain initiation is to ensure that the aminoacyl tRNA bearing the N-terminal amino acid residue in the nascent polypeptide chain enters the P site. In eukaryotes, methionine (Met), and in prokaryotes, formylMet (fMet), always serve as the N-terminal amino acid residue of newly initiated polypeptides. There are two different tRNA molecules for Met even though there is only one codon. The tRNA that has the unique property of entering the P site is called initiator tRNA. A Met bound to this tRNA can be formylated in the presence of an enzyme, as it always is in prokaryotes, and is designated $tRNA_f^{Met}$. Although the mechanism of chain initiation in both types of cell is similar, eukaryotes lack the formylating enzyme so the N-terminal amino acid residue is Met rather than fMet. The formylating enzyme is present in mitochondria, so chain initiation resembles that in prokaryotes. In prokaryotes, the formyl group is removed, as is the Met if it is not to be the N-terminal amino acid residue of the mature protein. In eukaryotes the Met is similarly removed in appropriate cases when about 30 amino acids have been added to the chain.

Initiation factors in eukaryotes

Many proteins serve as initiation factors, which ensure the correct location of the $Met-tRNA_f^{Met}$ in the P site of the ribosome. Those for eukaryotes are designated eIFs. As shown in Fig. 3.50, these factors associate with mRNA and are joined by the small ribosomal subunit (40S) and GTP to give a complex with the AUG correctly aligned. This complex is then joined by the large ribosomal subunit (60S) with the release of GDP, to give the ribosome (80S) initiation complex. The process in prokaryotes is essentially similar, although with fewer initiation factors (designated IFs).

Chain termination

When UAA or one of the other nonsense codons (UAG, UGA) in mRNA occupies

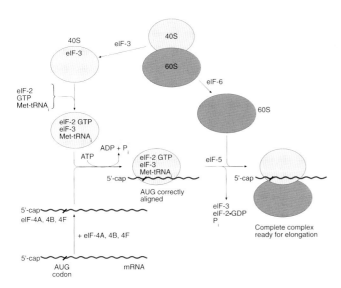

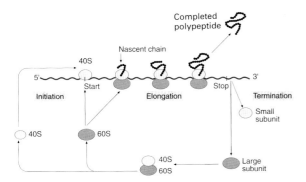

Fig. 3.50 Factors involved in chain initiation.

Fig. 3.51 The ribosome cycle and chain termination.

is worth recalling that, whereas bacteria are prokaryotes and animal cells are eukaryotes, fungi (e.g. *Candida albicans*, a pathogenic yeast) are eukaryotes. Consequently, it is difficult to find an antibiotic that is effective against the growth of fungi that is at the same time not toxic to humans.

Action of specific antibiotics

The first antibiotic to be used in experimental work was puromycin, which has a structure that resembles the 3′ terminus of tRNA with an amino acid residue attached. Puromycin prematurely terminates polypeptide synthesis, but because it is active on all types of cell it is not a useful antibiotic in therapy.

As an example of the action of antibiotics, two are shown in Fig. 3.52. Chloramphenicol inhibits peptidyltransferase in prokaryotes and in mitochondria. This accounts for the toxic effect of chloramphenicol in humans – it sometimes causes aplastic anemia. Cycloheximide inhibits translocase but it is specific for eukaryotes and is thus only useful experimentally.

Figure 3.53 shows the site of action of many commonly used antibiotics for the treatment of bacterial infection. Resistance to a wide range of chemotherapeutic agents is commonly associated with high expression levels of a single protein, the 170-kDa P-glycoprotein encoded in humans by the *MDR1* gene. The protein pumps drugs out of cells by an ATP-dependent process.

The atomic structure of the ribosome

The atomic structure of the large ribosomal subunit of an archaeal was determined recently by X-ray crystallography. This has permitted the

site A on the ribosome, a protein, known as a release factor, binds to site A in the presence of GTP and catalyses the termination reaction. The reaction involves the hydrolysis of the peptidyl tRNA ester bond, the hydrolysis of GTP and the release of the completed polypeptide chain, the de-aminoacylated tRNA and the ribosome from mRNA. In prokaryotes, there are three release factors, two of which are codon-specific, whereas in eukaryotes there are just two. Following the release of the polypeptide chain, the ribosome dissociates into its two subunits, ready for the next round of protein synthesis. A ribosome recycling factor has been identified in prokaryotes for this. The sequence of steps in the cycle is shown in Fig. 3.51.

CLINICAL IMPLICATIONS – THE ACTION OF ANTIBIOTICS ON PROTEIN SYNTHESIS

General principles

Although the mechanism of protein synthesis in prokaryotes and eukaryotes is basically similar, there are subtle differences,

such as the use of formylation of the amino acid residue in initiation mentioned above. Such differences explain the differential action of some antibiotics, which has been exploited by the pharmaceutical industry for the production of useful drugs. Penicillin is not in this category because its role is to inhibit an essential step in the synthesis of the cell-wall peptide in susceptible bacteria; it does not inhibit protein synthesis. Vancomycin binds to the terminal D-alanyl-D-alanine group on the peptide side chain of the membrane-bound intermediates in peptidoglycan synthesis. It

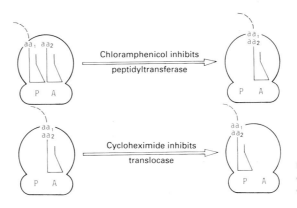

Fig. 3.52 The site of action of chloramphenicol and cycloheximide.

pinpointing of the many activities of the ribosome that have been described, e.g. the three sites of the attachment of tRNA have been visualized. The site of peptide bond synthesis turns out to be composed entirely of RNA, so that it is a ribozyme name for RNA with enzyme activity. The crystal structure of 12 complexes between the large ribosomal subunit and various antibiotics has shown that there are at least two modes by which they inhibit protein synthesis: they either block the exit of nascent polypeptides from the ribosome or bind to either the A or P site. This information should render possible the design of novel antibiotics.

THE ORIGIN OF MOLECULAR VARIANTS OF PROTEINS

Molecular variants of proteins arise by point mutations. Examples of the primary structure of such molecular variants are shown in Fig. 3.54, which are taken from the numerous hemoglobinopathies (see p. 62), serum albumin and insulin (see p. 69). In (2) there is a single amino acid change (a missense mutation), as already described for sickle-cell hemoglobin. In (3) there is a mutation that has given rise to a Term codon and so the normal chain is shortened; in summary, a sense codon has been converted to a nonsense codon. In (4), a nonsense codon has been converted to a sense codon so that an abnormally long chain is synthesized towards the C-terminus. In (5) there has been a mutation at the N-terminus, which has meant that the propeptide that is normally attached by two basic amino acids has not been removed. This occurs in some insulinopathies and in the formation of proalbumin Christchurch. The result is an abnormal extension at the N-terminus.

THE PRIMARY TRANSCRIPT OF THE GENE

Methods for demonstrating split genes

When the structure of the mRNA for ovomucoid was aligned with that of the strand of DNA from which it had been transcribed, the mRNA corresponded with a mosaic of separate segments of DNA. This is illustrated in Fig. 3.55, which is an electron micrograph of the mRNA hybridized to its genome and subsequently visualized. The DNA is shown in black and the mRNA in red. The loops of the DNA are lettered and show the sections of DNA that do not hybridize, the intervening sequences, and those that do hybridize.

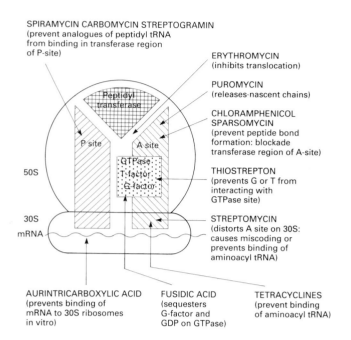

Fig. 3.53 The site of action of a range of antibiotics. Ciprofloxacin and nalidixic acid are members of the quinolone antibiotics that interact with DNA topoisomerase in the unwinding of DNA (see p. 20).

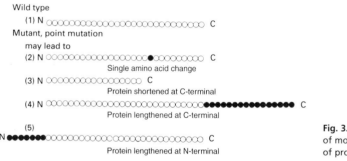

Fig. 3.54 The origin of molecular variants of proteins.

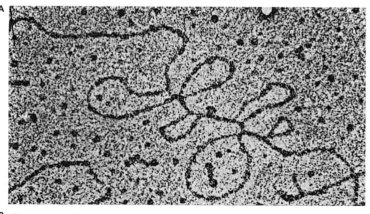

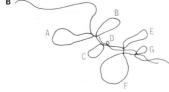

Fig. 3.55 Electron micrograph and line visualization revealing intervening sequences in a gene.

Introns and exons

Transcription gives rise to pre-mRNA (also called heterogeneous RNA or Hn-RNA). Figure 3.56 shows how the primary transcript pre-mRNA of the ovomucoid gene is modified to produce the mature mRNA, which is subsequently translated into protein. At the top of the figure is the template strand of the DNA with the loops labelled as in Fig. 3.55. The black blocks indicate the nucleotides that will subsequently be translated. These are known as exons, the intervening sequences being known as introns. The introns are excised and the exons are spliced together to give the mature mRNA, which is translated into protein. Nearly all eukaryotic genes contain introns, but they are not found in prokaryotes. Human genes are mostly composed of relatively short exons (average 146 base pairs) separated by much longer non-coding introns (average 3000 base pairs). This has complicated the search for human genes even with a knowledge of the structure of the entire human genome (see p. 218).

Excision of introns and splicing of exons

It is important that the introns should be excised from the pre-mRNA very accurately and that the exons are correctly spliced together. The essential basis for this process is the consensus sequences of bases of the introns; some of these are shown in Fig. 3.57. Thus, at the 5′ end of the introns there is AGGUAAGU, whereas at the 3′ end there is a stretch of ten pyrimidines (U or C) followed by any base (N) and by C and ending with AG. There is also a site between 20 and 50 nucleotides upstream of the 3′ splice site called the branch site.

Figure 3.58 shows how the excision and splicing is achieved and in particular how the branch site is used for the formation of a lariat. The process occurs in two transesterification reactions. First there is the formation of a 2′,5′-phosphodiester group with the concomitant release of the 5′ exon. Then the free 3′-hydroxyl group of the 5′ exon forms a phosphodiester bond with the 5′-terminal phosphate of the 3′ exon, yielding the spliced product. The intron is released in its lariat form and is rapidly degraded. The splice junctions are recognized and the two exons to be joined are brought together by means of small nuclear RNAs (snRNAs), which form protein complexes called small nuclear ribonucleoproteins (snRNPs, pronounced 'snurps'). The complex is known as a

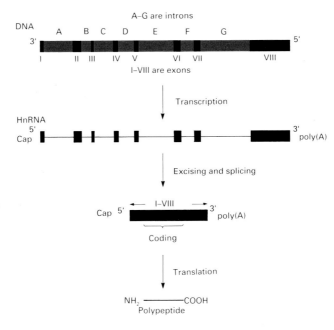

Fig. 3.56 Scheme for the maturation of pre-mRNA by the removal of introns and the splicing of exons.

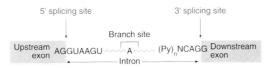

Fig. 3.57 Splicing signals. Consensus sequences for the 5′ splice site and the 39 splice site are shown.

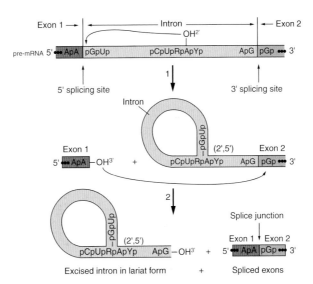

Fig. 3.58 The formation of a lariat in the splicing of exons in mRNA.

spliceosome, which is a very large structure of 50–60S. Antibodies obtained from patients with systemic lupus erythematosus played a crucial role in the discovery of snRNPs. In this autoimmune disease the patients possess a wide range of antibodies to nuclear components. It was shown that specific antibodies to snRNPs blocked splicing.

In the protozoan *Tetrahymena*, the removal of the intron does not require proteins; an RNA is formed from the excised intron. This RNA is known as a ribozyme, which has both nuclease and polymerase activities.

Alternative splicing to give different proteins

It is generally the case that exons are collinear with the domains of proteins. Thus, by selecting the exons in a given pre-mRNA, it should be possible to generate different mRNAs from the same

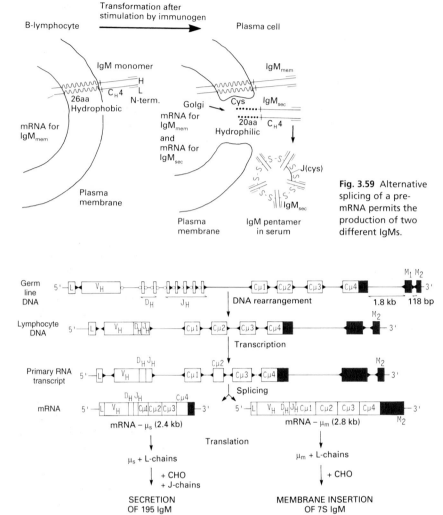

Fig. 3.59 Alternative splicing of a pre-mRNA permits the production of two different IgMs.

Fig. 3.60 Alternative splicing of the gene for IgM. V_H, $C\mu1$, etc, represent the different domains of IgM shown on p. 75. The red blocks indicate the exons that are distributed to the two mature mRNAs.

The generation of antibody diversity

An animal can synthesize many millions of different antibodies, each with the ability to interact with a specific antigen; this is explained in Chapter 5 (p. 73). The way that this is achieved represents a useful summary of the means whereby different proteins can be generated from the genome. There are three sources of such diversity:

1. A large repertoire of variable-region genes.
2. Somatic recombination, for example, any of several hundred V genes can become linked to any of five J genes.
3. Somatic mutation (e.g. in the formation of light chains).
4. Deamination of C→U (see p. 19).

Figure 3.61 depicts the way in which the numerous antibodies arise. The stem cell genome contains multiple variants of the L-chain V and J genes and the H-chain V, J and D (diversity) genes. The V genes are preceded by a small S segment coding for the signal peptide (see p. 45). As lymphocytes mature, each differentiating cell constructs particular L and H genes of virtually unique structure by a recombination process that randomly selects one out of each set of gene segments and assembles them together with a C gene. The pre-mRNA is spliced to give a mature mRNA, which is translated and the signal peptide removed. There is then oxidative formation of S–S bridges.

section of genomic DNA. Alternative splicing happens quite often, and an example is shown in Figs 3.59 and 3.60 for the generation of two different immunoglobulins (Ig). The B lymphocyte bears a monomer of IgM (see p. 73) on its surface. When such a lymphocyte is recognized by an immunogen it is stimulated to form a clone of plasma cells, which synthesize and secrete the IgM pentamer. The C-terminal region of the H (heavy) chain accounts for the monomer IgM being a membrane protein (see p. 74); the IgM pentamer is secreted. The monomer H-chain possesses a hydrophobic peptide of 26 amino acid residues, which has an affinity for the plasma membrane, whereas the H-chains of the pentamer have instead a hydrophilic peptide of 20 amino acids. Figure 3.59 shows the general plan for the generation of IgM_{mem} and IgM_{sec}, and Fig. 3.60 the details of the selection of the exons.

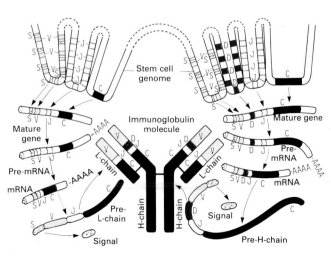

Fig. 3.61 The generation of antibody diversity.

THE CONTROL OF PROTEIN SYNTHESIS

The *lac* operon

It has previously been explained that, although all cells in an individual possess the same DNA, the nature of the proteins synthesized within the differentiated cells varies. This applies not only to the eukaryotic cells of multicellular organisms but also to bacteria under changing nutritional and environmental circumstances. The most obvious way for differential protein synthesis to result is by the control of the transcription of DNA in the production of mRNA.

The first demonstration of the control of transcription was by Jacob and Monod for the *lac* operon. An operon is defined as a group of contiguous genes that are transcribed into a single mRNA. The essential features are shown in Fig. 3.62. The operon is controlling the transcription of the mRNA for three proteins. The segment of DNA that contains all the information for the production of a single polypeptide is called a cistron, and the *lac* operon is called a polycistronic RNA.

The demonstration of the control of protein synthesis by the interaction of a specific protein with a segment of DNA sets the scene for all subsequent studies aimed at our understanding of the control of transcription in all types of cells. The repressor protein is shown as R, to which the galactoside inducer (shown in red) is bound. If the inducer is not bound to R then R assumes a different structure, labelled T, which can bind to the operator 'o' segment of the DNA; 'i' is the regulator gene that governs the synthesis of R; 'p' is the promoter segment of the DNA and is the point of initiation for the synthesis of the polycistronic mRNA. G_1, G_2, G_3 are structural genes governing the synthesis of the three proteins in the system marked P_1, P_2, P_3; one of these proteins is β-galactosidase, the others are permease and transacetylase. The polycistronic mRNA contains Shine–Dalgarno sequences (see p. 36) 5′ upstream before each coding sequence for the three proteins. This allows for the ribosomes to leave the mRNA and rejoin for the translation of each mRNA.

Transcription cannot occur while the repressor (protein) is bound to DNA because the site of initiation of transcription is at the promoter segment. The action of the β-galactoside inducer is to cause the repressor to leave the DNA so that transcription, and subsequently translation, can occur. Because the normal state is one in which the *lac* operon is inhibited, the phenomenon as described here is known as negative control.

The *lac* operon is, however, also subject to positive control. Thus, cyclic AMP (cAMP) binds to a catabolite gene activation protein (CAP) and the complex stimulates transcription by enhancing the tightness of binding of RNA polymerase to the promoter. The circumstance whereby glucose is the preferred energy source, and in its presence there are only very low levels of β-galactosidase and other catabolic enzymes, is explained by the phenomenon of catabolite repression. The presence of glucose lowers the concentration of cyclic AMP and hence there is an absence of the positive control referred to above.

Although an understanding of the *lac* operon was a seminal discovery, the characteristics of many other operons in prokaryotes with unique features have since been elucidated, but these will not be described here.

The control of protein synthesis in eukaryotes

The role of polyribosomes in the synthesis of proteins has been explained. In most tissues all the ribosomes are linked to mRNA and are involved in protein synthesis. In some tissues, such as the mammary gland of pregnant animals, some of the ribosomes are not associated with mRNA. The protein synthetic activity of a cell can, therefore, be changed either by the formation of polyribosomes from the existing ribosomes or by the production of additional polyribosomes. In either event, the process is described as global control. This contrasts with the situation whereby the synthesis of a particular protein is changed; this is known as specific control.

Protein synthesis in eukaryotes can be controlled in many ways. Thus the structure of chromatin undergoes changes probably due to the modification of the histones in the nucleosomes. There is also increasing evidence for control at the level of translation by the phosphorylation of initiation factors. Nevertheless, the primary control is at the level of transcription. As described for the *lac* operon, this specific control is effected by the DNA upstream from the start site of transcription and by the presence of many different proteins. The key enzyme in the transcription of the genes for structural proteins is RNA polymerase II, as previously described (see p. 28). This is a very large multisubunit enzyme.

The promoters recognized by this enzyme are considerably longer and more diverse than those of the *lac* operon. The general features of these promoters are shown in Fig. 3.63. The first nucleotide (the start site) of a DNA sequence is denoted +1, followed by +2, etc. The nucleotide preceding the start site is denoted −1. These refer to the coding (sense) strand, not to the template (antisense) strand. The coding strand has the same sequence as the mRNA, except for T in place of U. Promoters for RNA

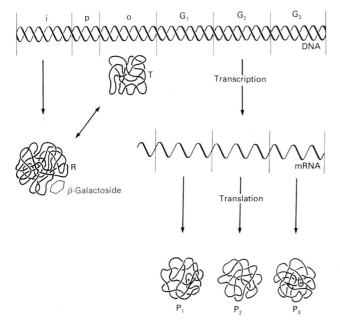

Fig. 3.62 The *lac* operon and its control by a repressor.

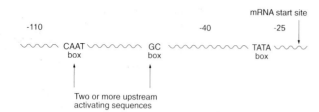

mRNA start site

-110   -40   -25

∿∿ CAAT ∿∿∿∿∿ GC ∿∿∿∿∿∿∿∿ TATA ∿∿∿
     box   box   box

Two or more upstream
activating sequences

Fig. 3.63 General features of promoters for mRNA precursors in eukaryotic cells.

polymerase are on the 5′ side of the start (upstream). There are several of these; the TATA and CAAT boxes are very common, as is the GC box. The activities of many promoters are increased by enhancers, which are sequences in DNA up to several thousand base pairs from the promoter. The binding might be on the 5′ side (upstream), or on the 3′ side (downstream) or even within a gene. Such enhancers are often tissue specific. Enhancers are recognized by specific proteins, called transcription factors, which stimulate RNA polymerase II to bind to a nearby promoter. The fact that enhancers are often, in terms of the linear DNA, so far from the promoters they control is explained on the basis of the folding of DNA to provide a tertiary structure that brings the two elements close together (see Fig. 13.15).

Factors that are the product of genes other than that which they control, which is the usual case, are termed *trans*-acting. Factors that are products of the gene they control, as shown for the *lac* operon, are termed *cis*-acting.

In prokaryotes, when several genes encoding particular proteins are expressed as a response to a particular signal, the genes are tightly linked together in an operon, as shown for the *lac* operon, so that there is a coordinate production of the proteins encoded by the individual genes. In higher organisms this does not occur because there are no polycistronic RNAs and the individual genes are transcribed into individual monocistronic RNAs encoding single proteins. Thus there must be other means to achieve coordination, particularly as the genes involved are often on different chromosomes. Thus the production of a functional antibody molecule requires the synthesis of both immunoglobulin heavy- and light-chain proteins. Whereas the heavy-chain locus is on chromosome 14 in humans, the light-chain genes are on both chromosomes 2 and 22. A similar situation exists in the case of hemoglobin, where the α-globin family is on chromosome 16 in humans and the β-gene globins are on chromosome 11.

Transcription factors

Although the base sequences in the promoter region of DNA play a critical role in positioning the start site of transcription, proteins are also involved. The TATA box is bound by a complex of proteins known as TFIID (transcription factor D for RNA polymerase II). Within this complex only one protein, known as TBP (TATA-binding protein), binds directly to the DNA, with the other proteins in the complex binding via association with TBP. A number of genes do not contain a TATA box but still require TBP for transcription, and it is postulated that yet another factor is involved, which binds to DNA before TBP.

Protein DNA recognition

Much effort is being devoted to discovering precisely how transcription factors recognize regulatory sequences in genes. Three important such protein motifs have been recognized: the helix-turn-helix motif, zinc-finger proteins and leucine zipper proteins. The first to be discovered was the helix-turn-helix motif, which is present in the proteins that bind to homeotic genes (those that control the architectural plan of the embryo). This motif is shown in Fig. 3.64 and is so called because it contains a short region that conforms to an α helix followed by a β turn and then another α helix. This motif is present not only in the homeobox of *Drosophila* but also in the DNA of bacteria that express regulatory proteins such as Cro. The figure shows that in the binding to DNA one helix lies across the major

groove whereas the second helix lies partly within the major groove where it can make specific contacts with the bases of DNA.

The zinc finger

Another motif is known as the zinc finger. The structure as shown in Fig. 3.65 contains a pair of cysteine residues followed by about 12 amino acid residues followed by another pair of cysteine or histidine residues. The cysteine pairs coordinate with Zn^{2+} so that the other amino acids form a finger-like protrusion. This structure is repeated nine times in the transcription factor TFIIIA (transcription factor for RNA polymerase III), which binds to the gene for 5S RNA as shown in Fig. 3.66, each finger binding in the major groove of the DNA helix. The motif has been shown to be present in several RNA polymerase II transcription factors.

The leucine zipper

The transcription factor C/EBP, which is involved in stimulating the expression of several liver-specific genes, was shown to contain a region of 35 amino acids in which every seventh was a leucine. Such a structure was also found in the proto-oncogene proteins Myc, Fos and Jun (see p. 222). The interaction with DNA is depicted in Fig. 3.67, in which it will be seen that the leucine zipper does not bind directly to DNA; rather, it facilitates the dimerization of the protein and provides the correct protein structure for DNA binding by the DNA-binding domains which are rich in arginine and lysine residues. To act as transcription factors the proteins must dimerize either as parallel homodimers (e.g. Fos : Fos) or as heterodimers (e.g. Fos : Jun) via the leucine zipper.

The basic DNA-binding domain of the leucine zipper has also been found in other proteins that do not contain a leucine

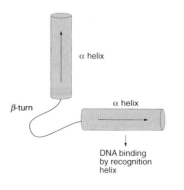

α helix

β-turn

α helix

DNA binding by recognition helix

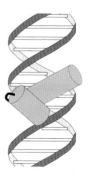

Fig. 3.64 The helix-turn-helix: a protein motif for DNA-binding proteins.

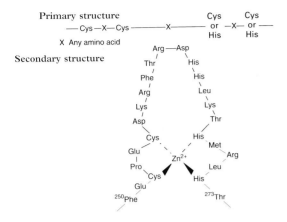

Primary structure
— Cys—X—Cys ————X———— Cys or His —X— Cys or His

X Any amino acid

Secondary structure

Fig. 3.65 The zinc finger: another important protein motif for binding to DNA.

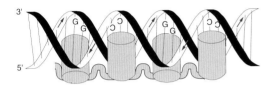

Fig. 3.66 Model of the binding of the zinc fingers in TFIIIA to the gene for 5S DNA.

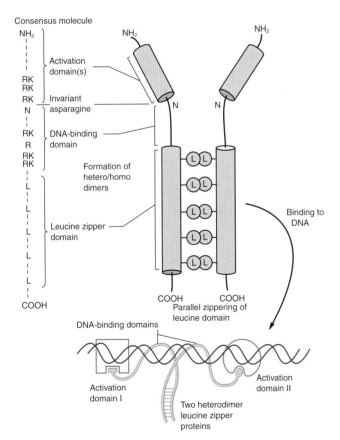

Fig. 3.67 Model of leucine zipper interactions. The conserved amino acids that are common to basic leucine zipper proteins are leucine (L), arginine (R), lysine (K) and asparagine (N).

Control of transcription by hormones

As will be shown in later chapters, many hormones exert their biological effect by binding to cell-surface receptors that activate second messengers such as cyclic AMP. The steroid hormones and thyroxine act in a different manner. They enter target cells and bind to specific receptor proteins in the cytosol. These migrate to the nucleus and control transcription by binding to DNA and controlling the expression of some 50–100 genes. The various receptor proteins possess a similar architecture and represent a superfamily. Their layout is depicted in Fig. 3.68. There is a highly conserved DNA-binding domain (red), a hormone-binding domain (pink) and a highly variable N-terminal domain that interacts with other transcriptional regulators (in black). When the hormone binds to the receptor, the DNA-binding domain is prevented from binding to DNA.

Figure 3.69 shows the structure of the conserved DNA-binding domain of the estrogen receptor. Eight critical cysteine residues bind to two zinc ions (Zn^{2+}). Substances that reduce the activity of hormones act by binding to the receptors. The structures of several such compounds (anti-estrogens and anti-progestins) are compared with the structures of the corresponding hormones in Fig. 3.70. Diethylstilbestrol was the first non-steroid compound shown to have estrogen activity. Tamoxifen is an anti-estrogen that is much used in the prevention and treatment of breast cancer. RU 486 (mifepristone) is used in combination with prostaglandin analogues for the termination of pregnancy.

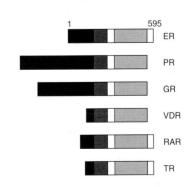

Fig. 3.68 The structure of hormone receptors. ER, estrogen; PR, progesterone; GR, glucocorticoid; VDR, vitamin D_3; RAR, retinoic acid; TR, thyroxine.

zipper. In this structure the basic domain is associated with an adjacent region that can form a helix-loop-helix structure, which is distinct from the helix-turn motif. It consists of two amphipathic helices (containing all the charged amino acids on one side of the helix) separated by a non-helical loop. This DNA-binding domain plays a similar role to the leucine zipper in mediating protein dimerization and facilitating DNA binding by the adjacent basic DNA-binding motif.

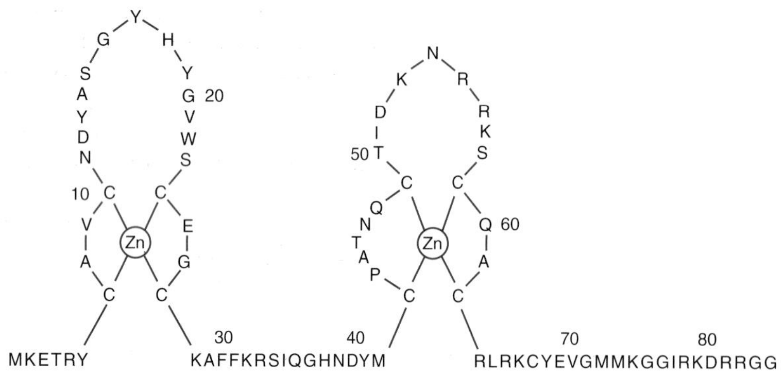

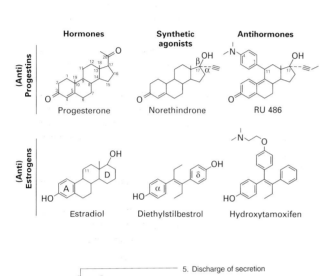

Fig. 3.69 The structure of the conserved DNA-binding domain of the estrogen receptor.

MKETRY   KAFFKRSIQGHNDYM   RLRKCYEVGMMKGGIRKDRRGG

Fig. 3.70 Comparison of the structures of steroid hormones and antihormones.

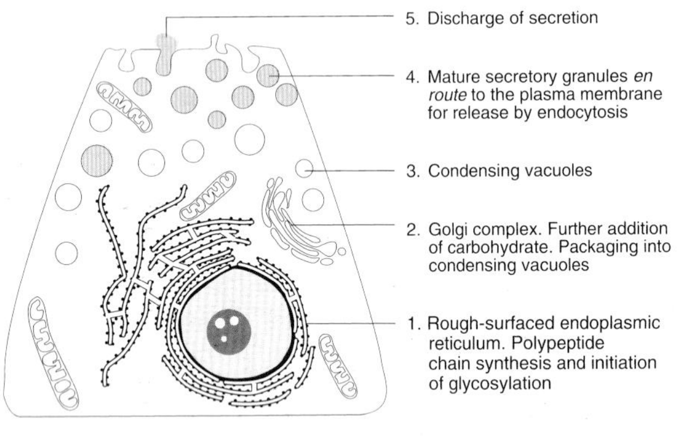

Fig. 3.71 A cartoon of a pancreatic cell showing the movement of proteins synthesized on the rough-surfaced endoplasmic reticulum to the plasma membrane.

5. Discharge of secretion

4. Mature secretory granules *en route* to the plasma membrane for release by endocytosis

3. Condensing vacuoles

2. Golgi complex. Further addition of carbohydrate. Packaging into condensing vacuoles

1. Rough-surfaced endoplasmic reticulum. Polypeptide chain synthesis and initiation of glycosylation

MOLECULAR CELL BIOLOGY

PROTEIN KINESIS

Role of organelles

Irrespective of the type of cell, the newly synthesized proteins have to be despatched to their correct destination where they fulfill their biological function. The means by which this is achieved has come to be known as protein kinesis. The process is particularly complex in eukaryotic cells that contain many different membrane-bound organelles. As an example, Fig. 3.71 is a cartoon of a pancreatic cell. Proteins destined for secretion from the cell are synthesized on the rough-surfaced endoplasmic reticulum (RER), from which they move through the cell to pass through the plasma membrane. During their passage they might be modified either by the attachment of prosthetic groups or by partial proteolytic cleavage (examples of post-translational modification). The RER also synthesizes proteins for various other destinations. These include the lysosomal proteins and those that are retained within the cisternae of the endoplasmic reticulum, as well as the proteins that comprise the Golgi complex. The proteins destined for the nucleus, peroxisomes and mitochondria (and chloroplasts) are synthesized in the cytosol, as are the proteins that constitute components of the cytosol itself, the so-called housekeeping proteins. Protein kinesis is achieved by the possession by the proteins of identification labels, which are usually either a peptide sequence contained within the protein or an additional peptide at either the N- or the C-terminus. These characteristic sequences are termed topogenic sequences.

Membrane-bound and free ribosomes

Although all the ribosomes in eukaryotic cells have a very similar composition, some are present in the cytosol unattached to membrane (free ribosomes) and some are attached to the endoplasmic reticulum (bound ribosomes). The mRNA in the cytoplasm associates with free ribosomes to form polyribosomes (see p. 37). If the mRNA is for a secretory protein, the first 20–25 amino acids from the N-terminus form a signal peptide. The polyribosomes then become membrane bound. The structure of many signal peptides is known. Their structure has little in common except for a hydrophobic region towards the middle. The general principles of these events are shown in Fig. 3.72.

The signal peptide hypothesis

In the original scheme it was proposed that the signal peptide interacted directly with the membrane of the endoplasmic reticulum. It is now clear that the interaction is with the signal recognition particle (SRP). SRP consists of several different proteins and a 7S RNA. As the signal peptide emerges from the ribosome following translation of the mRNA, it binds to SRP. Further translation is arrested until the SRP docks with the membrane of the endoplasmic reticulum, as shown in Fig. 3.73. The SRP is released to the cytosol and translation is resumed. Several proteins contribute to an aqueous, protein-conducting channel, known as a translocon, through which the nascent protein passes to the cisternae. As the signal peptide emerges it is removed by signal peptidase. The primary translation products containing the signal peptides are termed preproteins, hence preproinsulin, preproparathyroid hormone, etc., as explained on p. 32.

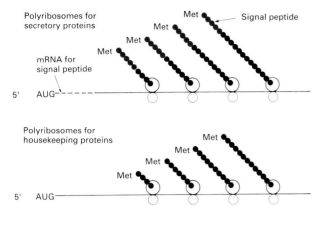

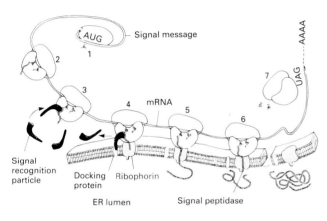

Fig. 3.72 Most eukaryotic cells possess two types of ribosomes: 'free' and 'membrane-bound'.

Fig. 3.73 The signal hypothesis for the synthesis of proteins that enter the cisternae of the rough-surfaced endoplasmic reticulum (ER).

are galactosyltransferase (see p. 197), which serves as a marker for the *trans* membranes, and *N*-acetylglucosaminyl-transferase, an enzyme involved in complex carbohydrate biosynthesis, for the *medial* membranes. These enzymes are synthesized in the rough-surfaced endoplasmic reticulum and are anchored in the Golgi membranes by their membrane-spanning domain.

Lysosomal enzymes and the mucolipidoses

The lysosomal enzymes are synthesized in the endoplasmic reticulum as large precursor proteins that are *N*-glycosylated in the Golgi apparatus as described above. For such enzymes to be delivered to the lysosomes from the *trans*-Golgi network, *N*-acetylglucosamine phosphate has to be transferred to mannose residues by a specific enzyme. This enzyme is missing in certain mucolipidoses (I-cell disease and pseudo-Hurler's polydystrophy), in which the fibroblasts from affected individuals show dense inclusion bodies (hence I-cells) and multiple lysosomal enzymes are secreted into the medium. Patients have abnormally high levels of lysosomal enzymes in the serum and other body fluids (see Fig. 3.75).

The role of the Golgi apparatus

The Golgi apparatus is highly specialized for a variety of functions, including protein glycosylation and subsequent transport of glycoproteins to their final destinations. Three compartments have been identified in the Golgi apparatus; these are termed *cis*, *medial* and *trans*, as shown in Fig. 3.74. Each compartment is involved in a different stage of protein processing. The last station is named the *trans*-Golgi network (TGN), which plays a pivotal role in directing proteins to their appropriate cellular destination, as indicated in the figure. The sorting involves the assembly of cytosol-oriented coat structures. The elucidation of these has been greatly aided by the use of a fungal antibiotic, brefeldin, which reversibly arrests protein export from the TGN.

It is now realized that the Golgi apparatus is concerned not only with proteins passing from the endoplasmic reticulum towards the plasma membrane but also with proteins entering the cell by endocytosis.

Two enzymes present in fractions of disrupted cells containing Golgi membranes

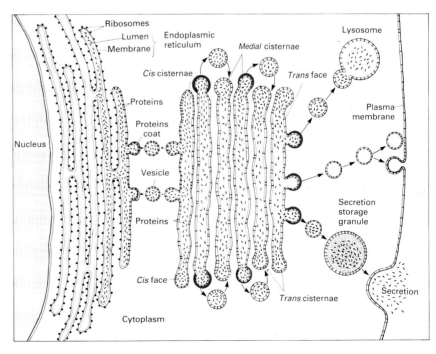

Fig. 3.74 A cartoon to illustrate the passage of proteins from the rough-surfaced reticulum. through the Golgi apparatus. The red circles indicate the site of formation of granules.

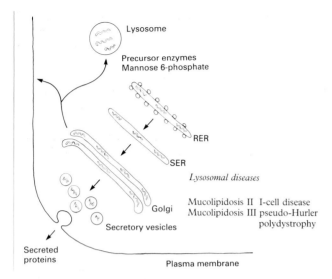

Fig. 3.75 The formation of lysosomal enzymes: the mucolipidoses.

Lysosomal diseases

Mucolipidosis II I-cell disease
Mucolipidosis III pseudo-Hurler polydystrophy

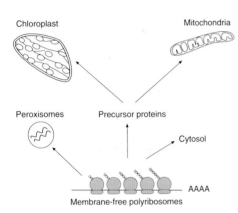

Fig. 3.76 The synthesis of proteins on 'free' ribosomes.

Luminal proteins

Certain proteins that are synthesized by the rough endoplasmic reticulum are not exported from the cell but are to be found in the cisternae. Such luminal proteins possess a four-residue peptide at the C-terminus that has the composition Lys-Asp-Glu-Leu (KDEL). These proteins pass along the membrane system to the Golgi apparatus, where they interact with a receptor and are then returned to the cisternae of the endoplasmic reticulum. Examples are peptide disulfide isomerase and immunoglobulin-binding protein, both of which are important in ensuring that nascent proteins possess the correct tertiary structure.

Nuclear proteins

No proteins are synthesized in the nucleus; the nuclear proteins are derived from the cytosol. Whereas small proteins can pass freely through the nuclear pores, the passage of larger proteins is controlled. The nuclear pores, which are complex

structures (see p. 3) containing at least 100 different proteins, have a receptor for the selected proteins and then a mechanism for the utilization of energy for their passage to the interior of the nucleus. Such proteins contain a characteristic peptide of the nuclear localization sequence (NLS), within their structure that is essential for their passage. Whereas proteins enter through the pores, RNA, possibly in the form of ribonucleoprotein, passes out of the nucleus to the cytosol through the pores.

Peroxisomes

These organelles are present in all eukaryotic cells and are rich in enzymes that generate hydrogen peroxide, and the enzyme catalase, which degrades it (see p. 84). Peroxisomes are present principally in liver and kidney. Unlike the import of proteins into mitochondria, proteins are imported into peroxisomes at their mature size, a tripeptide at the C-terminus acting as the targeting sequence. Figure 3.76 summarizes the role of the free ribosomes

in this respect and for the synthesis of the proteins destined for the mitochondria and chloroplasts as described below.

CLINICAL IMPLICATIONS – PEROXISOMAL ENZYME DEFICIENCY DISORDERS

There are many diseases related to the malfunctioning of the peroxisomes. Zellweger syndrome is an autosomal recessive disease caused by a failure of protein import into peroxisomes, which remain in the cell only as empty 'ghosts'. In Zellweger patients, mutations have been found in many different genes, including those located in the cytosol and peroxisomal membrane. There are at least four rare diseases of peroxisome biogenesis, which are characterized by multiple metabolic defects and mental retardation. Some diseases affect only a single metabolic pathway, one of which is primary hyperoxaluria type 1. This is a rare calcium oxalate kidney stone disease in which mutations in a single gene encoding a metabolic enzyme causes it to be mistargeted to the mitochondria. Some diseases are caused by the failure to oxidize fatty acids; e.g. peroxisomal enzymes catalyse α-oxidation of fatty acids in which the β position is blocked, as in phytanic acid, an acid formed by gut bacteria from components of chlorophyll. Accumulation of this acid in Refsum's disease causes a variety of neurological symptoms. Failure by acyl CoA oxidase to oxidize very long chain fatty acids causes their accumulation in pseudoneonatal adrenoleukodystrophy. A summary of some of the peroxisomal diseases is shown in Table 3.7.

The origin of mitochondrial proteins

In many respects, mitochondria resemble the prokaryotic bacteria, and this has given rise to the concept that they arose in evolution by the incorporation of bacteria into eukaryotic cells. Their similarity to bacteria in terms of the protein synthesis (see p. 36) that takes place within mitochondria has been explained. Mitochondrial DNA is derived solely from the mother because only the head of the spermatozoon, which is devoid of mitochondria, enters an oocyte at fertilization. Thus those proteins encoded by the mitochondrial genome will come from the mother. This fact is of significance when the origin of various populations is being traced – a subject known as molecular anthropology. Complications

Table 3.7 Peroxisomal disorders

Disorder	Biochemical defect
Zellweger – neonatal ALD	Peroxisomal biogenesis
Infantile Refsum	Peroxisome target receptor protein (peroxins)
Rhizomelic chondrodysplasia type I	Receptor protein (peroxins)
Rhizomelic chondrodysplasia type II	Dihydroxyacetone phosphate acyltransferase
X linked ALD	ATP target binding protein
Refsum disease	Phytanoyl CoA hydroxylase
Pseudoneonatal ALD	Acyl CoA oxidase deficiency, bifunctional enzyme and thiolase
Hyperoxaluria type 1	Alanine-glyoxylate aminotransferase
Acatalasemia	Catalase

ALD, adrenoleukodystrophy, in which there is progressive demyelination of cerebral white matter.

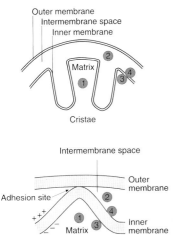

Fig. 3.77 The origin of mitochondrial proteins.

are synthesized with a cleavable N-terminal targeting sequence. This is usually basic, is 15–20 amino acids long and can form an amphiphilic α helix or β strand. The nascent polypeptides interact with chaperones (see p. 15), which ensures that they remain unfolded, and are then transferred to proteins that act as 'protein import receptors' at the outer membrane. These receptors deliver the precursor, N-terminal first, to a protein-conducting channel in the outer membrane. In appropriate cases it inserts it into a protein-conducting channel in the inner membrane. This occurs in response to the pull of the electric potential across the membrane and by an ATP-driven translocator motor that is attached to the inner side of the inner-membrane transport channel. The Tom and Tim

systems possess various crucial proteins, of which at least one plays a role in both systems. A chaperone is also present in the matrix. As shown in Fig. 3.77 (bottom), passage across the two membranes is aided by the close juxtaposition of the two membranes at attachment sites.

SUMMARY OF PROTEIN SYNTHESIS WITHIN THE EUKARYOTIC CELL

Figure 3.78 summarizes the steps in the expression of DNA to produce mature proteins located in the correct sites within the cell to enable them to fulfil their biological function. Any obstacles to the achievement of this architecture are likely to have a seriously detrimental effect on the functioning of the body. Such defects can be caused by mutations, as in the case of α_1-antitrypsin and emphysema (see p. 70). Some drugs, such as phenobarbital, cause an increase in the amount of smooth-surfaced endoplasmic reticulum. Ingested organic solvents such as carbon tetrachloride and trichlorethylene have a markedly bad effect on the rough-surfaced endoplasmic reticulum.

PROTEIN DEGRADATION

General principles

Ultimately, the breakdown of all proteins depends on the action of proteolytic enzymes, the action of which is explained elsewhere (see p. 155). Our present concern is the way in which proteins are

arise because each cell in the body carries hundreds of mitochondria and the DNA of each mitochondrion is subject to mutation.

A typical eukaryotic cell contains roughly 10 000 different proteins, of which about 10% are in the mitochondria. Because mitochondria synthesize only a dozen proteins, they must import 99% of their proteins from the cytoplasm. In the transfer of such proteins to the mitochondria the proteins need to be located in one of four positions: in the intermembrane space, on the outside of the inner membrane, on the matrix side of the inner membrane and in the matrix (Fig. 3.77, top).

The outer and inner membranes contain distinct protein transport systems; that for the outer membrane is termed Tom (translocase of the outer mitochondrial membrane) and that for the inner membrane Tim (translocase of the inner mitochondrial membrane). Most proteins imported into the mitochondria

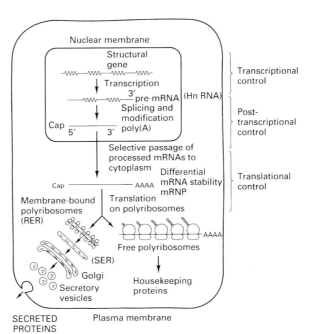

Fig. 3.78 A summary of the steps in the synthesis of proteins within the eukaryotic cell.

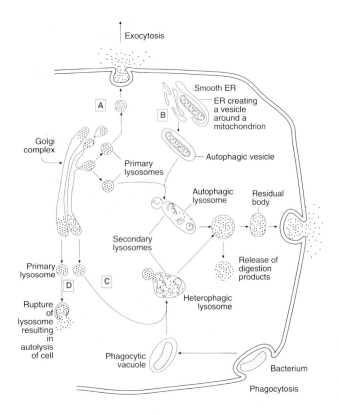

Fig. 3.79 The lysosomal system for the degradation of proteins and other macromolecules such as polysaccharides and nucleic acids.

selected for intracellular breakdown. The working hypothesis is that cells contain no useless proteins, so those that are not required have to be degraded to free amino acids, which can be recycled. Two general methods have been identified for the intracellular degradation of proteins: the lysosomal system and the ubiquitin system.

The lysosomal system

Figure 3.79 shows the formation of primary and secondary lysosomes and their role in cellular digestive processes. The primary lysosomes, which bud from the Golgi apparatus, can take several pathways: exocytosis (A), the transport of proteins out

of the cell; phagocytosis (B and C), the formation of phagic lysosomes for digesting organelles or ingested matter; autolysis (D), destruction of the cell itself.

Clinical implications – lysosomal diseases

Some 50 different enzymes have been detected in the primary lysosomes. These encompass those that degrade proteins, peptides, lipids, glycolipids, polysaccharides and glycoproteins. The enzymes have acid pH optima and the interior of the lysosomes is maintained at a pH of 4–6, probably by a proton pump mechanism. A wide variety of genetic enzyme deficiency diseases have been reported that result in severe damage to the central nervous

system, cardiac muscle, liver, bone marrow and vascular tissue (see Table 3.8). The substrate for the missing enzyme gradually accumulates within secondary lysosomes, leading to their increased fragility and eventual disruption with intracellular release of their contents, especially cathepsins, which causes severe cellular dysfunction and raised plasma levels of lysosomal acid phosphatase. Diagnosis is usually based on sensitive assays using fluorometric substrates in cultured fibroblasts prepared from the skin biopsy of patients, or for antenatal diagnosis amniotic or chorionic villous cells. Treatment, apart from organ transplantation, can involve enzyme replacement therapy in some disorders, e.g. Gaucher disease (β-glucosidase deficiency) and Fabry disease (α-galactosidase deficiency).

The ubiquitin system

Ubiquitin is a 76-amino acid polypeptide that is present in virtually all types of cell, hence its name. Ubiquitin is activated by the interaction of ATP and two enzymes. The resulting complex then becomes attached to the protein targeted for degradation. Just how proteins are selected for destruction is not fully understood, but there is a strong correlation between the nature of the N-terminal amino acid and those immediately following and the length of the survival time of a protein in a cell. In yeast, ubiquitin is synthesized as a polypeptide that contains five sequences of ubiquitin and which is then processed to form ubiquitin. Figure 3.80 shows the programmed destruction of cytosolic proteins by the ubiquitin-marking system. E_2 is an enzyme involved in the transfer of ubiquitin to lysine residues on target proteins. These events take place on a multiprotein complex known as a proteasome, the structure of which is now known for yeast.

Table 3.8 Examples of lysosomal deficiency disorders

Disease	Accumulating substrate (principal organ affected)	Enzyme deficiency
Pompe disease	Glycogen (heart/liver)	α-Glucosidase (acid maltase)
Metachromatic leukodystrophy	Cerebroside sulfate (nervous system)	Aryl sulfatase A
Krabbe leukodystrophy (3 types)	Galactosylsphingosine (brain, peripheral nervous system)	β-Galactosidase
Gaucher disease (4 types)	Glucosylceramide (brain, spleen, bone marrow, liver)	β-Glucosidase
Tay–Sachs disease (5 types)	Gangliosides (brain, spinal cord, peripheral nerves, retina)	Hexosaminidase(s)
Fabry disease	Ceramide trihexoside (kidney, peripheral nerves, heart)	α-Galactosidase
Niemann–Pick disease (5 types)	Sphingomyelin (brain, bone marrow)	Sphingomyelinase
Hurler disease	Mucopolysaccharides (liver, spleen, brain, bone, cornea, connective tissues)	α-Iduronidase

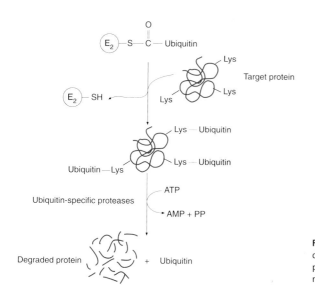

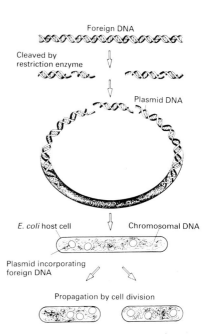

Fig. 3.80 The programmed destruction of cytosolic proteins by the ubiquitin-marking system.

Fig. 3.82 The basic principles for the formation of a recombinant DNA.

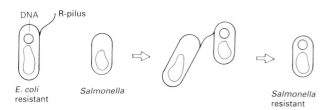

Fig. 3.81 The transfer of antibiotic resistance between bacteria by a plasmid vector.

RECOMBINANT DNA (GENETIC ENGINEERING)

GENERAL PRINCIPLES

An early demonstration of the transfer of DNA from one cell type to another concerned drug resistance of bacteria. The property of the antibiotic resistance of certain strains of *E. coli* could be transferred to a pathogenic bacterium such as *Salmonella*. The explanation of this phenomenon led to the discovery of the plasmid, whereby the gene conferring antibiotic resistance resides in a form of extrachromosomal DNA. The resistance is due to an enzyme that causes the degradation of the antibiotic. Figure 3.81 illustrates the phenomenon.

The use of plasmids and other vectors

By inserting a foreign gene into the plasmid it can be used as a vector, resulting in a recombinant DNA that then replicates in a suitable host. The organism containing the modified vector is allowed to multiply so that eventually an increased quantity of the vector can be recovered and the foreign DNA released. Alternatively, the

foreign DNA can be expressed to give rise to protein that can be recovered either by lysing the cells or from the extracellular medium. The cells containing the foreign DNA are known as clones, and so the technique is described as cloning. The general principles of the procedure are shown in Fig. 3.82.

Alternative vectors

Although *E. coli* and its plasmids have been the preferred vectors, there is increasing interest in alternative systems. Thus λ phage can be used as a vector in *E. coli*, which allows for the use of larger inserts. Eukaryotes such as yeast and baby hamster kidney cells are also useful in that, unlike bacteria, they effect the glycosylation of the foreign protein. Foreign DNA can be inserted into animal cells in culture either directly as a calcium precipitate or as a modified virus. Sometimes gold particles with the foreign DNA adsorbed can be shot into the cells.

Procedures for the insertion of foreign DNA

Two general methods for the construction of recombinant molecules are illustrated in

Fig. 3.83. The method on the left starts with a partially purified mRNA and forms double-stranded complementary DNA (cDNA) with oligo(dC) tails. On the right, genomic DNA is degraded by a restriction enzyme into roughly 'gene-sized' pieces. The plasmid has two antibiotic-resistant sites, one of which is cleaved by the same restriction enzyme used in the degradation of the DNA. The gene-sized piece can be annealed into the cleaved plasmid DNA. In the other approach, the cleaved DNA is tailed with oligo(dG) by means of terminal transferase (see p. 24) and annealed to the cDNA. The host is transformed and cells selected for the appropriate insert. Antibiotic resistance is useful in this case, since, if the bacterial colonies are grown on a medium containing tetracycline, only those colonies (clones) that contain the plasmid will grow.

THE USE OF GENE PROBES

The Southern blot

To detect fragments of DNA in an agarose gel that are complementary to a given RNA or DNA sequence, Southern devised a method for transferring denatured DNA to cellulose nitrate (nitrocellulose). The DNA fragments can be permanently fixed to the cellulose nitrate by heating at 80°C. Subsequently, a radioactive probe can be hybridized to the cDNA on the cellulose nitrate. The method, known as the Southern blot, is illustrated in Fig. 3.84. The dry filter paper draws the buffer

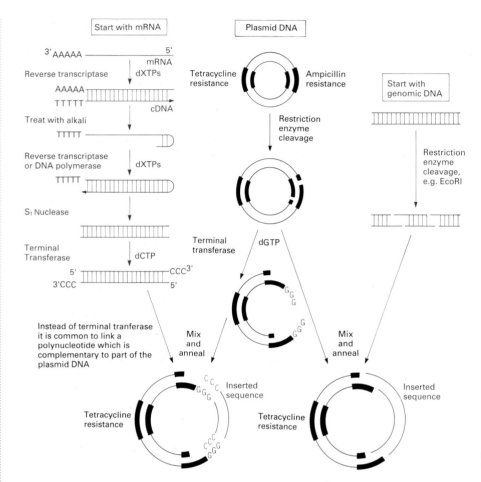

Fig. 3.83 The methods used to insert foreign DNA.

solution up from the gel, carrying the DNA with it into the cellulose nitrate. A similar method for RNA is known as the Northern blot. When antibodies are used to detect proteins after separation on two-dimensional gels, the procedure is known as the Western blot.

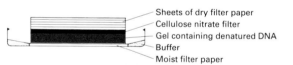

Fig. 3.84 The Southern blot technique for the transfer of DNA fragments from gel to nitrocellulose sheet.

Mapping restriction sites around a gene

Provided the base sequence of at least part of the gene of interest (gene X in Fig. 3.85) is known, a radioactive probe can be prepared and used to hybridize with fragments of DNA separated by gel electrophoresis, as illustrated in Fig. 3.85. Such probes can also be used with tissue sections to locate the site of the nucleic acid. This is known as in vitro hybridization.

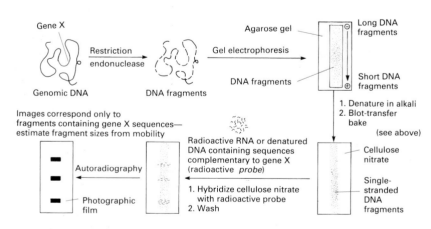

Fig. 3.85 Use of a radioactive probe for in vitro hybridization.

CLINICAL IMPLICATIONS OF DNA TECHNOLOGY

Antenatal diagnosis

Recombinant DNA techniques can make it possible to determine the genetic make-up of the fetus being carried by the mother. With certain knowledge of the status of the fetus, the mother might, in some societies, be able to choose to have an abortion. Formerly, it was necessary to obtain a sample of fetal blood by fetoscopy, but this could not be done until the second trimester, which meant that the diagnosis was late in the pregnancy. Samples of DNA can be obtained much

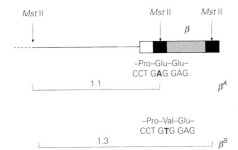

Fig. 3.86 The use of restriction enzymes for the diagnosis of sickle-cell anemia.

earlier from either the amniotic fluid or the chorion villus, the safety of the fetus being paramount. The use of PCR (see p. 27) has also enabled radioisotopes to be avoided as will be explained.

Diagnosis of sickle-cell anemia

An example is the problem of sickle-cell anemia, for which methods have been developed to determine whether the fetus is homozygous for the sickle-cell trait. As will be explained in Chapter 4 (p. 63), the genetic change is located in the β chain of HbA, and, as was shown in the section on the genetic code (p. 34), the mutation causes a change of A for U. Figure 3.86 shows the use of the restriction enzyme *Mst*II. The base substitution that causes HbS removes an *Mst*II site. In normal DNA, an *Mst*II fragment of 1.1 kb is generated. The absence of the *Mst*II site in those with HbS generates a longer *Mst*II fragment of 1.3 kb. Heterozygotes show both fragments, homozygotes only one.

Oligonucleotide probes can, therefore, be used to detect the presence of specific genes that are responsible for a particular disease. There are problems, however, in that a phenotype might arise as a result of many different mutations as has been found for phenylketonuria (see p. 123). In such a case, many different probes would be required to provide a definitive result.

Use of the polymerase chain reaction

The development of the PCR (see p. 27) has greatly facilitated the identification of mutations that alter restriction enzyme sites. In the case of the sickle-cell mutation, an appropriate fragment of the β globin gene is amplified some 30 times, after which the DNA fragments are digested with the restriction enzyme *Dde*I, which has a recognition site that is abolished by the A→T mutation at codon 6. Normal DNA is cleaved into two fragments of about 150 and 201 bp,

whereas DNA from patients yields a 351-bp fragment. Because PCR produces so much DNA, these fragments can be detected by either ethidium bromide or silver staining of DNA bands on gels; no radioactive probes are required.

TRANSGENESIS

There are three major ways of introducing DNA into mammalian germ tissue such that the progeny of the recipient will carry the gene. The first involves microinjection of DNA solutions into the nucleus of an egg by means of a fine needle. The second involves the use of retrovirus-based vectors. The gene to be introduced is ligated into the genome of the retrovirus. The retrovirus DNA (or strictly cDNA) is then introduced into a cultured cell line that is capable of producing all the components of the retrovirus except for the viral RNA. Recombinant virus stock is then used to infect an early embryo, which is then placed into a donor mother. The third method depends on the existence of cultured cell lines, which become germ cells if injected into early embryos. A variation on this method is to inject nuclei from cultured cells to enucleated unfertilized eggs, particular attention being paid to the cell-cycle stage of both donor and host cells; the eggs are then artificially stimulated to develop. The usual method is to use nuclei from fetal cells but there are attempts to use nuclei from adult cells, which would be of more significance in terms of possible human clones.

One use of transgenic animals such as goats and sheep is to introduce human proteins, which can subsequently be extracted from the milk. Examples are factor IX (for blood coagulation, see p. 191) and α_1-antitrypsin (see p. 70). The methods can also be applied to plants. Thus bananas can be used to produce an oral vaccine against hepatitis and cowpeas for a vaccine against parvovirus in dogs. Mice do not produce practical amounts of drug but are easier to use and help in proving the

technology. Another use of transgenesis is to inactivate or remove a particular gene and hence study the role of the gene in the physiology of the so-called knock-out mouse. A common way of obtaining knock-out mice is to use embryonic stem (ES) cells, which are derived from embryos 3.5 days postcoitum and arise from the inner cell mass of the blastocyst. The ES cells can be grown in vitro and retain the potential to contribute extensively to all of the tissues of an animal when injected back into a host blastocyst, which is allowed to develop in a foster mother. The injected cells become established in the mouse germ line. Such ES cells can be modified by the introduction of exogenous DNA for gene targeting. This depends on the fact that the cells are able to recombine the introduced vector DNA with a homologous chromosomal target. As both alleles can be relatively easily disrupted, a null mutant can be generated. An example is the removal of the gene for the prion protein that plays a role in the infection of animals that results in bovine spongiform encephalopathies. The resulting mice appeared to be normal. An alternative, and now preferred method, of producing a knock-out animal is to use RNAi (see p. 31).

MONOGENIC AND POLYGENIC DISEASES

Some diseases, such as sickle-cell anemia and Huntington's disease, are due to a defect in a single gene and are hence known as monogenic diseases. The hereditary basis for other diseases, such as schizophrenia and type 2 diabetes, depends on the contribution of several genes and hence these are known as polygenic diseases. In such diseases the alleles of multiple genes, acting together within an individual, contribute to both the occurrence and the severity of the disease. The same applies to the hereditary aspects of ability such as that to play a violin or a game.

CLINICAL IMPLICATIONS – REVERSE GENETICS

The case of sickle-cell anemia is a good example of functional cloning in that the function of the aberrant gene is known. In many genetic diseases, such as the autosomal dominant Huntington's disease, the function of the aberrant gene is unknown. In such cases, the strategy is to correlate the phenotype with a

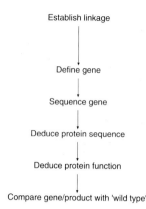

Establish linkage

↓

Define gene

↓

Sequence gene

↓

Deduce protein sequence

↓

Deduce protein function

↓

Compare gene/product with 'wild type'

Fig. 3.87 Reverse genetics.

Table 3.9 Trinucleotide repeats in human genetic diseases

Disease	Repeat	Location of gene	Normal length	Full disease length
Fragile-X site A	CGG	5'UT	6–54	200 → 1000
Fragile-X site E	CCG	Promoter	6–25	> 200
Freidreich's ataxia	GAA	Intron 1	7–22	200–1700
Myotonic dystrophy	CTG	3'UT	5–35	50–4000
Spinocerebellar ataxia 8	CTG	Untranslated	16–37	110–500
Huntington's disease	CAG	Coding	6–35	36–100
Haw River syndrome	CAG	Coding	7–25	49–75
Spinocerebellar ataxia 1	CAG	Coding	6–38	39–83
Spinocerebellar ataxia 2	CAG	Coding	14–31	32–77
Spinocerebellar ataxia 6	CAG	Coding	4–17	21–30
Spinocerebellar ataxia 7	CAG	Coding	7–35	37–200
Machado Joseph disease	CAG	Coding	12–39	62–86
Kennedy Disease	CAG	Coding	9–35	38–62

chromosome deletion. The missing gene, present in normal subjects, is then sequenced, the amino acid sequence deduced and the function of the gene predicted. Figure 3.87 shows the steps in the application of this procedure. This strategy is called positional cloning. One success of this strategy is the genetic basis of cystic fibrosis. By the use of standard linkage markers the gene was located on chromosome 7. A candidate gene was located and sequenced. Comparison of the sequence with existing proteins provided clues as to the function. The gene codes for the cystic fibrosis transmembrane conductance regulator (CFTR), a chloride channel requiring both cyclic AMP-dependent phosphorylation and ATP hydrolysis to open. The cause of Duchenne muscular dystrophy has also been studied. The gene involved was located on the X chromosome and codes for a sarcolemmal protein of M_r 400 000, named dystrophin. The precise function of this protein is not at present clear.

The cause of Huntington's disease is an example of another phenomenon that is increasingly commonly found, namely the occurrence of unstable expansions of trinucleotide and other repeats (see Table 3.9). The length of the repeat correlates with the age of onset of the disease, or, in the case of fragile X syndrome (the fragile sites are identified as non-staining gaps on chromosomes that are inducible by certain conditions of tissue culture), to the risk of having affected children. The repeats can occur normally within the genome and can be either perfect repeats (i.e. with no variation in the base composition) or imperfect repeats. When located within or near transcribed sequences, the expanded repeat can have an effect on either the gene transcript or gene product that might cause the disease. In Huntington's disease the repeat is CAG and in fragile X CGG. The process whereby the repeats are generated is called dynamic mutation.

INTERPLAY BETWEEN PROTEIN STRUCTURE AND THE SEARCH FOR GENES – DNA LIBRARIES

In Fig. 3.83 the use of restriction enzymes to break down a genome into 'gene-sized' pieces is described. The resulting product is known as a 'genomic DNA library' which can be probed for many purposes. One example might be the following: the primary structures of a polypeptide component of a protein is known so that a complementary DNA strand (cDNA) can be synthesized based on the genetic code. This cDNA can be used to probe the DNA library for a polynucleotide containing a complementary strand, which may well be much longer than the probe, possibly the length of the complete gene. This can be cloned. In this way the gene for the protein of interest can be identified and its function studied in cell systems. Even though the complete structure of the protein was not known its structure may be deduced from the structure of the protein was not known its structure may be deduced from the structure of the gene by use of the genetic code. In a similar way the frequency of the occurrence of protein domains may be studied by probing the DNA libraries.

In species for which the structure of the entire genome has been determined, it is possible to search the database for base sequences corresponding to any amino acid sequence that may be of interest, and thereby identify genes in which it occurs. The assumption is that the human genome database provides information concerning the primary structure of every human protein.

A BRIEF GLOSSARY OF TERMS NOT PREVIOUSLY EXPLAINED

ARF protein

GTPase responsible for regulating coat assembly and clathrin coat assembly at Golgi membranes.

Cosmid cloning

A technique for cloning large eukaryotic fragments in *Escherichia coli*. It employs the single-stranded 'cos' sites at each end of λ phage, which are required for packaging in phage heads.

Frame shift mutation

A mutation that is caused by the insertion or deletion of one, two or multiples of, paired nucleotides, the effect of which is to change the reading frame of codons during protein synthesis, yielding a different amino acid sequence beginning at the mutated codon.

Fusion proteins

Hybrid proteins containing both bacterial and eukaryotic amino acid sequences. They are particularly useful for the purification of proteins expressed by rDNA because one of the proteins can be subjected to affinity chromatography.

Heat shock genes

High temperatures and other stress-inducing treatments evoke the expression of heat shock genes in yeasts and other eukaryotes giving rise to heat shock proteins.

Hedgehog (Hb)

A family of secreted signalling proteins that are used for the development of most tissues in nearly all animals. Mutations in Hb signal transduction components are implicated in human cancer and birth defects.

Heteroduplex

A DNA molecule, the two strands of which come from different individuals so that there might be some base pairs or runs of base pairs that do not match.

Holliday junction

X-shaped structure observed in DNA undergoing recombination, in which two DNA molecules are held together at the site of crossing-over.

Homeobox

Short conserved DNA sequence that encodes the homeodomain.

Homeodomain

Conserved DNA-binding motif found in many developmentally important transcription factors.

Hox genes

Group of developmentally important genes that encode homeodomain-containing transcription factors and help determine the body plan in animals.

Inversion

The alteration of a DNA molecule made by removing a fragment, reversing its orientation and putting it back into place.

Kinetochore

Complex structure formed from proteins on a mitotic chromosome to which microtubules attach and which plays an active part in the movement of chromosomes to the poles.

Linker

A small fragment of synthetic DNA that has a restriction site that is useful for gene splicing because it can be added as an extension to the foreign DNA.

Long terminal repeat (LTR)

Direct repeat sequence, containing up to 600 base pairs, that flanks the coding region of integrated retroviral DNA.

M13 phage

A single-stranded DNA phage. The double-stranded replicative form can be used as a cloning vector.

Metallothionein (MMT)

A metal-binding protein that is induced in animal cells by a variety of metals (e.g. zinc). The expression of the fusion protein can be regulated by using the MMT gene promoter fused to the coding region of the protein of interest.

Mitosis-promoting factor (MPF)

A heterodimeric protein, composed of a mitotic cyclin and cyclin-dependent kinase (CDK), that triggers entrance of a cell into mitosis by phosphorylating multiple specific proteins, resulting in chromosome condensation, assembly of the mitotic apparatus, and nuclear breakdown.

Nick translation procedure

Procedure for labelling DNA in vitro using DNA polymerase 1 first to create a gap in one strand of DNA and then to fill by the synthesis of a labelled nucleotide.

Open reading frames

Long stretches of triplex codons in DNA that are not interrupted by a translation stop codon.

Palindrome

A self-complementary nucleic acid sequence, i.e. a sequence identical to that of its complementary strand (both read in the same 5′→3′ direction).

Pseudogenes

DNA sequences that are similar to functional genes but do not express a functional product.

Rab protein

A large family of GTPases present in the plasma membrane and other organelle membranes that are involved in conferring specificity on vesicle docking.

Ran

A GTPase present in both cytosol and nucleus that is required for the active transport of macromolecules into and out of the nucleus through nuclear pores complexes.

Ras protein

A GTP-binding protein that is tethered to the plasma membrane by a lipid anchor and functions in intracellular signalling pathways. Activation of Ras is induced by surface receptors.

Restriction maps

The location of the multiple sites within a DNA that are susceptible to cleavage by a variety of restriction enzymes. Such a map will indicate the degree of homology of different DNA molecules.

SNAREs

A large family of transmembrane proteins present in organelle membranes and in vesicles derived from them. They are involved in guiding vesicles to their correct destination. They exist in pairs – a v-SNARE in the vesicle membrane binds specifically to a complementary t-SNARE in the target membrane.

Src family

A family of cytoplasmic tyrosine kinases that associate with the cytoplasmic domains of some enzyme-linked receptors that lack intrinsic tyrosine kinase activity. They transmit a signal by phosphorylating the receptor itself and other signalling proteins.

Toll-like receptor family (TLR)

Family of mammalian pattern-recognition receptors abundant on macrophages, neutrophils and the epithelial cells of the gut.

Transfection

Infection of a cell with isolated DNA or RNA from a virus or viral vector.

Transformation

The introduction of an exogenous DNA preparation (transforming agent) into a cell.

Transposon DNA

A mobile DNA element within the genome.

Wnt

A family of secreted signalling proteins that are usually used in the development of most tissues. Mutations in Wnt signal proteins are implicated in human cancer.

Yeast artificial chromosomes (YACs)

A cloning vector formed from bacterial plasmids, two yeast telomeres, a yeast centromere and other elements that allow for the accommodation of human DNA fragments. The vector can be introduced into yeast, where it functions as an artificial chromosome.

Protein structure and function with hemoglobin as an example

4

The characteristics of globular and fibrous proteins is first described, followed by the distribution of amino acids in a globular protein and the nature of the peptide bond. The presence of α helices and β sheets are described as important components not only of fibrous proteins but also of globular proteins. The general principles of protein folding are explained, followed by a consideration of the tertiary structure of proteins, the identification of domains and motifs, and the concept of protein families and superfamilies, e.g. the serpins, and homologous proteins. The relationship between protein structure and function and the concept of homologous proteins and ancestral genes are described. The conformational diversity of proteins is described, especially with respect to transmissible dementias, followed by a description of proteomics. The structure of myoglobin and hemoglobin is described and the interaction of the subunits of the latter in the quaternary structure. The importance of polymorphism in hemoglobin both in respect to normal and abnormal proteins is described with particular mention of sickle-cell hemoglobin. The properties of myoglobin and hemoglobin are outlined, in particular the sigmoidal saturation curve of hemoglobin by oxygen and its modulation by bisphosphoglycerate. The physiological role of this modulator and the characteristics of some abnormal hemoglobins are described.

THE PROPERTIES OF PROTEINS

Living cells depend for their existence on the presence of thousands of different proteins that combine with other molecules with great precision. The combination might involve other proteins as, for example, in muscle contraction, or a whole range of other substances. Thus enzymes, which are usually proteins, combine with their substrates at the active site of the protein, the extent of the combination often depending on the binding of another substance at another site. The control of gene expression, as has been shown in Chapter 3, depends on the binding of protein and DNA, and control by hormones involves the interaction between the hormone and the receptors either on the plasma membrane or in the cytoplasm. Transport across membranes depends on protein–solute interactions, nerve activity involves transmitter substance-protein interactions, and immune protection involves antibody–antigen interactions. These specific interactions will be described in Chapters 5 and 15 and later in the text.

THE FOLDING OF GLOBULAR PROTEINS

GENERAL PRINCIPLES

Characteristics of globular and fibrous proteins

In Chapter 2, the fundamental characteristics of proteins were described with the emphasis on primary structure. From the known properties of proteins it is obvious that they cannot merely consist of long polypeptide chains but must be more sophisticated. In terms of the polypeptide component, proteins can be divided into two main groups: fibrous and globular proteins. The fibrous proteins are physically tough and insoluble in water or dilute salt solution. They have polypeptide chains arranged along a long axis to give fibres or sheets. Some typical fibrous proteins will be described in Chapter 5, but examples are actin and keratin. Globular proteins have their polypeptide chains tightly folded into compact spherical or globular shapes. Most are soluble in aqueous solutions. In this chapter hemoglobin will be used as an example; other globular proteins, such as those found in serum and the antibodies, will be described in Chapter 5.

Some proteins fall into a category between fibrous and globular. Like the fibrous proteins they are rod-like but, like

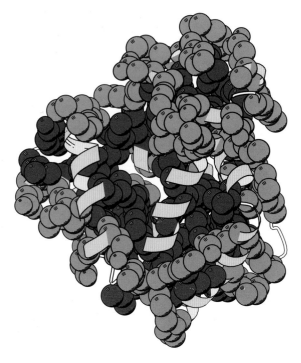

Fig. 4.1 The polypeptide chain of a globular protein folds so that apolar residues tend to be buried to form a hydrophobic interior with polar groups situated at the hydrophilic surface of the protein.

the globular proteins, they are soluble in aqueous solutions. Examples in this category are myosin and fibrinogen.

The distribution of amino acids within a globular protein

The polypeptide of a globular protein folds so that apolar residues tend to be buried to form a hydrophobic interior with polar groups situated at the hydrophilic surface of the protein. Figure 4.1 shows the general characteristics of a globular protein as represented by myoglobin. The hydrophobic residues (Val, Ile, Leu, Phe, Tyr, Trp) are in red and charged residues are in black.

A characteristic of enzymes (see Chapter 6) is that often they have a cleft extending into the protein interior; this cleft might contain some polar groupings.

Hydrogen bonds (see p. 12) play an important role in the folding of proteins. The α helix is particularly prominent in fibrous proteins, but it also plays an important role in globular proteins. The same considerations apply to the other conformation, namely the β-pleated sheet.

The nature of the peptide bond

In Chapter 2 it was mentioned that the peptide bond is rigid with only limited rotation. This is illustrated in Fig. 4.2. It will be seen that, in a peptide chain, rotation is possible only between certain atoms. The $C_\alpha CONHC_\alpha$ is planar.

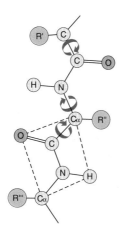

Fig. 4.2 The characteristics of the peptide bond showing that rotation about the bonds is limited.

The α helix

In the α helix the maximum number of hydrogen bonds is present; thus, as indicated in Fig. 4.3, there are 3.6 amino acid residues per turn. For this to be achieved, the polypeptide chain is twisted into a right-handed helix.

The β conformation

A polypeptide chain in which there are no hydrogen bonds within the chain is described as being in the β conformation. A single chain in the β conformation is referred to as a β strand. Such chains can interact with one another, as shown in

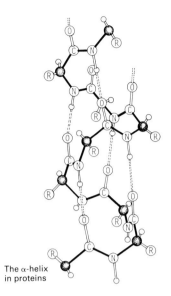

The α-helix
in proteins

Fig. 4.3 The α helix. Hydrogen bonds help to maintain its conformation.

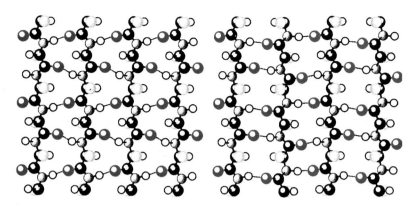

Fig. 4.4 The β-pleated sheet in which the hydrogen bonds link the chains. The chains are parallel on the left and antiparallel on the right. The oxygens (red) of the peptide bonds are shown forming hydrogen bonds.

Fig. 4.4. The R groups are in the opposite plane to the hydrogen bonds and so do not interact. The chains can be either parallel (i.e. with the chains NH_2 to COOH running in the same direction, left) or antiparallel (right). These are referred to as a β-pleated sheet, a structure that is not only found in fibrous proteins but is also present in the tertiary structure of globular proteins, as will be illustrated.

Within proteins the α helices and β strands are connected by so-called loop regions. Globular proteins that possess pleated sheets are said to be in the β conformation.

Representation of α helices and β sheets

To simplify the structural diagrams of proteins, conventions have been adopted to depict secondary structures. An α helix is represented either as a solid cylinder, sometimes with a helix inside it, or more often as a helical ribbon, as shown in Fig. 4.5A. The individual sections of the β strands that participate in β-pleated sheet formation are represented as broad arrows (Fig. 4.5B). The unstructured chains shown at either end are referred to as loops when connecting either α helices or β strands (Fig. 4.5C). Two antiparallel β strands (Fig. 4.5C) are described as a β hairpin. An extended polypeptide chain in the β configuration always twists slightly to the right so that the arrows are usually drawn with this twist in protein structures.

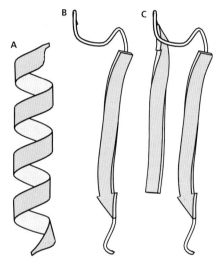

Fig. 4.5 The conventions used to denote the different types of structure. (A) α helix, (B) β strand, (C) antiparallel β strands, the β hairpin.

GENERAL PRINCIPLES OF PROTEIN FOLDING

THE DERIVATION OF GENERAL PRINCIPLES

The primary structure of some 500 000 proteins has so far been achieved, with new structures continuously being reported. As indicated previously, these structures are either determined directly or are deduced from the gene structure. Determination of the tertiary structure is much more difficult. The traditional way of doing this has been by crystallization of the protein followed by X-ray crystallography. Even though the application of computers has made this method much less time-consuming, it is still necessary to prepare suitable crystals, which is not always easy. In addition to X-ray crystallography, the application of NMR spectroscopy (see below) has proved effective, especially with

respect to smaller proteins. In total, the tertiary structure of some 6000 proteins has been achieved. In view of this small number compared with that for the primary structure, there have been many attempts to create computer systems that will allow the prediction of the tertiary structure from the primary structure. An example of the difficulty of doing this is seen in hemoglobin, all the molecules of which have very similar secondary and tertiary structures, yet there are few invariant amino acid residues. Moreover, we so far lack an understanding of the rules that govern the folding of proteins, so that it is not surprising that computer modelling of tertiary structure prediction has proved difficult.

NMR spectroscopy

NMR (nuclear magnetic resonance) or MRI (magnetic resonance imaging) depends on the nuclei of atoms having a spin that can be controlled by a powerful magnetic field. The spinning nuclei orientate themselves in the magnetic field and can absorb radio energy. The method works because the body is largely composed of water; the hydrogen atoms contained being good resonators. Different organs contain different amounts of water and, therefore, show up in contrast in the images.

COMMON PATTERNS OF TERTIARY STRUCTURE

Comparison of the tertiary structure of proteins with respect to the relative order of α helices and β strands along the peptide chain has allowed for the grouping of proteins. This is shown in Fig. 4.6. It will be seen that some proteins contain mainly α helices and few or no β sheets, whereas

all-α
**Hemoglobin
β-subunit**

all-β
**Immunoglobin IgG
constant domain**

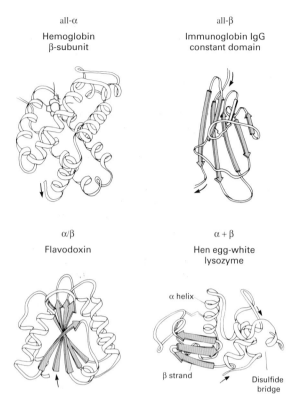

α/β
Flavodoxin

α + β
**Hen egg-white
lysozyme**

Fig. 4.6 Types of structure of globular proteins.

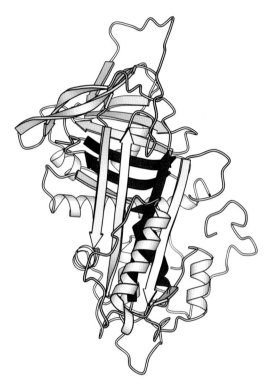

Fig. 4.7 Protein families: the structure of a typical serpin, antithrombin. For an explanation of the red strands, see the text.

in others there are several β strands but few or no α helices. In IgG there are two β sheets, which pack together but are twisted. In αβ structures, α helices and β strands tend to alternate. Often, the β strands form a parallel sheet that is surrounded by α helices, whereas in others there are α helices and β strands that tend to segregate into different regions of the polypeptide chain.

IDENTIFICATION OF DOMAINS AND MOTIFS

In larger proteins, with a size in excess of about 200 amino acid residues, there are often regions that form compact islands of folded structure, usually linked together by unstructured polypeptide. Such a structure is found in hen egg-white lysozyme, as seen in Fig. 4.6; these structures are known as domains. A protein domain is a well-defined modular unit within a protein that either performs a specific biochemical function (functional domain) or constitutes a stable structural component within a protein structure (structural domain). A motif is defined as typically small segments of a protein sequence or fragments of a protein structure, which are well conserved and can occur in different contexts. They are often important for the stability or

function of a protein; they can be likened to a stitch in a fabric. Protein domains and motifs are often associated with different partial activities of a protein; this is especially so for enzymes, several examples of which will be described. Thus, the nicotinamide adenine dinucleotide (NAD) dehydrogenases are typical in that they must bind NAD^+ and also the substrate to be oxidized. Different NAD^+ dehydrogenases all bind NAD^+ but each binds a different substrate. This occurs on a separate domain from that of the substrate; however, all the NAD^+ domains have a similar structure (see p. 99).

Chapter 3 described the presence of exons in eukaryotic genes. There is some evidence that exons are collinear with the polypeptides of the domains. This is an attractive idea in that it supports the concept of exon-domain shuffling in evolution whereby the genes for larger proteins might have evolved by the accidental juxtaposition of exons.

THE CONCEPT OF PROTEIN FAMILIES

As mentioned earlier, the dehydrogenases are similar in structure in respect to their NAD^+ domains. In other words, these enzymes constitute a family. In most cases, protein families have been detected by a

comparison of primary structure, taking into account conservative replacement of amino acids that would be unlikely to seriously affect protein structure. By such means a consensus sequence of amino acid residues might be detected, which represents a functional domain, the biological role of which has already been identified. In other cases, families have been conjectured from a similarity of tertiary structure but the proteins have a rather wide range of functions. The lipocalins, which are composed of proteins that bind a wide range of small hydrophobic ligands, are one such family; serpins (*ser*ine *p*roteinase *in*hibitors) are another. The structure of the serpins will be described as an example.

The serpins are a family of proteins of medical importance because their dysfunction can lead to blood-clotting disorders, emphysema and cirrhosis. Prominent members are two plasma proteins, α_1-antitrypsin, which inhibits elastase (see p. 70), and antithrombin, which is an inhibitor of thrombin, a protein that, among other actions promotes blood coagulation. The structure of antithrombin is shown in Fig. 4.7. The helix shown in red is helix B, the upper of the two short β strands (also in red) is 4B, the lower is 5B and the long vertical strand

	Helix B	Sheet 3A	Sheet 4B	Sheet 5B
Human antitrypsin	-PVSIATAFAMLSLGT-	-LVNYIFFKGKW-	-KPFVFLMI-	-FMGKVVNPT-
Heparin cofactor II	-PVGISTAMGMISLGL-	-INLCIYFKGSW-	-RPFLFLIY-	-FMGRVANPS-
Antithrombin	-PLSISTAFAMTKLGA-	-LVNTIYFKGLW-	-RPFLVFIR-	-FMGRVANPC-
C1 inhibitor	-PFSIASLLTQVLLGA-	-LVNAIYLSAKW-	-QPFLFVLW-	-FMGRVYDPR-
Protein C inhibitor	-PVSISMALAMLSLGT-	-LVNYIFFKGTW-	-QPFIIMIF-	-FLARVMNPV-
Corticosteroid BG	-PVSISMALAMLSLGA-	-MVNYIFFKAKW-	-RPFLMFIV-	-FLGKVNRP

Fig. 4.8 A comparison of the primary structure of members of the serpin superfamily; the conserved residues are shown in heavy type.

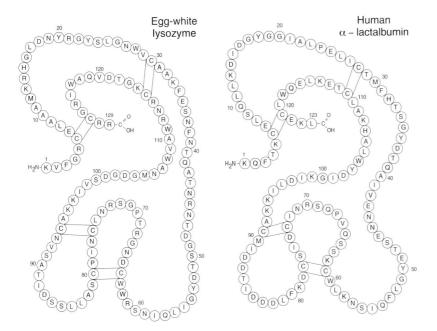

Fig. 4.9 Comparison of the primary structure of α-lactalbumin and egg-white lysozyme: two proteins with a similar primary structure but different biological activities.

is 3A. The actual amino acid sequences of these regions are shown in Fig. 4.8, with the conserved residues in heavy type.

The serpins are thought to have developed by divergent evolution over a period of some 500 million years. The original ancestral protein is presumed to have had the function of a serine proteinase inhibitor, but some members of the family that are currently included on the grounds of similarity of structure have lost this function and developed specialized roles (e.g. corticosteroid-binding globulin – corticosteroid BG in Fig. 4.8), or have no recognized function apart from nutrition (e.g. ovalbumin). Others retain this function, including the inhibitors of C1 (the first component of complement; see p. 76) and protein C (a normal plasma serine proteinase that is inactivated by thrombin and cleaves clotting factors Va and VIIIa (see p. 191) to inactive forms). Hard and fast rules do not exist for allocating proteins to superfamilies; it is done by general consensus. The serpins are unique in their mode of action in that it probably involves the initial formation of a Michaelis complex between the serpin and protease, followed by a cleaved inhibitor–proteinase complex so that the serpins are suicidal inhibitors that are destroyed as a result of their inhibitory action.

The term 'superfamily' is used to distinguish between closely related and distantly related proteins. Thus the α and β globins of hemoglobin are classified as two separate families and, together with the myoglobins, form the globin superfamily.

THE RELATIONSHIP BETWEEN PROTEIN STRUCTURE AND FUNCTION

Once the primary structure of a protein has been determined, it is now common to ascertain by means of the database whether the primary structure resembles that of any protein family. It is sometimes possible to infer the function of a protein in this manner. An example is the protein identified from the gene responsible for cystic fibrosis. It was explained in Chapter 3 (p. 52) that the gene codes for the cystic fibrosis transmembrane conductance regulator, which is a chloride channel protein. The prediction of the function of this protein has been amply supported by subsequent work.

HOMOLOGOUS PROTEINS AND ANCESTRAL GENES

Having determined the primary structure of a protein and detected similarities in excess of about 30%, it has been common to state that the proteins are homologous. There are those who would confine this term to those proteins that have been shown from both their primary structure and the organization of their genes to have been derived by the duplication of a common ancestral gene. An example of two such homologous proteins is shown by α-lactalbumin and egg-white lysozyme. These are both involved in the breakage and formation of β1–4-glycosidic bonds but their properties differ.

Lysozyme is a naturally occurring antibiotic, being found in virtually all tissue secretions (see Fig. 4.6). It hydrolyses the β-glycosidic bond between C-1 of N-acetylmuramic acid and C-4 of N-acetylglucosamine and thereby degrades the cell wall of bacteria. As explained on p. 197, α-lactalbumin plays a part in the formation of lactose, a β1–4 disaccharide.

Figure 4.9 shows the primary structure of lysozyme and α-lactalbumin. They are strikingly similar, particularly with respect to the location of the S–S bonds. Many residues play a part in the action of lysozyme, but particularly Glu-35 and Asp-52. In α-lactalbumin, its Ca^{2+}-binding properties are important, and Asp-82, Asp-83, Asp-87 and Asp-88 are particularly significant in this respect. A mutant of α-lactalbumin, involving a change of 6 amino acids, has created a protein with lysozyme activity.

Figure 4.10 shows the organization of the genes for α-lactalbumin from several species compared with the gene for egg-white lysozyme. The number of base pairs in the exons and introns is indicated. There is a striking similarity in the size of the first three exons. The variation in the size of exon 4 can be accounted for on the basis that this exon contains several untranslated nucleotides (see p. 39).

Thus, in the case of lysozyme and α-lactalbumin, both the primary structure of the proteins and the organization of their genes support the concept that they arose by duplication of a common ancestral gene and are, therefore, truly homologous. During the course of evolution, the

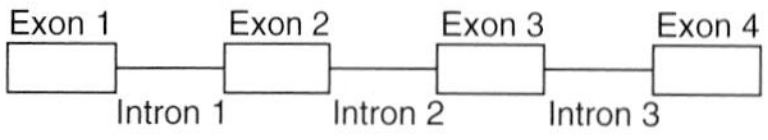

	Exon 1	Intron 1	Exon 2	Intron 2	Exon 3	Intron 3	Exon 4
Human α-lactalbumin	159	648	159	489	76	499	333
Guinea-pig α-lactalbumin	165	335	159	481	76	507	314
Rat α-lactalbumin	165	341	159	429	76	1016	328
Chick lysozyme	165	1270	162	1810	79	79	180

Fig. 4.10 The organization of the genes of α-lactalbumin and lysozyme lends support to their common origin from an ancestral gene.

Table 4.1 Some conformational diseases

Disease	Protein affected	Site of folding
Hypercholesterolemia	Low-density lipoprotein receptor	ER
Cystic fibrosis	Cystic fibrosis transmembrane regulator	ER
Phenylketonuria	Phenylalanine hydroxylase	Cytosol
Huntington disease	Huntingtin	Cytosol
Marfan syndrome	Fibrillin	ER
Osteogenesis imperfecta	Procollagen	ER
Sickle cell anemia	Hemoglobin	Cytosol
Alpha-1-antitrypsin deficiency	Alpha-1-antitrypsin	ER
Tay–Sachs disease	Beta-hexosaminidase	ER
Scurvy	Collagen	ER
Alzheimer disease	Beta-amyloid/presenilin	ER
Scrapie/Creutzfeldt–Jakob disease	Prion protein	ER
Parkinson disease	Alpha-synuclein	Cytosol
Familial amyloidoses	Transthyretin/lysozyme	ER
Retinitis pigmentosa	Rhodopsin	ER
Cataract	Crystallin	Cytosol
Cancer	P53	Cytosol

ER, endoplasmic reticulum.

Table 4.2 The occurrence of transmissible dementia

Species	Name of dementia
Sheep	Scrapie
Humans	Kuru in New Guinea
	Creutzfeldt–Jakob disease (CJD)
	Gerstmann–Straussler–Scheinker disease (GSS)
	Fatal familial insomnia (FFI)
Cows	Bovine spongiform encephalopathy (BSE)

properties of the two proteins have diverged, α-lactalbumin having virtually no enzymic activity and lysozyme, no activity with respect to lactose synthesis.

CONFORMATIONAL DIVERSITY

Reference has already been made to our ability to reverse the denaturation of an enzyme and recover its activity (see p. 15). This experiment was taken to show that once the primary structure had been achieved in a cell, a single, specific tertiary structure would arise, possessing the appropriate biological function; the structure of a protein would change only after a ligand was bound (see Induced fit of enzymes, p. 85 and Allosteric properties of enzymes, p. 94). This concept was reinforced by the protein crystallographers, because crystallization is a purification process leading to the isolation of conformationally homogeneous molecules. It has long been realized that the crystal structure of a protein might not be its only conformation in the cell. It is now accepted that a protein can exist in an ensemble of different conformations in equilibrium before encountering a substrate or hapten. This provides a mechanism for controlling activation and permitting multifunctionality. The conformational diversity ranges from fluctuation of side chains to the movement of loops and secondary structures. NMR analysis has proved particularly effective in revealing conformational diversity. Often this is controlled through interaction with another protein called a 'molecular chaperone' (see Chapter 2).

CLINICAL IMPLICATIONS – CONFORMATIONAL DISEASES

The above concepts are now being used to understand the basis for a group of diseases known by several names including the 'conformational diseases' or 'misfolding diseases', which are characterized by the deposition of proteinaceous aggregates in a variety of organs such as liver, heart and brain. Many of these diseases are described as 'amyloidoses' because the aggregated material stains with dyes such as Congo red in a manner similar to starch (page 111), the aggregates are referred to as 'amyloid fibrils'. The diseases, some of which are listed in Table 4.1, include Alzheimer disease, Creutzfeldt–Jakob disease, cystic fibrosis and Parkinson disease. In some cases the aggregate is intracellular (Parkinson) rather than extracellular in the typical amyloidoses. The basic concept is that a normal protein is either present in a partially unfolded state or becomes so and is then transformed into fibrils. At this stage it is not known whether the fibrillar aggregates themselves give rise to the clinical manifestations or whether they are merely present in a disease. There seems to be an inherent propensity for proteins to aggregate and so this is one of the primary issues that living systems have to control to survive. The development of molecular chaperones is one example of a strategy to minimize the effects of aggregation.

Transmissible dementias

Table 4.2 shows some of the common diseases of the brain that cause dementia, and which result from misfolding caused by a transmissible agent. The diseases are transmitted by the preparation of extracts of the brains of affected individuals, which are either fed to other members of the same species or to other species. The active agent in all cases appears to be a protein named prion proteinaceous infective particle, designated PrP^{sc}; a nucleic acid does not seem to be involved. The tissues of the body contain a protein with the same primary structure as PrP^{sc}, designated PrP^c, the function of which is unknown. The difference in structure between the proteins resides in the tertiary structures, PrP^{sc} possessing much more β-pleated sheet than PrP^c. The onset of the disease involves the conversion of the normal protein into PrP^{sc} by a conformational change, which might have been expected to involve a molecular chaperone but so far none has been detected. It now seems certain that bovine spongiform encephalopathy (BSE) has been transferred to patients to give them new variant Creutzfeldt–Jakob disease (CJD), which is invariably fatal. It is presumed that the source of the infection was contaminated beef.

Polymorphism at codon 129 in the human prion gene encoding either Met or Val has been identified and might contribute to CJD susceptibility or incubation time. The human distribution among Caucasians is 37% Met/Met, 51% Met/Val and 12% Val/Val. All the cases of new variant CJD so far reported are homozygous for Met, so it remains possible that those expressing Val at codon 129 might occur in the future and the clinicopathologic phenotype might be different from the cases already identified.

PROTEOMICS

The entire complement of proteins produced in a cell or organism is called the proteome, derived from the genome, which is the entire complement of genetic information. To study the proteome, which might well comprise hundreds or thousands of different proteins, it has been necessary to develop large-scale and high-throughput protein analysis techniques, and these techniques essentially define the discipline of proteomics. The most common technique is 2D-gel electrophoresis. A protein mixture is loaded onto a polyacrylamide gel and the proteins separated by isoelectric focusing, which means the proteins migrate in a pH gradient until they reach their isoelectric point. The gel is then equilibrated in a detergent (see p. 12) and the proteins separated in the second dimension according to their M_r. The gel is then stained and the proteins revealed as a pattern of spots. The structure of the proteins can be determined by such methods as mass spectrometry. The differences between proteomes can be revealed, e.g. the difference between the proteomes of liver and hepatoma, and protein disease markers can be devised. An example of the use of proteomics is the differentiation between types of bladder cancer, which can be difficult to distinguish by histological examination. In the Western world, bladder cancers are usually transitional cell carcinomas, whereas those in Africa are often squamous cell carcinomas. The techniques are also useful to the pharmaceutical industry to check for the toxic effects of drugs.

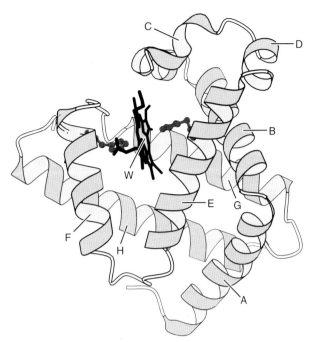

Fig. 4.11 The architecture of myoglobin involves eight helical regions. The histidines interacting with heme are shown in red.

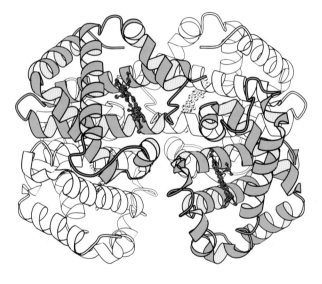

Fig. 4.12 The arrangement of the four chains of hemoglobin.

STRUCTURE AND PROPERTIES OF MYOGLOBIN AND HEMOGLOBIN

STRUCTURE OF MYOGLOBIN

The architecture of myoglobin involves eight helical regions as shown in Fig. 4.11. These are denoted by the letters A–H; the regions joining the helices are denoted by pairs of letters (e.g. FG, joining helices F and G, not shown in the figure).

Histidines in helices E and F interact with heme on either side. The oxygen (O_2) molecule sits at W. Helices E and F form the walls of a box for the heme; B, G and H are the floor and the CD corner closes the open end. The heme pocket consists in the main of non-polar (group 1) amino acids.

Myoglobin carries charged amino acid residues at positions that are hydrophobic in hemoglobin and which are important in bonding the hemoglobin subunits together, as will be explained. For this reason myoglobin molecules do not associate together.

STRUCTURE OF HEMOGLOBIN

Comparison of subunits with myoglobin

Hemoglobin (Fig. 4.12) consists of four chains comprising two pairs of identical chains; these are designated $\alpha_1\alpha_2$ and $\beta_1\beta_2$. There are few bonds between the two α chains or between the two β chains. However, there are strong hydrophobic bonds between unlike chains (e.g. $\alpha_1\beta_1$, $\alpha_1\beta_2$, $\alpha_2\beta_1$ or $\alpha_2\beta_2$). The bonds between an α and a β monomer are stronger than α–α or β–β bonds or those between one $\alpha\beta$ dimer and another. Thus, if hemoglobin is dissociated by treatment with 8-M urea, $\alpha\beta$ dimers always result, rather than $\alpha\alpha$ or $\beta\beta$ dimers. This is shown in Fig. 4.13.

The α chain of hemoglobin differs from the β chain by the deletion of one residue in the NA segment, the addition of two residues in the AB corner and the deletion of six residues in the CD segment and the D helix.

The binding of oxygen to hemoglobin results in the movements of α_1 and β_1 chains as a unit relative to the α_2 and β_2 chains. Deoxyhemoglobin is denoted as having the T (tense) form, and oxyhemoglobin the R (relaxed) form.

The formation of the quaternary structure of hemoglobin

This is shown in Fig. 4.14; the four chains interact to give a compact structure, which is essential for correct protein function. If there is any change in the primary structure of the chains that affects the quaternary structure, the properties of the hemoglobin will be changed. Although this folding is common to the hemoglobin of every species possessing this type of molecule, only about ten amino acid residues are invariant (i.e. present in every case). Some changes in the primary structure make little difference to the tertiary structure, whereas others have a profound effect, as in sickle-cell hemoglobin (see below).

HEMOGLOBIN POLYMORPHISM IN THE HUMAN

In the normal human

Figure 4.15 shows the different types of hemoglobin that are present in the normal human and which arise from the expression of the gene loci. In particular, it should be noted that fetal hemoglobin differs from adult hemoglobin.

CLINICAL IMPLICATIONS – HEMOGLOBINOPATHIES

The inherited disorders of hemoglobin fall into three groups. First, there are the structural hemoglobin variants described below. Second, there are the thalassemias, which are characterized by a reduced rate of production of either the α or β globin chains and which are, therefore, divided into the α and β thalassemias. Finally, there

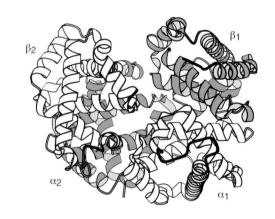

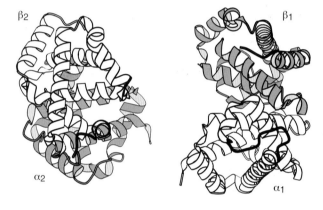

Fig. 4.13 The dissociation of hemoglobin by urea causes the formation of mixed-chain dimers.

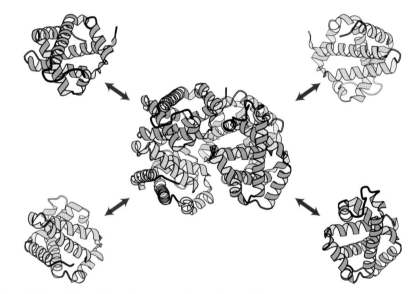

Fig. 4.14 Formation of the quaternary structure of hemoglobin.

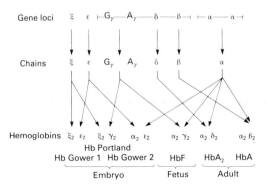

Fig. 4.15 Hemoglobin polymorphism in the human arises as the result of expression of different gene loci.

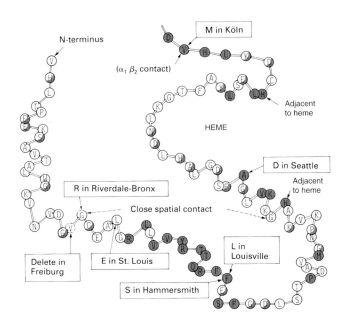

Fig. 4.16 Variation in the primary structure of the β-globin chains of human hemoglobin.

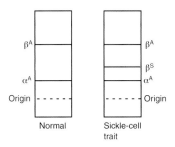

Fig. 4.18 The β chain of sickle-cell hemoglobin can be separated from the β chain of normal hemoglobin by electrophoresis.

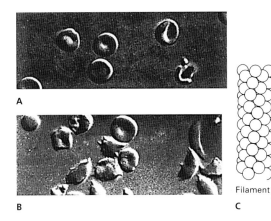

Fig. 4.17 Sickle-cell hemoglobin has a profound effect on the shape of deoxygenated red cells and causes the formation of filaments of protein.

are defects in the normal switch from fetal to adult hemoglobin.

Examples of some replacements in primary structure

In Fig. 4.16, the residues participating in $\alpha_1\beta_1$ and $\alpha_1\beta_2$ contacts are shown in red; the position of other variants that do not produce clinical symptoms are denoted as half red. As mentioned above, an invariant amino acid is one that has never been found to vary in any hemoglobin so far sequenced. There are only two amino acid residues that are common to all hemoglobins: histidine, which forms a covalent link with the heme iron; and a phenylalanine in position 1 of the loop made by helices C and D, which wedges the heme into its pocket. All other residues are replaceable, but in 33 specific positions replacements are restricted to non-polar residues.

Sickle-cell hemoglobin (HbS)

As shown in Chapter 3 (p. 51), sickle-cell anemia is an excellent example of a monogenic molecular disease in that the mutant hemoglobin is caused by a single point mutation whereby a change in one nucleotide in the gene causes the replacement of a glutamic acid in the β chain by a valine. This has little effect on the physiological properties of oxygenated HbS and the red blood cells appear normal as shown at (a) in Fig. 4.17; however, deoxygenated HbS forms rod-like filaments (c), which cause the red cells to sickle (b). Patients homozygous for the sickle gene have only HbS, whereas those with the sickle-cell trait (heterozygous for the gene) have both kinds of hemoglobin in about equal amounts. The frequency of the sickle-cell gene is as high as 40% in certain parts of Africa. This is no doubt because it confers a small but highly

significant degree of protection against most lethal forms of malaria. Glucose 6-phosphate dehydrogenase deficiency – caused by a mutation leading to a defective enzyme – also protects against falciparum malaria, because the parasite requires reduced glutathione and the products of the pentose phosphate pathway to survive.

Electrophoresis of sickle-cell hemoglobin chains

If hemoglobin is treated with a buffer containing urea and dithiothreitol at pH 8.9, the chains separate and can be subjected to electrophoresis on paper. As shown in Fig. 4.18, this is a useful way of identifying heterozygotes of the sickle-cell hemoglobin gene.

Thalassemias

Mutations of the genes encoding the α and β chains can lead to imbalance in the relative amounts of the chains synthesized, a condition known as thalassemia. In α thalassemia there is reduced or total lack of the α chain, and in β thalassemia a partial or total lack of the β chain. The severity of the disease, which occurs more especially in people originating from Mediterranean regions, varies with the amount of chain synthesized, resulting in varying degrees of erythrocyte microcytosis and anemia.

THE BINDING OF OXYGEN AND BISPHOSPHOGLYCERATE

Oxygen

Oxygen binds to Fe^{2+} and this triggers the change in conformation from T to R as previously mentioned. It should be noted that oxygen does not bind when the Fe^{2+} is oxidized to Fe^{3+}, as is found in methemoglobin.

The binding of oxygen to the iron atom reduces the diameter of the iron atom and it moves into the plane of the porphyrin ring.

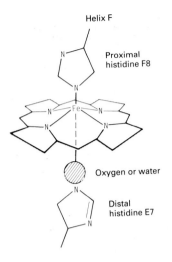

Fig. 4.19 The link between the iron-containing porphyrin ring and the globin chains in hemoglobin.

2,3–Bisphosphoglycerate

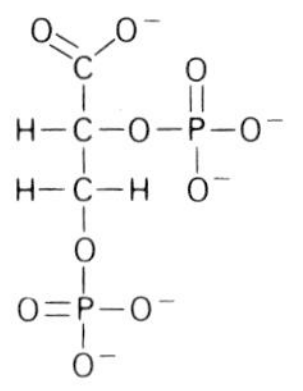

Fig. 4.20 The structure of 2,3-bisphosphoglycerate (BPG).

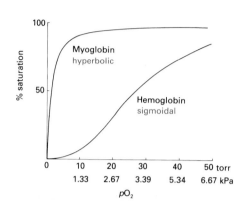

Fig. 4.22 The oxygen saturation curves of myoglobin and hemoglobin are significantly different.

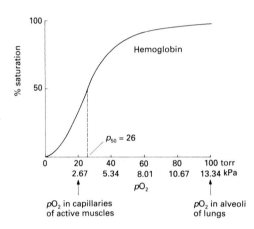

$p_{50} = 26$

pO_2 in capillaries of active muscles

pO_2 in alveoli of lungs

Fig. 4.23 The extent of the oxygen saturation of hemoglobin in the lungs and muscle capillaries.

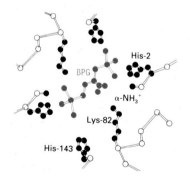

His-2

BPG

α-NH$_3^+$

Lys-82

His-143

Fig. 4.21 The site at which 2,3-bisphosphoglycerate (BPG) binds to deoxyhemoglobin.

The oxygen binds at a site near the distal histidine on helix E (see p. 61) (Fig. 4.19). The movement of the iron atom moves the proximal histidine F8 and produces a conformational change in that subunit. This is transmitted to the other subunits.

Bisphosphoglycerate

Bisphosphoglycerate (BPG; Fig. 4.20, the older term for this compound is diphosphoglycerate, DPG), which, as will be seen, has an important physiological role, binds specifically to deoxyhemoglobin. It binds to the central

cavity created by the four subunits of deoxyhemoglobin. It is extruded on oxygenation because this cavity becomes too small but tends to reduce the affinity for oxygen. As shown in Fig. 4.21, the mode of binding of BPG to human deoxyhemoglobin is by the interaction of BPG with three positively charged groups on each β chain.

PROPERTIES OF MYOGLOBIN AND HEMOGLOBIN

Hyperbolic and sigmoidal curves

The difference in subunit structure of myoglobin and hemoglobin is reflected in their oxygen saturation curves, as shown in Fig. 4.22. The sigmoidal curve of hemoglobin is indicative of cooperative interactions between protein subunits; the affinity for oxygen becomes progressively greater as successive oxygen sites are filled. Cooperative phenomena are dealt with more fully in Chapter 6.

Effect of pO_2

The effect of the partial pressure of oxygen (pO_2) in the capillaries and lungs is such

that in the lungs hemoglobin becomes virtually fully saturated, whereas in the muscle capillaries it loses over 50% of its oxygen. This is illustrated in Fig. 4.23.

Effect of pH

Lowering the pH from 7.6 to 7.2 results in the release of oxygen from oxyhemoglobin, as shown in Fig. 4.24.

The role of bisphosphoglycerate

BPG is present in human red cells. It reduces the affinity of hemoglobin for oxygen by binding to deoxygenated hemoglobin but not to the oxygenated form. The affinity of BPG for fetal hemoglobin is much weaker than for adult hemoglobin, so oxygen combines preferentially with fetal hemoglobin. The degree of reduction in the affinity of oxygen for hemoglobin depends on the BPG/hemoglobin ratio. This is shown in Fig. 4.25. To the extent that the binding of oxygen to hemoglobin is to be likened to the interaction of a substrate with an enzyme, BPG can be regarded as an allosteric effector, as will be explained in Chapter 6 (p. 94).

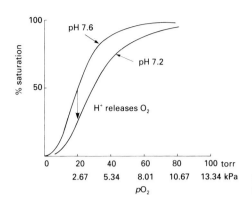

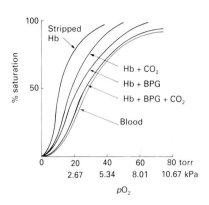

Fig. 4.24 The effect of pH on the saturation of hemoglobin with oxygen.

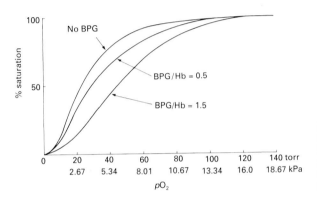

Fig. 4.25 The effect of the 2,3-bisphosphoglycerate/hemoglobin (BPG/Hb) ratio in human red cells on the extent of the oxygen saturation of hemoglobin.

Fig. 4.26 The effect of carbon dioxide (CO_2) on the saturation of hemoglobin with oxygen and the cumulative effect of 2,3-bisphosphoglycerate (BPG).

Effect of carbon dioxide

The effect of carbon dioxide (CO_2) is to decrease the amount of hemoglobin that is present in the oxygenated form. The effects of carbon dioxide and BPG are cumulative; this is shown in Fig. 4.26.

Glycated hemoglobin

Glucose can react with the N-terminal amino acid residues (valine in the human) of the β chains of hemoglobin A (HbA) to produce a so-called 'fast' HbA_1. The means of attachment is through a non-enzymic reaction so that a ketoamine is formed (glucose-CH_2-NH-βA), as shown in Fig. 4.27. The reaction is a continuous process that occurs slowly during the lifespan of the red blood cell. The concentration of HbA_1 is correlated to the degree of diabetic control, so the assay of HbA_1 reflects the patient's average blood glucose concentration over a long period. Because the carbohydrate link is not the same as in glycoproteins (see p. 196), the name glycated hemoglobin is preferred. The phenomenon is not confined to hemoglobin and a number of other glycated proteins have been reported. The unglycated HbA_0 can be separated from HbA_1, either by column chromatography or by electrophoresis on agar gel, as shown in Fig. 4.27. The charged groups of agar interact with A_0 to a greater degree than A_1, thus retarding the migration of A_0.

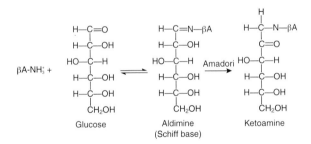

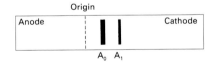

Fig. 4.27 The steps in the glycation of proteins. Fructosamine is the ketoamine produced and can be measured to indicate the extent of glycation. Most of the fructosamine measured derives from albumin, which is also glycated, as this is the most abundant plasma protein. It has a half-life of 3 weeks, in contrast to the 2 months of hemoglobin, so that fructosamine measurements reflect changes in glycation more rapidly than those of HbA_1, and thus give complementary information. The glycated hemoglobin can be separated from unglycated protein by electrophoresis (bottom).

Proteins: specialized functions

5

The structure and function of groups of proteins that are of particular interest in medical science are described. Plasma proteins are clearly relevant in this respect and the electrophoretic profiles of such proteins are of diagnostic use. Serum albumin is the most abundant of the serum proteins and its structure and role are described. α_1-Antitrypsin plays an important role in inhibiting the action of elastase and this has relevance to emphysema, particularly for smokers with a ZZ mutation.

The role of the various iron-binding proteins and the metabolism of iron are described. This is followed by a description of the clinical implications of defective iron metabolism. The structure of collagen, the most abundant protein in the body, and its biosynthesis are described. There follows a summary of the defects in collagen synthesis. The structure of the most common immunoglobulins is described, followed by the major histocompatibility complexes (MHC) and their receptors. A comparison is made of the structures of all these proteins in the superfamily. The production of polyclonal and monoclonal antibodies is followed by a description of the function of complement and of C1q as a typical complement protein. Differences between humoral and cell-mediated immunity are indicated. The uses of immunoassay and of antibodies in diagnosis with radioactive ligands and by ELISA are described, followed by their use in immunoaffinity chromatography, Western blotting and immunocytochemistry.

The chapter ends with a description of the proteins of molecular motors: striated muscle and the sliding-filament model of muscle contraction, smooth muscle and the non-muscle systems. The last includes a description of the role of tubulin, dynein and kinesin in the cytoskeleton and the movement of chromosomes, cilia and organelles. A number of conditions resulting from defects in the structure of muscle and other motor proteins, and associated metabolism, are summarized.

PLASMA PROTEINS

DEFINITIONS AND GENERAL MATTERS

Plasma can be defined as the content of the blood apart from the formed elements, by which is meant the cells such as the red blood cells. To obtain plasma from freshly drawn blood, clotting must be prevented either by the addition of compounds that neutralize or remove Ca^{2+}, such as EDTA (ethylenediaminetetraacetic acid) or oxalic acid, which removes the calcium as insoluble calcium oxalate, or by the addition of heparin (see p. 113). The blood is then centrifuged and the plasma removed by decantation. In contrast to plasma, serum is the fluid that is obtained after the blood has clotted and separated by centrifugation. As far as specific proteins are concerned, the main difference between plasma and serum is that plasma contains fibrinogen; this is removed by clotting and is therefore absent from serum.

Globular proteins, especially those in the plasma, have by tradition been separated into albumins and globulins. Albumin is soluble in pure water whereas the globulins are insoluble in pure water but soluble in iso-osmotic NaCl (saline). Globulins are usually precipitated by half-saturated $(NH_4)_2SO_4$ whereas albumin is only precipitated by fully saturated $(NH_4)_2SO_4$.

All the plasma proteins are synthesized in the liver except for the antibodies, represented by γ-globulin. This fact is the basis for the so-called liver function tests, in which the ratio of albumin (the most abundant of the plasma proteins) to γ-globulin (the most abundant of the globulins) is determined. A low ratio is indicative of a poorly functioning liver; however, this is a rather crude measure of liver function, especially as the basis of the methods used is often unclear.

As explained in Chapter 2 (p. 12), the proportions of the serum proteins can be roughly assessed by paper or gel electrophoresis, bearing in mind that each separated globulin band contains many different proteins with similar electrophoretic mobilities. It is still common to subject a patient's serum to electrophoretic analysis and the patterns shown in Fig. 5.1 are typical. The major proteins contained in the various globulin bands are indicated in Table 5.1.

The measurement of a number of specific proteins gives useful information in the diagnosis and management of disease.

GLOBULINS

ALB α_1 α_2 β γ

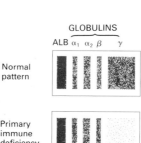

Normal pattern

Primary immune deficiency — Impaired synthesis of immunoglobulins. Usually familial

Multiple myeloma — A monoclonal band, referred to as a paraprotein, which is due to production of a specific immunoglobulin by a malignant clone of cells. Paraproteins are also found rarely in other diseases

Nephrotic syndrome — Albumin lost into urine, and sometimes γ-globulin. Increase in α_2-globulin

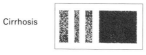

Cirrhosis — A polyclonal gammopathy with increase in many different immunoglobulins of all classes

Infection — Elevated α_1 and α_2 proteins. Usually decreased albumin. So-called 'acute-phase' response

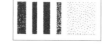

Chronic lymphatic leukaemia — Quite often associated with decreased γ-globulin

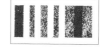

Plasma should not be used: — If plasma is used instead of serum, fibrinogen band gives the appearance of a paraprotein, leading to misleading diagnosis

α_1 Antitrypsin deficiency — α_1-antitrypsin deficiency associated with emphysema of the lung in adults, and juvenile cirrhosis

Fig. 5.1 Electrophoresis of serum proteins on cellulose acetate membrane using a buffer at pH 8.6 can be used to diagnose abnormalities in a patient's serum. The protein bands are visualized by staining with a dye. Table 5.1 lists the principal protein constituents of the various bands of globulin. ALB, albumin.

Table 5.1 The principal constituents of the serum globulin bands separated by electrophoresis

Globulin	Representative constituents
α_1	Thyroxine-binding globulin
	Transcortin
	Glycoprotein
	Lipoprotein
	Antitrypsin
α_2	Haptoglobin
	Glycoprotein
	Macroglobulin
	Ceruloplasmin
β	Transferrin
	Lipoprotein
	Glycoprotein
γ	γG, γD, γM, γE, γA

These are listed in Table 5.2. More information about the significance of some of the proteins will be found later in the text. Diagnosis is also assisted by the measurement of various enzymes in the serum, as explained in Table 6.1 (p. 89). Thyroxine-binding globulin (TBG) carries 70% of the thyroid hormone (T_4 and T_3) in plasma. About 25% is carried on albumin and the rest is bound to transthyretin, formerly known as pre-albumin. Four transthyretin molecules may transform into amyloid fibrils that deposit in cardiac and other tissues, giving rise to the condition known as senile systemic amyloidosis in some elderly individuals. Patients suffering from familial amyloidotic polyneuropathy inherit a single-point mutation, valine to methionine, which causes the soluble, globular transthyretin to polymerize and gradually deposit as fibrous material in the

Table 5.2 Measurement of specific proteins that aid diagnosis

Protein	Function	Reason for assay
α_1-Antitrypsin	Inhibits trypsin and elastase	See text
β_2-Microglobulin	Part of HLA antigen	Raised in tubular dysfunction
α-Fetoprotein	Synthesis in fetal liver	In serum of adult patients with hepatoma
		In amniotic fluid for diagnosis of neural tube defects
Amylase	Breakdown of sugars	Acute pancreatitis
Ceruloplasmin	Oxidizing enzyme	Reduced in Wilson's disease
C-reactive protein (CRP)	Immune and inflammatory responses	Increased in acute illness, diabetes, etc.
Ferritin	Tissue iron storage protein	Indication of body iron stores
		Also acute-phase protein
Haptoglobulin	Binds hemoglobin	Reduced in hemolysis
Prostate specific antigen (PSA)	Prostate physiology	Raised level with enlarged prostate either benign or, particularly, malignant
Thyroxine-binding globulin (TBG)	Thyroid hormone binding	Investigation of thyroid disease
Transferrin	Iron transport	Response to nutritional status and iron stores
Troponin	Muscle thin filament	TNT rapid increase after myocardial infarction

HLA, human leucocyte antigen.

heart or eye. The resulting amyloid fibres (see p. 60) have been shown to consist of long, straight, unbranched rods about 100 Å in diameter.

SERUM ALBUMIN

Serum albumin is a single molecule with an M_r of 65 000 in the human, comprising some 585 amino acid residues. In humans, about 60% of serum protein is serum albumin. It makes an important contribution to the osmolarity of the serum but it is also important because of its ability to bind many different substances, in particular free fatty acids. Its binding properties are indicated in Fig. 5.2. A substance that is bound to another compound is known as a ligand. Our ability to understand the molecular basis for the ligand binding of serum albumin has awaited knowledge of the tertiary structure of the protein; this has recently been elucidated. The main features are shown in Fig. 5.3, which depicts two very similar wings. Having stressed the biological properties of this protein, there is an enigma, because there are some people who virtually lack serum albumin, a condition known as analbuminemia, and yet appear to be normal.

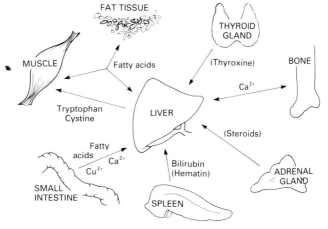

Fig. 5.2 Serum albumin binds many ligands. The ligands in between parentheses are transported by albumin when the primary carriers are filled.

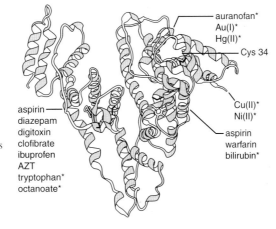

Fig. 5.3 The structure of human serum albumin. This protein has an M_r of 65 000; it consists of 585 amino acid residues and contains 17 disulfide bridges, one free thiol (Cys 34) and one tryptophan. The various ligand-binding sites are indicated: the asterisks denote binding sites that can be inferred; all the others have been determined by X-ray crystallography. The overall distribution, metabolism and efficacy of many drugs can be altered based on their affinity for serum albumin. In some cases, a putative drug is ineffective because of its high affinity for this abundant protein.

α_1-ANTITRYPSIN

Normals

The main component of the α_1-globulin band (see p. 12) from the electrophoresis of serum proteins consists of a protein called α_1-antitrypsin. It is wrongly named because it is active against elastase rather than trypsin and is a member of a group of serine proteinase inhibitors or serpins (see p. 58). In normal liver the destructive power of elastase released from the neutrophils is held in check by α_1-antitrypsin.

Effect of smoking and emphysema

Cigarette smoking increases the number and activity of lung neutrophils and consequently the amount of elastase. Moreover, oxidation by hydrogen peroxide reduces the protection afforded by a given

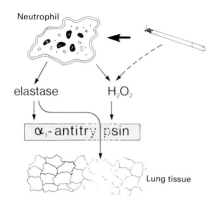

Fig. 5.4 Smoking increases the amount of elastase and reduces the efficacy of α_1-antitrypsin.

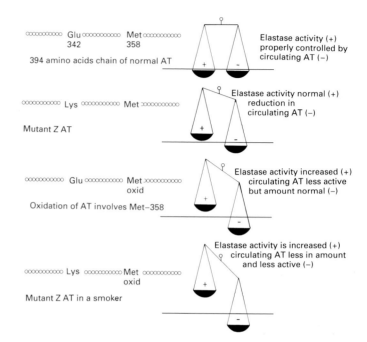

Fig. 5.5 The effects of mutations of α_1-antitrypsin (AT) and smoking on the activity of elastase and amount of α_1-antitrypsin. The horizontal line indicates the situation in the normal person where the elastase activity (left) is counterbalanced by the amount of α_1-antitrypsin (right). The effect of smoking and mutations is explained in the text.

amount of circulating α_1-antitrypsin. α_1-Antitrypsin is less active after oxidation, and elastase then causes tissue breakdown and loss of elasticity in the lungs (i.e. emphysema). These effects are summarized in Fig. 5.4.

Effect of mutants

Two mutants of α_1-antitrypsin occur, both are confined to people of European descent: the S-variant in 5–8% (genotype MS) and the Z-variant in 4% (genotype MZ). The tissue specificity of α_1-antitrypsin depends on position 358 in the polypeptide chain of 394 amino acids being occupied by either methionine or valine. The methionine residue is susceptible to oxidation, as previously mentioned.

The various effects of the mutations are indicated in Fig. 5.5. In normals, the critical positions in the chain are occupied by glutamate and methionine or valine. In non-smokers, emphysema is unusual. The scales at the top of Fig. 5.5 show that the elastase activity is properly controlled by α_1-antitrypsin. In normal smokers, the methionine is oxidized and the amount of elastase is raised. Although the amount of α_1-antitrypsin secreted is normal, it is less active against the elastase. Hence smoking, even in normals, leads to a tendency to emphysema. In the ZZ mutant, glutamate is replaced by lysine, which results in only 15% of the normal amount of α_1-antitrypsin being secreted. The retained α_1-antitrypsin accumulates in the endoplasmic reticulum of the hepatocytes where much of it is degraded, but some aggregates to form insoluble intracellular inclusions, which are associated with the liver disease of ZZ children. If ZZ individuals smoke, the effects are cumulative; the amount of elastase is raised,

there is less α_1-antitrypsin and what there is is less active. Hence the occurrence of emphysema is probable.

IRON-BINDING PROTEINS

Transferrin

Transferrin transports iron and regulates intestinal iron absorption. It is synthesized in the liver and is present in the β-globulin band of the serum proteins (see p. 12). It is a glycoprotein with two iron (ferric) binding sites. Many cells possess transferrin receptors on which the cells depend for their essential supply of iron. Transferrin is taken up by receptor-mediated endocytosis (see p. 210). In non-erythroid cells, uptake is regulated by control of receptor protein synthesis by cellular iron, which regulates the metabolic stability of the mRNA which has iron-responsive elements (IRE) at the untranslated 3' end of the molecule. These have AU-rich destabilizing sequences that are masked by active iron-response element-binding protein (IRE-BP). At high Fe concentration the IRE-BP is inactive and the AU-rich sequences promote degradation of transferrin receptor (TfR) mRNA. This reduces Fe input thus protecting the cell. At low Fe concentration, IRE-BP is active and binds to the TfR mRNA, which blocks the destabilizing AU-

rich sequences, allowing translation of the mRNA. Transferrin receptor increases and more Fe enters the cell.

Ferritin

Ferritin is the iron store in the liver and spleen. Apoferritin is the iron-free form. Ferritin consists of 24 subunits of a varying mixture of H subunits (178 amino acids) and L subunits (171 amino acids), M_r about 450 000. A thin coat of aggregated polypeptide monomers surrounds an inorganic core of up to 4500 iron atoms. Its level in liver and spleen is controlled at the level of translation, and depends on the amount of iron available. The control of intracellular iron concentration by the IRE-BP is an elegant example of a single protein that regulates the translation of one mRNA and degrades another. The 5' untranslated region of ferritin mRNA contains an IRE to which IRE-BP binds, thus blocking the 40S ribosomal subunit from scanning the mRNA when the Fe concentration is low. This means that there is less ferritin to bind Fe and so the Fe is available for Fe-requiring enzymes. At high Fe concentration the IRE-BP is inactive and does not bind to the mRNA. Thus more ferritin is produced, and binds more iron.

Hemosiderin

Hemosiderin is iron-loaded ferritin that has undergone partial proteolysis, probably within lysosomes, rendering it insoluble and reducing the availability and thus the potential toxicity of its iron.

Hepcidin

Hepcidin is an acute antimicrobial peptide synthesized by liver. It inhibits intestinal iron absorption. Hepcidin is currently considered to be the principal regulator of intestinal iron absorption (see below), altering expression of duodenal ferric reductase and divalent metal transporter (DMTI) in crypt cells and mature enterocytes.

General metabolism of iron

There is no excretory mechanism for iron, which slowly accumulates in the body throughout life, some 10% of dietary iron being absorbed. Frequent loss of blood, such as in menstruation, can cause anemia if dietary iron is inadequate because iron is essential for hemoglobin synthesis and thus red cell formation. When the red cells are destroyed, the iron is removed from hemoglobin by reticuloendothelial cells, where it remains until taken up by transferrin for utilization elsewhere. If excessive amounts of iron are absorbed, it can accumulate in the reticuloendothelial cells, such as the Kupffer cells of the liver; this condition is known as iron overload or hemosiderosis due to the deposits of hemosiderin. The problem of iron overload commonly arises when those with thalassemia receive blood transfusions. The excretion of some iron through the kidneys can be induced by the chelating agent desferrioxamine but removal of blood (venesection) is the only really effective method of removing iron from the body.

Intestinal iron absorption

Dietary iron exists in the ferric form either as relatively insoluble salts or in heme. Some ferric iron is reduced and solubilized within the acid environment of the stomach but most absorption takes place in the proximal small intestine (duodenum). At least two steps are independently regulated, i.e. uptake across the luminal brush border membrane and exit across the basolateral membrane of the enterocytes en route to the body iron stores. The precise

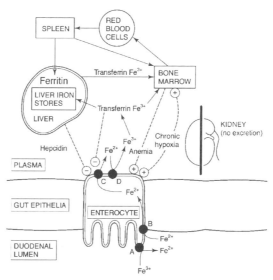

Erratum

Please note that Figure 5.6 on page 71 is incorrect. The correct Figure 5.6 is shown here.

Fig. 5.6 The absorption and subsequent metabolism of iron. Letters against closed circles indicate proteins as follows: (A) Intestinal ferri-reductase (D Cyt*b*). (B) Divalent metal transporter (DTMI). (C) Ferroportin (iron-regulated transporter 1 – Ireg1). (D) Intestinal ferroxidase (hephaestin). See text for protein functions. Broken lines indicate stimulation (+) or inhibition (–) of intestinal iron absorption.

mechanisms of these regulatory steps are not fully understood. Iron absorption is increased by iron deficiency, chronic hypoxia, pregnancy and erythroid hyperplasia, and normally decreased in iron overload.

Ascorbic acid (vitamin C) strongly increases the absorption of iron through its role in the conversion of dietary Fe^{3+} to Fe^{2+}. A surface membrane ferric reductase, duodenal cytochrome *b* (Dcytb), is present in the microvilli of the duodenal enterocytes. This enzyme is up-regulated by iron deficiency, e.g. by anemia and chronic hypoxia. Closely associated with the reductase is the DMTI. This carrier is proton-coupled and requires a pH gradient for activity. DMTI can transport a variety of divalent transition elements as well as Cd^{2+} and Pb^{2+}. It cannot transport Fe^{3+} and is up-regulated by iron deficiency. Heme iron can be released within the duodenal lumen facilitated by acid-reducing conditions but heme can also be taken up by the duodenal enterocytes. Release of iron is mediated by heme oxygenase, the iron entering an ill-defined intracellular pool. Enterocyte apoferritin acts as an intracellular iron sink but is not an essential part of the absorption process itself. At the basolateral membrane a further transporter, ferroportin or iron regulatory protein 1 (Ireg1), is involved. Oxidation of the exported Fe^{2+} is mediated by an intestinal ferro-oxidase (hephaestin) and by plasma ceruloplasmin (Fig. 5.6). The extent to which transferrin in the plasma is saturated with iron is a major regulator of iron absorption.

CLINICAL IMPLICATIONS OF IRON METABOLISM

In genetic (idiopathic) hemochromatosis, the regulation of iron absorption is disrupted and enhanced absorption occurs in the face of a massive accumulation of iron in the tissues (hepatic, cardiac, pituitary and pancreatic islet cells). The consequences of this iron overload are severe and treatment is required by regular venesection to remove the iron excess. The defect in genetic hemochromatosis has been located to a gene *HFE*. Inheritance of this variant, one of the most common genetic defects, is not invariably associated with the full clinical syndrome. Genotyping patients for the C282Y and H66D mutations of *HFE* is clinically useful. Atransferrinemia, a rare genetic disorder, is accompanied by hepatic iron overload with iron deficient anemia. Regular injections of transferrin partially reverses the iron overload and corrects the anemia.

Fragments of the erythroid transferrin receptor are found circulating in the plasma. Assays of soluble transferrin receptor are a useful measure of iron deficiency and of total erythroid mass. Serum ferritin is a useful measure of iron stores and iron overload. It is an acute-phase protein and misleading elevated levels, independent of iron stores, can be found in malignant disease, chronic inflammation, e.g. rheumatoid arthritis and, particularly, acute hepatitis.

Levels of hepcidin are decreased in iron deficiency, chronic hypoxia and anemia. Levels are increased in iron overload,

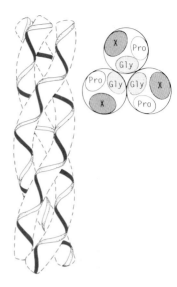

Fig. 5.7 A model of the triple-stranded tropocollagen. To the right is a cross-section showing the outline of each strand and the position of glycine.

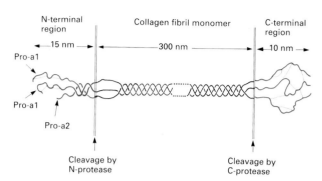

Fig 5.8 The synthesis of collagen. The red dotted lines indicate the S–S bonds.

–C=O groups of residues on other chains. Thus the direction of the hydrogen bonds is transverse to the long axis of the collagen rod.

Collagen biosynthesis

Collagen is synthesized in the form of a precursor protein, procollagen. The collagens have large genes with some 42 exons in the case of the α chains of type I collagen. The biosynthetic route has many processing steps. The initial transcript is termed preprocollagen, which enters the rough endoplasmic reticulum where the N-terminal signal peptide is removed to form procollagen as shown in Fig. 5.8. This contains unfolded chains with N- and C-terminal peptides. Some prolines and lysines are hydroxylated and enzymes add sugars to the lysines. The C terminal peptides of the three chains form a globular structure stabilized by disulfide bonds catalysed by the enzyme disulfide isomerase. This has three consequences. First, the correct chains are selected. Second, it aligns the three polypeptide chains with their first Gly–X–Y repeats in register so that the triple helix is formed with all three chains in phase. Third, the propeptides prevent the assembly of procollagen into fibrils, which would prevent its secretion. Correct folding of the chains requires the enzyme prolyl–peptide isomerase. Procollagen is secreted through the plasma membrane. The procollagen proteases then cleave the propeptides to form the collagen fibre monomer, formerly called tropocollagen, which retains short peptide sequences at each end of the chains. Thus for each rod-like molecule 95% of its length is in the triple-helical conformation but the 2–3% at each end is non-helical – these are the telopeptides. The importance of the telopeptides, which are around 10–20 amino acids in length, relates to the cross-linking of individual monomers within a collagen fibril. The fibril monomers assemble to form insoluble fibres and microfibrils (see

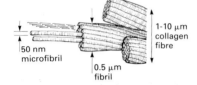

Fig. 5.9 Microfibrils consist of staggered arrays of collagen molecules.

Fig. 5.9). The telopeptides have lysine or hydroxylysine residues. These can be oxidized by lysyl oxidase to aldehydes, which then form Schiff bases with other lysines or hydroxylysines in the body of the adjacent triple-helical monomers within the fibre. The telopeptides are critical in covalent cross-link formation, which stabilizes the collagen fibrils and gives them the high-tensile strength characteristic of the fibres in skin, bone, etc. Antibodies to the cross-linked telopeptide fragments permit the recognition of specific collagen types. Whereas the collagens described above form fibrils, others polymerize into sheets, which surround the organs, epithelia or even whole animals.

Gelatin is formed from a mixture of collagen chains without propeptides, which have been removed by treatment with acid or gelatinase. Boiling dissociates the chains from each other and when cold the chains randomly associate out of register forming a network that solidifies into a gel.

CLINICAL IMPLICATIONS – DISEASES DUE TO DEFECTS IN COLLAGEN SYNTHESIS

There are a number of diseases due to defects in collagen synthesis. A summary of these is shown in Table 5.3. Scurvy results from dietary deficiency of ascorbic acid leading to reduced proline hydroxylation, as described on p. 106. Collagen containing insufficient hydroxyproline loses temperature stability. Clinical manifestations are suppression of the

chronic inflammation and animal models of genetic hemochromatosis. Mutations of hepcidin occur in early onset (juvenile) hemochromatosis.

COLLAGEN

Collagen structure

Collagen is the most abundant protein in mammals and is the major fibrous element of skin, bone, tendon, cartilage, blood vessels and teeth. To fulfil its many roles, the basic structure of collagen varies, having been classified into some 25 genetic types but all contain three polypeptide chains of about 1000 amino acid residues, each in a left-handed helical formation. This is shown in Fig. 5.7. In contrast to globular proteins, the amino acid sequence of the collagen chains is regular, except for about the last 20 amino acid residues at each end; every third residue is glycine, usually followed by proline (also shown in Fig. 5.7). Two unusual amino acid residues are also present: hydroxyproline (Hyp) and hydroxylysine, formed by post-translational hydroxylation of proline and lysine, respectively. Hence a typical sequence might be:

–Pro–Met–Gly–Pro–Arg–Gly–Leu–Hyp–

Each of the three strands is hydrogen bonded to the other two strands; there are no intrachain hydrogen bonds, which are a feature of the α helix. The hydrogen donors are the peptide–NH groups of glycine, and the acceptors are the peptide

Table 5.3 Selected disorders in collagen biosynthesis and structure

Disorder	Collagen defect	Clinical manifestation
Osteogenesis imperfecta 1	Decreased synthesis of type I collagen	Long bone fractures prior to puberty
Osteogenesis imperfecta 2	Point mutations and exon rearrangements in triple helical regions	Perinatal lethality; malformed and soft, fragile bones
Ehlers–Danlos IV	Poor secretion, premature degradation of Type III collagen	Translucent skin, easy bruising, arterial and colon rupture
Ehlers–-Danlos VI	Decreased hydroxylysine in types I and III collagen	Hyperextensive skin, joint hypermobility
Ehlers–Danlos VII	Type I collagen accumulation: N-terminal propeptide not cleaved	Joint hypermobility and dislocation
Cutis laxa	Decreased hydroxylysine due to poor Cu distribution	Lax, soft skin; occipital horn formation in adolescents

orderly growth process of bone in children; poor wound healing and increased capillary fragility with resulting hemorrhage.

THE IMMUNE SYSTEM AND THE IMMUNOGLOBULINS

GENERAL CONCEPTS

The immune system

There are two forms of immune system, innate and adaptive. The innate response involves the pre-existing defences of the body and hence provides immediate protection against exposure to a new pathogen. Such innate responses are not specific to a particular pathogen and depend on a group of small proteins or peptides and phagocytic cells that recognize conserved features of pathogens. Innate systems are found in both vertebrates and invertebrates, as well as in plants. The adaptive system remembers previous encounters with specific pathogens and destroys them when they attack again. The adaptive immune response system protects the body against invasion by all types of macromolecules, especially proteins and polysaccharides, but not directly against small molecules, although such molecules might elicit an immune response if they are bound to a protein of the body. The body has two different types of immune response: (1) if the response to an immunogen is the production of soluble antibodies in the body fluids, it is called humoral immunity (the body fluids used to be called humours); (2) if the response is through cytotoxic or killer T cells, then the immunity is known as cell-mediated. These two mechanisms complement each other.

The challenge for the immune system is to be able to provide antibodies to interact with the antigens that arise as a result of the presence of an immunogen or with foreign cells (both known as non-self) that invade the body, but not to react in this

way with the body's own proteins (known as self). This subject was briefly introduced in Chapter 3 (p. 40), where the production of two forms of IgM was described as an example of 'alternative splicing' and the generation of antibody diversity was described. It is not appropriate in this text to consider all aspects of immunity, but there follows a description of the proteins that play important roles in the two types of immunity.

Humoral immunity

Antibodies are produced by a class of lymphocytes called plasma cells, which develop when B lymphocytes, which originate in the bone marrow (hence the B), are stimulated by the presence of an antigen. Whereas an immunogen is a substance that causes the body to produce an antibody, an antigen is a substance, or a component of a substance (such as a motif of a protein, known as an epitope) that causes the formation of a specific antibody. Figure 5.10 shows the stages in this transformation. The antigen binds to a virgin B cell, where it meets the specific antibody in the form of an immunoglobulin, IgM, which, in its monomer form, is displayed on the cell surface, as previously described (p. 40). The antigen is degraded into peptides and enters the cleft in a class II major histocompatibility complex (MHC) glycoprotein. MHC molecules are expressed on the cells of all higher vertebrates, having been first demonstrated in mice. In humans they are called HLA antigens (human leukocyte-associated). These degraded pieces of antigen are displayed on the cell surface. The B cell then binds to a helper T cell (T for thymus), which possesses the CD4 protein (CD stands for cluster of differentiation) and which has been activated by the same antigen. When this happens, the B cell multiplies, due to the release of cytokines

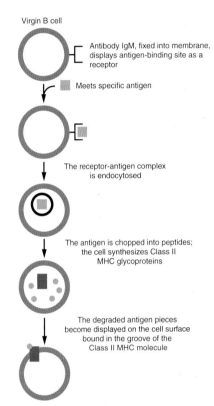

Virgin B cell

Antibody IgM, fixed into membrane, displays antigen-binding site as a receptor

Meets specific antigen

The receptor-antigen complex is endocytosed

The antigen is chopped into peptides; the cell synthesizes Class II MHC glycoproteins

The degraded antigen pieces become displayed on the cell surface bound in the groove of the Class II MHC molecule

Fig. 5.10 Steps in the conversion of a virgin B cell to an activated state ready for conversion to an antibody-producing plasma cell.

by the helper T cell, and matures into an antibody-secreting cell. The antibody is in the form of pentameter IgM. This phenomenon is known as clonal selection because the presence of the antigen has caused the selection of, rather than the de novo synthesis of, antibody from a library of billions of B cells, and multiplication of a clone of plasma cells devoted to the production and secretion of a single specific antibody. This is known as the acquired immune response and is depicted in Fig. 5.11. It also accounts for the fact that the secondary response to the presence of an antigen is more vigorous than the first, the clones of lymphocytes remaining from the first response being still present

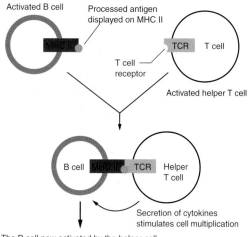

Fig. 5.11 A helper T cell activates an activated B cell to become a clone of plasma cells secreting antibody. TCR, T cell receptor.

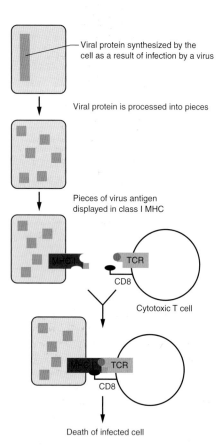

Fig. 5.12 The sequence of events in a cell-mediated immune reaction to a foreign antigen that was synthesized within a cell.

Cell-mediated immunity

It is the cytotoxic cells or killer T cells (which possess the CD8 protein) that are responsible for cell-mediated immunity, which leads to the removal of the offending virus. The protein of the infecting virus is processed into fragments, which combine with class I MHC and are brought to the surface by the MHC protein. There the complex is detected by a killer T cell, which expresses CD8 protein. The T cell then secretes compounds that destroy the infected cell. These events are illustrated in Fig. 5.12.

THE STRUCTURE OF THE MAJOR PROTEINS INVOLVED IN THE IMMUNE RESPONSE

The immunoglobulins

There are many different classes of immunoglobulin but they all have a common overall architecture, which is also found among the members of the so-called immunoglobulin superfamily of receptors. The structure of IgG is shown in Fig. 5.13. This is the protein that is produced in the largest amount after prolonged stimulation. It has two identical heavy (H) chains and two identical light (L) chains held together by S–S bonds. The antigen interacts with the hypervariable regions of the chains. The variability refers to the primary structure, which produces a tertiary structure that binds uniquely to each antigen. The constant regions are involved in the binding of complement, which will be described later. The structure is divided into the Fab antigen-binding domain and the Fc complement-binding domain. The molecule is cleaved by papain, which provides a crystallizable polypeptide that was important for structure determination. The three-dimensional structure of IgG is shown in Fig. 5.14. The structure is flexible so that the relative arrangement of the domains can change. Figure 5.15 summarizes the sites of movement. There are two regions involved in these changes: the hinge region at the junction of C_H1 and C_H2, and the switch region at the junction of the V and C domains in Fab.

Structure of IgM and IgA

The first response to an antigen is in the form of IgM, as described previously (see Fig. 3.59). IgM is a pentamer, the structure of which is shown in Fig. 5.16. In IgM, the hinge region in IgG is replaced by a rigid pair of extra domains (C_H2), whereas the C_H3 and C_H4 domains in IgM are structurally equivalent to the C_H2 and C_H3 regions, respectively, in IgG. IgM also contains the J chain, which is a polypeptide of M_r 15 000, rich in cysteine. The J chain links two heavy chains, thereby allowing for the formation of S–S bridges between the C_H3 and C_H4 domains of other monomers, so forming a pentamer. Similarly, the J chain is present in IgA. Each molecule of IgG has a valency of 2; that is, it has the potential to combine with two molecules of antigen (in theory, therefore, IgM has a valency of 10, but the effective valency is about 5).

Structure of MHC I and II

Figure 5.17 is a schematic representation of the structures. Class I proteins consist of a long α chain non-covalently bound to a small polypeptide called β_2-microglobulin. The α chain has three extracellular domains (α_1, α_2 and α_3), a transmembrane segment and a cytosolic tail. Differences

during the second challenge. They contribute to immunological memory.

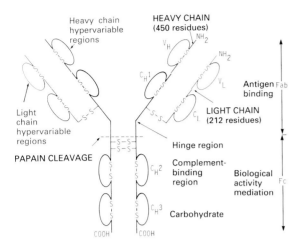

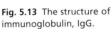

V_H and V_L — variable regions
C_L and C_H — constant regions

Fig. 5.13 The structure of immunoglobulin, IgG.

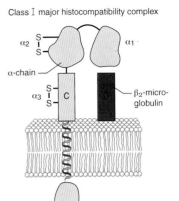

Class I major histocompatibility complex

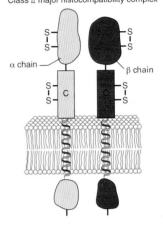

Class II major histocompatibility complex

Fig. 5.17 Schematic representation of the domain organization of class I and class II MHCs.

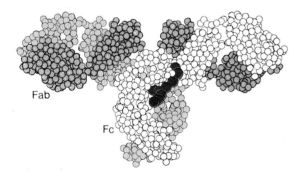

Fig. 5.14 Space-filling representation of the three-dimensional structure of human IgG Dob (Dob is human IgG₁ (κ) cryoglobulin). Dob has a 15-residue deletion in its hinge region compared to normal IgG. The two heavy chains are shown in white and in pink. Light chains are in grey. Carbohydrate is shown as red spheres.

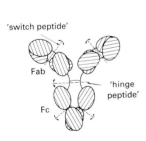

Fig. 5.15 The sites of movement of IgG. See text for explanation.

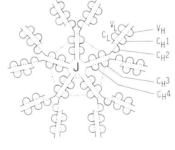

Fig. 5.16 The structure of IgM. The formation of IgM polymer depends on the presence of J chain.

between class I proteins are located mainly in the α_1 and α_2 domains, which form the peptide-binding site. The α_3 domain, which interacts with a constant β_2-microglobulin, is largely conserved. The overall plan of the class II MHC molecule is similar. The peptide-binding site is formed by the α and β domains.

Immunoglobulin superfamily

Figure 5.18 compares the domain organization of several prominent members of the family. Many receptors involved in the immune response and cell–cell recognition contain variable and constant regions related in sequence and structure to immunoglobulin domains.

PRODUCTION OF ANTIBODIES

Polyclonal antibodies

Polyclonal antibodies result from the administration of a protein or polysaccharide to an animal that is of a species unrelated to the source of the immunogen. The progress of immunization is assayed by the presence in the serum of antibodies that cause a precipitate when incubated with the immunogen. A large protein immunogen will usually have several antigen sites, each of which will give rise to an antibody; hence the name polyclonal antibodies. Such sites are called epitopes. As each antibody has two combining sites, the interaction between the antigens and the antibodies accounts for the precipitate, the so-called precipitin reaction. An excess of immunogen results in the re-solution of the precipitate.

MONOCLONAL ANTIBODIES

In contrast to polyclonal antibodies, a monoclonal antibody reacts only with a single epitope; hence there is no precipitation when the antibody and antigen are incubated together. The production of monoclonal antibodies has become a very important technique and will be described.

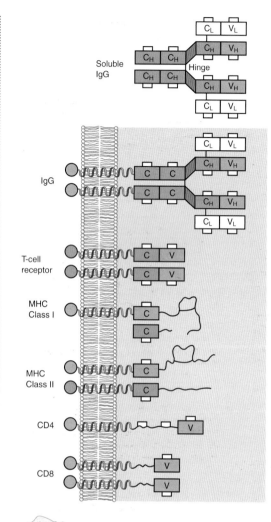

Fig. 5.18 Similarities in the domain organization of several prominent members of the immunoglobulin superfamily.

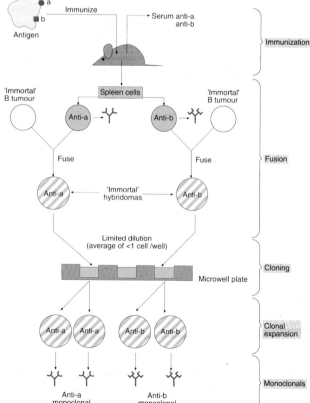

Fig. 5.19 Steps in the production of monoclonal antibodies.

In the example shown in Fig. 5.19, mice were immunized with an immunogen bearing two epitopes, a and b. The spleen cells make anti-a and anti-b, which appear as antibodies in the serum. The spleen is removed and the individual cells fused in polyethylene glycol with constantly dividing B-cell tumour cells selected for a purine enzyme deficiency (see below). The resulting cells are distributed into micro-well plates in HAT (hypoxanthine, aminopterin, thymidine) medium, which kills off all but the fused cells. Subsequent dilution of the medium ensures that each well contains one hybridoma cell or less. Each hybridoma, which is the fusion product of a single-antibody-forming cell and a tumour cell, will have the ability of the former to secrete a single species of antibody and the immortality of the latter, enabling it to proliferate continuously, with clonal progeny providing an unending supply of antibody with a single specificity - the monoclonal antibody.

The mutant cell line lacks hypoxanthine-guanine phosphoribosyltransferase (HGPRT). This enzyme catalyses the synthesis of inosinate (a precursor of AMP and GMP) in the salvage pathway (see p. 26). In the HAT medium, the aminopterin blocks de novo synthesis of nucleotides. Hypoxanthine cannot be used by the unfused myeloma cells because they lack HGPRT. Spleen cells contain HGPRT but are not 'immortal'. The hybridoma cells survive because they are both immortal and contain the HGPRT of the spleen cells.

COMPLEMENT

On p. 73 the general characteristics of the innate system of immunity were described. Another innate response is provided by a class of blood proteins known as complement; the name comes from their ability to assist, or complement, the activity of antibodies in fighting infection. Complement involves a complex series of some 20 proteins which, along with blood clotting, fibrinolysis and kinin formation, forms one of the triggered enzyme systems – in this case a series of proteases – found in plasma. These systems characteristically produce a rapid, highly amplified response to a trigger stimulus mediated by a cascade phenomenon where the product of one reaction is the enzyme catalyst of the next.

Complement can be triggered in three ways. One type of complement molecule, called C3, can bind to any protein, such as those in bacteria, and then attracts the

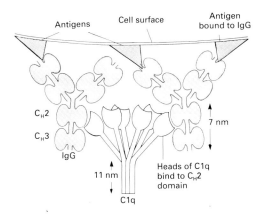

Fig. 5.20 The adaptive system of complement. This is initiated by the binding of antibodies to a bacterium which activates the complement protein C1q with the structure shown.

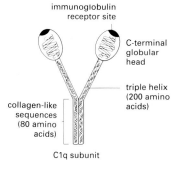

Fig. 5.21 The structure of the 'stalk' of C1q.

binding of other complement molecules. Another way is for a macrophage to secrete interleukin 6, which causes the liver to secrete mannose-binding protein; this binds to the capsule of a bacterium and triggers the complement cascade. These two ways involve the innate system.

The third type of complement action involves the adaptive system, illustrated in Fig. 5.20. The binding of antibodies to a bacterium activates a complement protein called C1q (M_r 400 000), which activates other complement molecules. C1q binds to the C_H2 domain of the IgG-antigen complex. As seen in Fig. 5.20, C1q structurally resembles a bunch of six tulips with three chains (subunits) in each tulip. In the subunit (shown in Fig. 5.21), the 'flower' is a globular structure, while the 'stalk' is elongated and resembles the triple-helical structure of collagen (see p. 72). Indeed, it even contains the Gly–X–Y triplet sequence with hydroxyproline. The result of the cascade of proteases is that the bacteria are destroyed by lysis.

IMMUNOASSAY AND AFFINITY CHROMATOGRAPHY

Radioimmunoassay

Antibodies, either polyclonal or monoclonal, can be used as specific analytical reagents to quantitate the amount of a protein or other antigen. In the original method, the substance to be analysed, called the analyte, is labelled with a radioactive isotope, usually [125]I. The principle of radioimmunoassay is shown in Fig. 5.22. First, a limiting and constant amount of antibody is incubated with a constant concentration of radioactive analyte such that, for example, 40–50% of the labelled analyte is bound by the antibody (A). When unlabelled analyte is added to the solution or extract being analysed, competition occurs between labelled and unlabelled analyte for the limiting concentration of binding sites on the antibody (B). The amount of labelled analyte remaining bound to the antibody can be measured after separation of the bound and unbound fractions of antibody. When no competing unlabelled analyte is present, the amount of labelled analyte bound will be high. When competing analyte is present, less labelled analyte will be bound to antibody. By mathematical analysis precise quantitation can be achieved of very low levels of analyte.

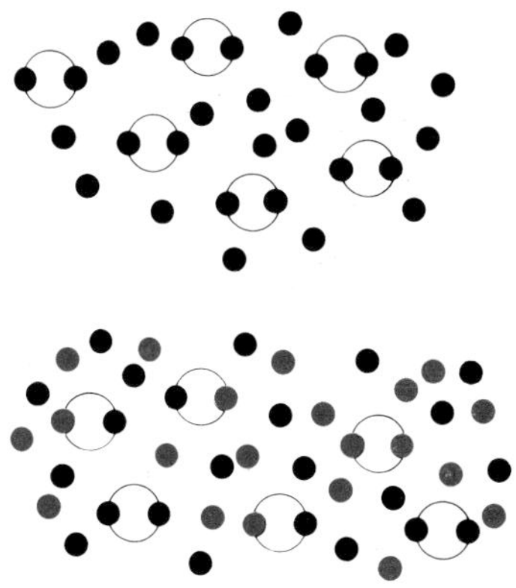

Enzyme-linked immunoassay (ELISA)

To overcome the disadvantages of using radioactivity, enzymes can be attached to the analyte and used in place of the radioactive analyte. The enzymes that are used catalyse a colour change in a chromogenic substrate, which is detected by spectrophotometry. The principle of the ELISA is shown in Fig. 5.23. Quantitative estimation of the enzyme reaction shows

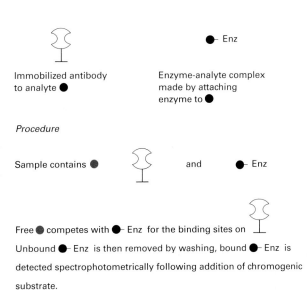

Fig. 5.22 The principles of radioimmunoassay illustrated. Black circles indicate labelled analyte, red circles unlabelled.

how much enzyme-labelled analyte was bound, this being inversely proportional to the amount of analyte in the solution being analysed. Commonly used enzyme–substrate combinations include alkaline phosphatase with *p*-nitrophenyl phosphate and horseradish peroxidase with tetramethylbenzidine.

Fig. 5.23 The principles of enzyme-linked immunosorbent assay (ELISA).

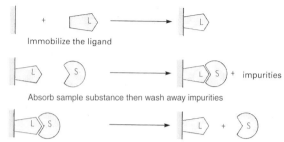

Immobilize the ligand

Absorb sample substance then wash away impurities

Desorb bound substance

Fig. 5.24 An illustration of the principle of immunoaffinity chromatography.

Enzyme:	Substrate analogue, inhibitor, cofactor
Antibody:	Antigen, virus, cell
Lectin:	Polysaccharide, glycoprotein, cell surface receptor, cell
Nucleic acid:	Complementary base sequence, histone, nucleic acid polymerase, binding protein
Hormone, vitamin:	Receptor, carrier protein
Cell:	Cell-surface-specific protein, lectin

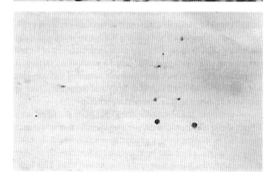

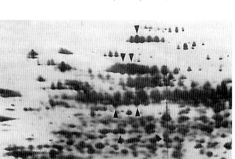

Fig. 5.25 Western blotting. At the top is the result of the separation in a two-dimensional gel of total protein from a tobacco leaf. At the bottom is the same gel blotted against antibody to proteins phosphorylated at threonine during mitosis.

Immunoaffinity chromatography

Antibodies can be used in the purification of proteins by affinity chromatography. The procedure is illustrated in Fig. 5.24. The specific ligand, in this case an antibody, is covalently attached to the column matrix, which is usually a dextran such as Sepharose. Substances that bind to the ligand, in this case antigens, are then passed down the column and are adsorbed. The antigens can be eluted by passing down the column solutions containing salts or other compounds that cause them to be desorbed. Examples of ligands that can be used are listed.

Western blotting

This is so called because of its resemblance to Southern blotting (see p. 49). It is a

method for detecting proteins that react to a specific antibody. The antibody-reactive proteins in a mixture are analysed by first resolving the proteins by two-dimensional denaturing gel electrophoresis. The gel then is placed in contact with a sheet of nitrocellulose and the proteins are transferred to the nitrocellulose by an electric current. After treatment of the nitrocellulose with antibody, the antigen–antibody reactions can be visualized either by the use of ^{125}I-labelled antibody or by the ELISA technique. An example is shown in Fig. 5.25.

Immunocytochemistry

Many techniques are now used to localize particular antigens in cytological preparations. The antibody is first conjugated with a fluorescent dye such as

fluorescein. A thin section of the tissue is then immersed in a solution of the labelled antibody and, after treatment, the bound antibody can be visualized by fluorescence microscopy. In other cases, the antibody is linked to ferritin and located by electron microscopy.

PROTEINS OF MOLECULAR MOTORS

INTRODUCTION

Coordinated movement, which is essential to life, is driven by molecular motors. Three systems can be identified in which various proteins play a critical role: (1) muscle contraction, which depends on myosin and actin; (2) the beating of cilia and flagella and the movement of chromosomes in cell division, which depend on dynein and tubulin; and (3) the movement of vesicles on microtubules, in which kinesin plays a role. In all of these systems, ATP is bound, causing conformational transitions in the proteins; these are reversed by the hydrolysis of ATP. Muscle will be considered first, followed by the non-muscle systems.

There are two main classes of muscle: striated and smooth. Striated muscle is typical of skeletal muscle, which is under voluntary nerve control and provides rapid contraction. Skeletal muscle fibres can be subdivided into two main types: slow-twitch fibres (type I Red) or fast-twitch fibres (type II White). A convenient histochemical method of determining the presence of the different fibres in a particular muscle is to visualize the presence of myosin ATPase after preincubation at pH 4.6. As shown by histochemistry in Fig. 5.26, the Red fibres appear dark in contrast to the White fibres. The Red fibres are mitochondria-rich using aerobic metabolism, and are well developed in endurance sportsmen. The White fibres lack mitochondria, are soon exhausted and rely on anaerobic metabolism; White fibres are prominent in sprinters and jumpers. In man, each striated muscle site has a mixture of the two types of fibre. Heart muscle is striated but has a different structure and is under involuntary nerve control. Smooth muscle is found in the intestine and blood vessels and is under involuntary nerve control. It is slow to act but contraction can be maintained for extended periods. In all muscle types, the reserve of ATP is low but can be boosted from a reservoir of creatine phosphate (see p. 126).

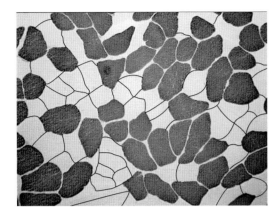

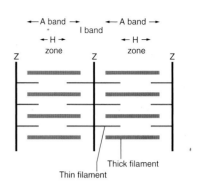

Fig. 5.29 The thick and thin filaments in muscle contraction. See the text for an explanation.

Fig. 5.26 Muscle biopsy from the human vastus lateralis muscle, processed for myosin ATPase histochemistry after preincubation at pH 4.6. The dark fibres are the slow (Type I Red) fibres and the light fibres (outlined in black) are the fast (Type IIa White) fibres.

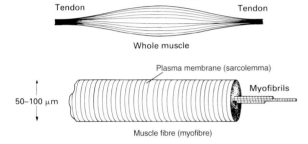

Fig. 5.27 The general architecture of striated muscle.

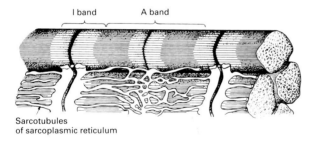

Fig. 5.28 Striated muscle under the microscope. The A and I bands are responsible for the striated appearance. The sarcoplasmic reticulum contains one major protein, a Ca^{2+}-stimulated ATPase. When the muscle is stimulated, the sarcoplasmic reticulum releases Ca^{2+}, which is needed for the contractile process. Ca^{2+} is then pumped back into the sarcoplasmic reticulum by the Ca^{2+}-stimulated ATPase.

STRIATED MUSCLE

General architecture

Striated muscle consists of fibres (myofibres), which contain myofibrils, each of which is surrounded by a membranous sac, the sarcoplasmic reticulum. These arrangements are shown in Fig. 5.27. The plasma membrane is called the sarcolemma, which is excited through its nerve endings; it encloses the cytoplasm, multiple nuclei and mitochondria. The functional unit is called a sarcomere, which repeats along the fibril axis. As seen in Fig. 5.28, a dark A band and a light I band alternate regularly. The central region of the A band, termed the H zone, is less dense than the rest of the band. The I band is bisected by a very

dense, narrow Z disc or Z line (Z for *Zwischen*, or division). On contraction of the muscle, the Z discs are pulled closer together, thus shortening the sarcomeres.

The thick and thin filaments in muscle contraction

There are two kinds of interacting protein filament in a sarcomere; their arrangement is shown in Fig. 5.29. The thick filaments, which are composed mainly of myosin, have a diameter of about 15 nm; the thin filaments, which are composed of actin, tropomyosin and troponin, have a diameter of about 9 nm. The thick and thin filaments interact by cross-bridges, which are domains of myosin molecules. Muscle shortens by as much as one-third of its

original length as it contracts. The sliding-filament model accounts for the shortening, which involves the thick and thin filaments sliding past each other. The force of contraction is generated by a process that actively moves one type of filament past neighbouring filaments of the other type.

Myosin

Myosin has three biological activities: (1) myosin molecules assemble spontaneously into filaments in physiological solutions; (2) it is an ATPase, which provides the free energy for contraction; (3) it binds to the polymerized form of actin (F-actin), the major constituent of the thin filaments. Actin and myosin form a complex called actomyosin, threads of which are capable of contraction. Actomyosin is dissociated by ATP.

Myosin is a large protein made up of six polypeptide chains: two identical heavy chains and two pairs of light chains. As seen in Fig. 5.30, the molecule consists of a double-headed globular region joined to a very long rod. The rod is a two-stranded α-helical coiled coil formed by the heavy chains. The heavy chain of each head binds two different light chains. Limited proteolysis of myosin has provided insight into its function. In Fig. 5.31, the red arrows indicate the points at which the myosin polypeptide chain can be cleaved by different agents into various components: HMM, heavy meromyosin; HMM-S_1, heavy meromyosin headpiece; LMM, light meromyosin; DTNB (dithionitrobenzene) light chain. LMM, like myosin, forms filaments but lacks ATPase activity and does not combine with actin. HMM catalyses the hydrolysis of ATP and binds to actin but does not form filaments. It can be split into two identical globular subfragments (each called S_1) and one rod-shaped subfragment

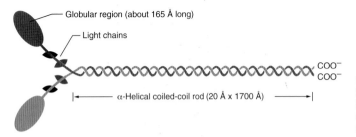

Globular region (about 165 Å long)

Light chains

α-Helical coiled-coil rod (20 Å x 1700 Å)

COO⁻
COO⁻

Fig. 5.30 Schematic illustration of a myosin molecule.

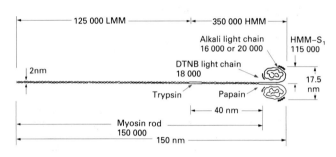

Fig. 5.31 The sites of cleavage (red arrows) of the various components of myosin by different reagents. See text for an explanation.

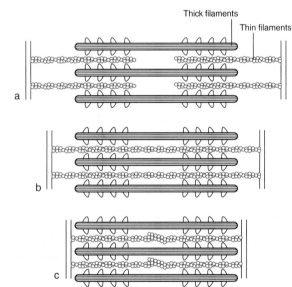

Thick filaments

Thin filaments

a

b

c

Fig. 5.32 The action of ATP and Ca²⁺ to initiate the contraction process. For explanation see text.

(called S_2). S_1 contains an ATPase site, an actin-binding site and two light-chain-binding sites. HMM-S_1 is the force-generating unit of myosin. The cyclic formation and dissociation of complexes between actin and S_1 leads to a sliding of the thin and thick filaments.

Actin

Actin is the major constituent of thin filaments (see below), the fibrous form being F-actin, which also is an ATPase. In electron micrographs, thin filaments appear rather like two strings of beads wound round each other. Each monomer in the filament makes contact with four others. As will be explained, actin is present in all eukaryotic cells.

The action of ATP and Ca²⁺

This is shown in Fig. 5.32. Under the action of ATP and Ca²⁺, the myosin headpieces interact with the actin–troponin–tropomyosin complex to initiate the contraction process. In resting muscle, when the cytosolic Ca²⁺ concentration is low, actin and myosin are held in check by tropomyosin and the troponin complex. During contraction, the thin filaments ('a' in Fig. 5.32) slide against the myosin headpiece until they meet (b) and overlap (c). Troponin is a complex of three subunits, troponin C (TNC), troponin T (TNT) and troponin I (TNI), each of which is expressed by more than one gene. The letters T, C, and I refer to the properties of the subunits. TNT binds tropomyosin (see Fig. 5.33), TNC binds calcium and TNI has an inhibitory role on the regulation of contraction by calcium ions. The complex of troponin subunits is an elongated structure with TNC and TNI forming a head and TNT forming a tail. The binding of TNT to tropomyosin positions troponin on the actin filament.

SMOOTH MUSCLE

Smooth muscle lacks striations and does not have the sarcomere structure that is characteristic of striated muscle. In response to signals that stimulate a contractile response, the myosin molecules polymerize into bipolar bundles and the actin molecules polymerize into filaments. In the absence of such signals, the polymers dissociate into single molecules. Smooth muscles have only a sparse sarcoplasmic reticulum network and depend on Ca²⁺ entering the cell from the extracellular space. Contraction is regulated by the degree of phosphorylation of its myosin light chains.

CLINICAL IMPLICATIONS – MUSCLE DISEASE

As muscle accounts for some 40% of body mass, muscle disorders have profound effects on whole body metabolism. The disorders can affect type I or type II fibres, causing wasting (atrophy) or more overt cellular damage, rhabdomyolysis. Examples of type I atrophy include inactivity, ageing and metabolic and inflammatory myopathies; examples of type II fibre atrophy include chronic alcoholism, steroid hormone excess and nutritional deficiencies. A variety of drugs and toxins damage muscle fibres leading to varying degrees of rhabdomyolysis. These include glucosteroids, statins, HIV treatments, autoimmune disorders (dermatomyositis)

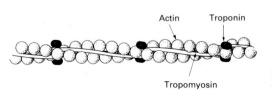

Actin   Troponin

Tropomyosin

Fig. 5.33 A model of a thin filament.

and hormone deficiencies or excess, e.g. thyroid hormone.

There is a large range of genetic-linked muscle disorders. These include defects in fat, carbohydrate or mitochondrial metabolism or in contractile or structural proteins. Examples include defects in fatty acid oxidation, muscle glycogen storage diseases, defects in the carnitine-mediated transport of fatty acids across the inner mitochondrial membrane and a variety of defects of the respiratory chain. Genetic disorders of the contractile mechanisms include muscular dystrophy and myotonic dystrophy where there are a variety of abnormalities of the dystrophin gene, the desmin myopathies, ion channel diseases including Na^+, Cl^- and Ca^{2+} channel myopathies and abnormalities of the neuromuscular junction, especially myasthenia gravis.

Muscle disease when there is cellular necrosis is accompanied by the release of creatine kinase into the circulation, which can increase 1000-fold. Other cytoplasmic enzymes, e.g. lactate dehydrogenase, aspartate aminotransferase, aldolase are also increased in the plasma. Creatine kinase is also released from damaged cardiac muscle, e.g. myocardial infarction, but skeletal and cardiac muscle have distinct isoenzymes, which can be distinguished electrophoretically and immunologically. More recently, assays of cardiac-specific tropinin have been developed as an early, sensitive and specific indication of cardiac damage. Severe muscle damage is accompanied by release of myoglobin and ions such as K^+ and PO^{3-}. The cardiac form of TNT in humans is about 31 amino acids longer than the skeletal muscle form, which makes it easy to detect. Serum levels of TNT and TNI increase within 4 hours of an acute myocardial infarction and remain high for about 7 days in many patients. Because the heart is so vital for survival, relatively minor molecular defects command attention. It is estimated that about 1 of 500 persons carries a mutation in a gene that compromises cardiac function. For example, many different point mutations in the myosin heavy chain can compromise its function. The heart attempts to compensate for the contractility defect through hypertophy, the so-called hypertrophic cardiomyopathies.

In contrast to the variety of circulating markers resulting from acute damage, there are none available for the muscle fibre atrophies or hypertrophies such as cardiomyopathy, alcoholic type II fibre atrophy or illicit anabolic steroid hypertrophy. Muscle biopsy with histochemical studies remains an important

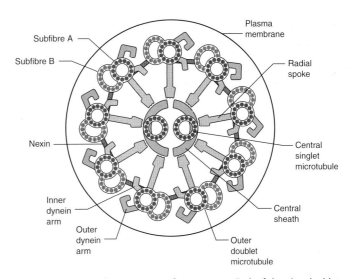

Fig. 5.34 Schematic diagram of the structure of an axoneme. Each of the nine doublets resembles a figure of eight, 37 nm × 25 nm. The smaller of the pair, subfibre A, is joined to a central sheath of the cilium by radial spokes. Microtubule doublets are also held together by nexin links. Two arms emerge from each subfibre A. All the arms in a given cilium point in the same direction.

diagnostic approach for these and other muscle disorders.

NON-MUSCLE SYSTEMS

Eukaryotic cells have an internal scaffolding called the cytoskeleton, which gives the cell its distinctive shape and enables it to transport vesicles, undergo changes in shape and migrate. There are three classes of filamentous assemblies: microfilaments, intermediate filaments and microtubules (see p. 4). Microfilaments (p. 211) are made of actin. The intermediate filaments (p. 212) contain two- or three-stranded α-helical coiled-coil cores flanked by diverse sequences; an example is the keratins of hair. Microtubules (p. 211) are hollow cylindrical structures built from two kinds of similar subunit: α and β tubulin. The rigid wall of a microtubule is made up of alternating α and β tubulin subunits.

Microtubules are major components of eukaryotic cilia and flagella, which are constructed from a bundle of fibres called an axoneme; this is surrounded by a membrane that is continuous with the plasma membrane. Figure 5.34 is a schematic diagram of the structure of an axoneme. An ATPase called dynein can be extracted, which is located in the arms of subfibre A. Dynein is a very large protein, being the mass of a ribosome; it has a similar ATPase cycle to myosin, but drives the sliding of parallel adjacent microtubules which causes bending of the axoneme.

During the separation of daughter chromosomes in mitosis, microtubules are

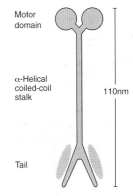

Fig. 5.35 Kinesin consists of two heads, an α-helical coiled-coil stalk and a bifurcated tail. Two 70-kDa light chains (grey) are associated with two 110-kDa heavy chains (red).

formed by the addition of α and β tubulin molecules to pre-existing filaments or nucleation centres. Most microtubules undergo rapid assembly and disassembly, a property called dynamic instability. Colchicine inhibits all processes that depend on functioning microtubules by blocking their polymerization. Taxol (palitaxel) has the opposite effect; it stabilizes tubulin in microtubules and promotes polymerization. and hence prevents cell division; Taxol is a valuable anti-cancer drug.

Vesicles and organelles are transported by kinesin, a large protein containing two large and two smaller subunits, as shown in Fig. 5.35. One end of the kinesin molecule interacts with a microtubule and the other end grabs the cargo to be transported. ATP hydrolysis by kinesin is tightly coupled to its binding to a microtubule and to the generation of force.

The structure and function of enzymes

Chemical transformations in biological systems are catalysed by enzymes. These are usually proteins but some nucleic acids (ribozymes) can catalyse chemical reactions (e.g. RNA splicing). Folding of the polypeptide chain of enzymes is important in creating the conformation or spatial organization of the active site, where compounds undergoing transformation bind forming the enzyme-substrate complex. Enzyme kinetics describe these interactions mathematically.

Factors affecting the ability of enzymes to catalyse reactions are discussed. Extremes of temperature or pH will denature proteins and inactivate enzymes. At temperatures up to about 50°C, enzyme activity increases with temperature. Enzymes show their own individual pH–activity profiles, which result from ionization effects on amino acid side chains, particularly those involved in the active site. The different mechanisms by which an inhibitor can affect an enzyme reaction are outlined. The assay of enzymes in plasma can be useful in diagnosis. Effectors that bind to sites other than the active site are referred to as allosteric and yield sigmoid kinetic plots. Allosteric behaviour usually occurs in proteins with more than one subunit. Enzymes can also be regulated by covalent modification, particularly by phosphorylation and dephosphorylation. Proteins with different structures catalysing the same reaction (isoenzymes) provide a further level of regulation.

Small molecules required for an enzyme reaction, but not consumed in the reaction, are called cofactors or coenzymes. They can be metal ions or organic chemicals and can form part of the active site or can be bound to the site just for the reaction sequence. A number of water-soluble vitamins act as precursors of these coenzymes.

THE PROPERTIES OF ENZYMES

GENERAL PROPERTIES

An enzyme accelerates the rate at which a reaction proceeds towards equilibrium. It does not change the position of equilibrium, nor does it affect the direction in which a reaction proceeds. These are determined by the laws of thermodynamics (see p. 89).

In common with other proteins, enzymes are sensitive to temperature change. Most enzymes start to denature at temperatures above 50°C, and their catalytic action diminishes (Fig. 6.1). Some enzymes are heat stable because they do not denature on heating. These are often small proteins without a great deal of tertiary structure. They are sometimes erroneously referred to as 'thermophilic enzymes', but the term thermophilic is reserved for certain bacteria that can grow at high temperatures. Enzymes are also affected by pH, first by direct effects on the structure of the enzyme protein, as in cases of extreme pH values that contribute to protein denaturation, but also because of changes in the ionization of charged amino acid residues that function in the active site (see below). Different enzymes vary in

their sensitivity to pH change, and some typical examples of different responses are shown in Fig. 6.2. The rate of the reaction is generally proportional to the amount of enzyme present and a linear relationship is often found (Fig. 6.3). Enzyme kinetics is a term embracing the study of enzyme properties by measuring the effect of different conditions on the rate constants. When we refer to the enzyme reaction rate, we imply a theoretical rate that occurs near the start of the reaction, when negligible amounts of product have been formed. This is known as the initial rate, often represented as v_i. It is only possible to measure this rate with the use of highly specialized techniques and, for many practical purposes, the rate measured over the first minute or two after adding the enzyme to a reaction mixture is nearly linear and will give an acceptable analysis. The reason that it is necessary to measure the initial rate of the reaction, rather than the rate at later points in time, is that the study of the reaction kinetics is simplified if carried out using an analysis that assumes that negligible amounts of product have been formed. Such an analysis was first proposed by Michaelis and Menten, whose names are always associated with the equation derived on p. 86.

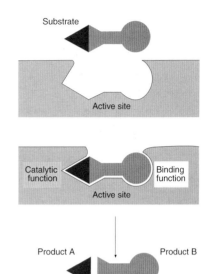

Fig. 6.4 The active site has binding and catalytic functions. Some enzymes have such a high catalytic efficiency that they must catalyse a reaction almost every time they encounter a substrate molecule, i.e. contact between substrate and enzyme is virtually always at the active site. Such an enzyme is catalase, that catalyses the conversion of two molecules of H_2O_2 to one molecule of O_2 and two of water.

THE NATURE OF THE ACTIVE SITE

The active site is a region of the enzyme in which the side-chains of some amino acid residues are tailored to binding the substrate, while others, which might also have a binding function, participate in the catalytic process; Fig. 6.4 summarizes this situation. Figure 6.5 shows in more detail how the active site can arise from the folding of the protein chains, using chymotrypsin as an example. The residues that function in the active site, which in this case include His–57 and Ser–195, can originate from widely separated positions in the polypeptide chain, and even from different peptide chains, His–57 being in chain B and Ser–195 in chain C. They are brought into juxtaposition by the way in which the chains fold. His–57 and Ser–195, together with Asp–102 (not shown in Fig. 6.5), are involved in the catalytic action of chymotrypsin. The same amino acid residues are found in a number of other proteolytic enzymes, including elastase, and participate in a mechanism known as the charge relay system, as shown in Fig. 6.6. This mechanism depends on the fact that His–57 lies sufficiently close to Ser–195 for one of its nitrogens to form a hydrogen bond with the hydroxyl of Ser–195. Asp–102 is able to form another hydrogen bond with the other ring

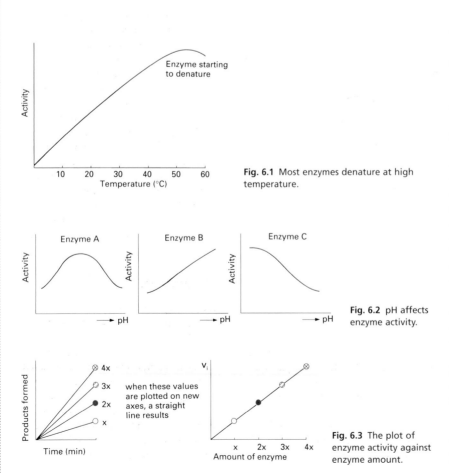

Fig. 6.1 Most enzymes denature at high temperature.

Fig. 6.2 pH affects enzyme activity.

Fig. 6.3 The plot of enzyme activity against enzyme amount.

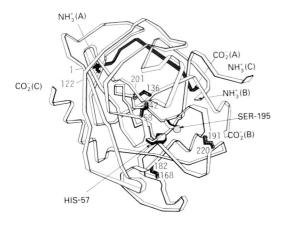

Fig. 6.5 The active site is formed by polypeptide chain folding.

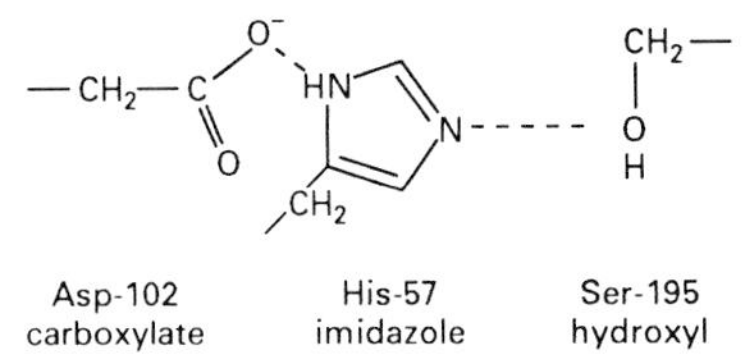

Fig. 6.6 The charge relay system.

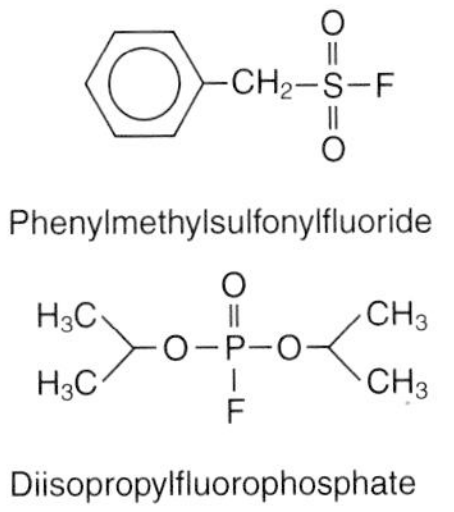

Asp-102 carboxylate

His-57 imidazole

Ser-195 hydroxyl

Fig. 6.7 The structures of diisopropylfluorophosphate and phenylmethylsulfonylfluoride.

Phenylmethylsulfonylfluoride

Diisopropylfluorophosphate

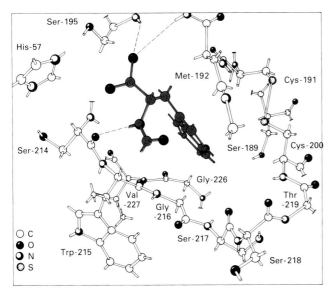

Fig. 6.8 The active site of chymotrypsin.

inhibitors. Thus the fluoride atom of diisopropylfluorophosphate (for structure, see Fig. 6.7) reacts with this hydroxyl to form a covalent bond with release of HF. Other inhibitors block His-57, one such being the much used protease inhibitor phenylmethylsulfonylfluoride (for structure, see Fig. 6.7), which attacks the histidine nitrogen and results in its sulfonation.

The serine endopeptidases comprise a large family with extensive sequence homologies. The active site of chymotrypsin is shown in greater detail in Fig. 6.8, and that of another serine endopeptidase, elastase, is shown in Fig. 6.9. Comparison of the two active sites reveals great similarity in the positioning of His-57 and Ser-195, but the binding region of elastase contains bulky side-chains of Val-216 and Thr-226 (coloured pink), which are not present in chymotrypsin, glycines being present in corresponding positions in that enzyme. Glycine is the smallest of the amino acids, having no side-chain, so the binding pocket of chymotrypsin can thus accommodate a more bulky substrate, *N*-formyl-L-tryptophan being shown, than that of elastase, shown here as binding *N*-formyl-L-alanine. The binding pocket of trypsin is very similar to that of chymotrypsin, except that residue 189 is an aspartate that promotes binding of positively charged side-chains.

Another aspect of enzyme tertiary structure that is important in function is the flexibility permitted by rotation at the α-carbons of the backbone. The enzyme conformation is affected by binding of the substrate, as shown in Fig. 6.10, where the change induced in hexokinase by binding of glucose is revealed by X-ray crystallography studies of the enzyme crystallized in the presence and absence of glucose. The red lines show that part of the backbone has a different conformation in the absence of the substrate. This phenomenon is known as induced fit.

ENZYME KINETICS

DERIVATION OF THE MICHAELIS–MENTEN EQUATION

A mathematical analysis of the kinetics of an enzyme-catalysed reaction was proposed by Michaelis and Menten. The derivation of the equation is based on a model of enzyme action in which the enzyme (E) binds to a single substrate (S) to form an enzyme–substrate complex (ES). This complex then breaks down to form

nitrogen of His-57. The term 'charge relay system' derives from the fact that a negative charge is displaced from Asp-102 towards the hydroxyl of Ser-195, making this hydroxyl highly reactive towards compounds with a centre that is electron-deficient (i.e. the hydroxyl becomes highly nucleophilic). The carbonyl carbon of the peptide bond being hydrolysed presents

such a centre, and is thus attacked by the serine hydroxyl. The activity of this serine residue gives to this class of enzyme the name serine endopeptidase, and any compound that can block this serine hydroxyl will inhibit these enzymes. Certain nerve gases, known as organophosphates because they contain a phosphate linked to carbon-containing groups, are such

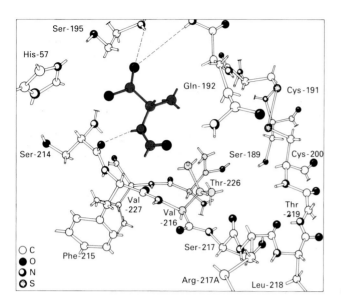

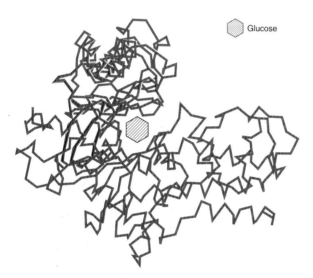

Fig. 6.9 The active site of elastase.

Glucose

Fig. 6.10 Induced fit of enzyme and substrate.

Strictly, this derivation is restricted to a single-substrate reaction. In multisubstrate reactions, if other factors are held constant and the concentration of only one substrate is varied, the initial rate plotted against the concentration of that substrate often produces a hyperbolic curve, which can also be analysed using the Michaelis–Menten equation. Indeed, a relationship of the Michaelis–Menten type is observed when many phenomena that involve binding are examined, including transport of molecules across membranes, binding of ligands (e.g. hormones) to receptors and drug-related effects.

k_2 is also referred to as k_{cat}. Thus, from the above, $v = k_{cat}[ES]$. At very high (saturating) substrate concentrations, v approximates to V_{max}, and [ES] to [E_t], so that under these conditions k_{cat} can be calculated from $V_{max} = k_{cat}[E_t]$ if the molar concentration of the enzyme is known.

GRAPHICAL TREATMENT OF THE MICHAELIS–MENTEN EQUATION

If the time course is plotted – i.e. the amount of product formed is plotted against time – the rate will slow as more products are formed (Fig. 6.11). This is because the products can combine with enzyme to reform the ES complex, leading to a reverse reaction. Note that equation 1 does not show this reaction because this would complicate the analysis (see above).

If, in a series of experiments, the substrate concentration is progressively increased but the same amount of enzyme and other reaction conditions are used, the initial rate found in each experiment can be plotted against the substrate concentration. A curve is obtained (similar in appearance to the time course but very different in meaning) that approaches a plateau at higher substrate concentrations. This curve, and the way it is derived, is illustrated in Fig. 6.12, where a series of initial rates is shown on the left and the plot of the 2-min points on the right. The

products (P) with the liberation of free enzyme (E).

$$E + S \underset{k_{-1}}{\overset{k_1}{\rightleftharpoons}} ES \overset{k_2}{\rightarrow} E + P \quad (1)$$

k_1, k_{-1} and k_2 are rate constants for the various reactions as indicated above.

It is assumed that the reaction is in the steady-state, in which the concentration of ES remains constant, and the analysis applies only to a period near the start of the reaction, at which point negligible amounts of products have been formed, so that the reverse reaction, $E + P \rightarrow ES$, can be ignored. Then:

$$\frac{d[ES]}{dt} = k_1([E_t] - [ES])[S] - k_{-1}[ES] - k_2[ES]$$

$$= 0 \text{ ([E}_t\text{] is the total amount of enzyme)}$$

$$k_1[E_t][S] - k_1[ES][S] - k_{-1}[ES] - k_2[ES] = 0$$
$$k_1[E_t][S] = [ES](k_1[S] + k_{-1} + k_2)$$

$$\frac{k_1[E_t][S]}{k_1[S] + k_{-1} + k_2} = [ES]$$

Divide LHS by k_1:

$$[ES] = \frac{[E_t][S]}{[S] + \frac{(k_{-1} + k_2)}{k_1}}$$

The initial rate (v) of formation of product $= k_2[ES]$ and when the enzyme is saturated with substrate, maximum rate (V_{max}) $= k_2[E_t]$ and the Michaelis constant

$$K_m = \frac{k_{-1} + k_2}{k_1}$$

So $v = k_2[ES] = \dfrac{k_2[E_t][S]}{[S] + K_m}$

$$= \frac{V_{max}[S]}{[S] + K_m} \quad (2)$$

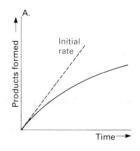

Fig. 6.11 Initial rate of reaction must be approximated.

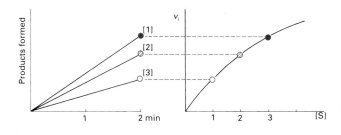

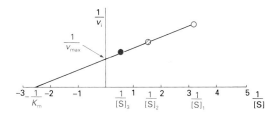

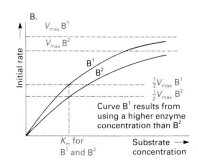

Fig. 6.12 The plot of activity against substrate concentration.

Fig. 6.13 As enzyme amount increases, V_{max} increases but K_m remains constant.

Fig. 6.14 The Lineweaver–Burk plot.

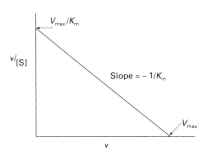

Fig. 6.15 The Eadie–Hofstee plot.

plateau level, which is obtained only at a theoretical (infinite) concentration, represents the maximal rate, or V_{max}, of the Michaelis–Menten equation, indicated as V_{max} B^2 on curve B^2 in Fig. 6.13. The Michaelis constant (K_m) corresponds to the substrate concentration at which the initial rate is half the maximal rate. If a different series of similar experiments is performed using a greater enzyme concentration, a similar curve with greater initial rates and a greater maximal rate will be derived. However, the K_m will remain the same (curve B^1 in Fig. 6.13). Curves such as this are inadequate for determining V_{max} and K_m. A graphical treatment for this purpose depends on a transformation of equation 2 to the form:

$$1/v = 1/V_{max} + (K_m/V_{max})(1/[S])$$

This is the equation of a straight line in which $1/v$ and $1/[S]$ are variables, the intercept on the ordinate represents $1/V_{max}$ and the intercept on the abscissa represents $-1/K_m$. This plot is known as the Lineweaver–Burk plot (Fig. 6.14). An alternative method utilizes a plot of $v/[S]$ against v, with intercepts as shown in Fig. 6.15. This is known as the Eadie–Hofstee plot.

ENZYME INHIBITION

Enzyme activity is inhibited by compounds that can compete with the substrate in binding to the active site, or alternatively compounds that can modify the active site by, for example, reacting covalently with one of the amino acid residues that contribute to activity. In the presence of such an inhibitor, the initial velocity is reduced, so $1/v$ is increased. This will influence the Lineweaver–Burk plot in a variety of ways, depending on the nature of the inhibition. In competitive inhibition, when both substrate and inhibitor can bind with the active site and compete for its occupation, the lines obtained in the presence of inhibitor intersect on the ordinate; hence V_{max} is unaltered (Fig. 6.16). This is interpretable in the sense that at infinite concentration of substrate the inhibitor will be effectively excluded from the active site. However, K_m is increased, because a higher concentration of substrate is needed to achieve half the maximal rate. In non-competitive inhibition, the effect of the inhibitor is the same as would be obtained by completely blocking a percentage of the active sites, giving a result similar to that found if the amount of enzyme is reduced (Fig. 6.17). V_{max} is reduced and K_m is unaffected. A third type of inhibition is known as uncompetitive inhibition. This occurs in certain cases in which the inhibitor can only bind after the substrate has been bound (i.e. it binds to the ES complex) and then inhibits formation of products (Fig. 6.18). In many cases, however, plots that do not precisely fit any of these types of inhibition are obtained, indicating more complex situations. Some more complex aspects of inhibition are related to the regulation of allosteric enzymes; this is discussed later (p. 94).

CLINICAL IMPLICATIONS – THE USE OF ENZYME ASSAY IN DIAGNOSIS

Principles of measurement

The assay of enzymes in the plasma is used as an important aid to diagnosis. The rate of enzyme activity depends on the composition of the solution in which the

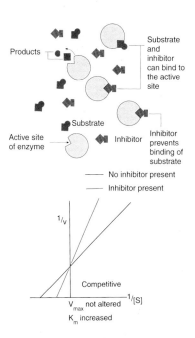

Fig. 6.16 Competitive inhibition.

reaction is conducted. Choice of buffer is important, as some salts from which buffers are prepared might be inhibitory to the enzyme. The Henderson–Hasselbalch equation, which relates the pH of a buffer solution to the pK of the weak acid from which it is prepared, is useful and is derived in Box 6.1. In the assay of a serum enzyme, inhibitors or activators may be present in the serum and affect the rate of reaction.

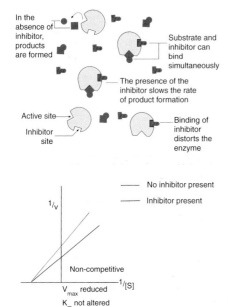

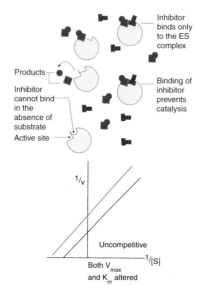

Fig. 6.17 Non-competitive inhibition.

Fig. 6.18 Uncompetitive inhibition.

BOX 6.1

DERIVATION OF THE HENDERSON-HASSELBALCH EQUATION

In general, for an equilibrium [AB] $\rightleftarrows$ [A] + [B]

$$\frac{[AB]}{[A][B]} = K_{association} \quad \text{and} \quad \frac{[A][B]}{[AB]} = K_{dissociation}$$

For pH equilibria, HA is a conjugate acid and A⁻ a conjugate base:

$$\frac{[H^+][A^-]}{[HA]} = K_a \quad (1a)$$

(K_a is the acid dissociation constant)
Taking logs:

$$\log[H^+] + \log[A^-] - \log[HA] = \log K_a \quad (2a)$$

pH is defined as $-\log[H^+]$, pK_a as $-\log K_a$

Thus, multiplying equation (2a) by −1 and rearranging:

$$pH = pK_a + \log \frac{[A^-]}{[HA]} \quad (3a)$$

This is the Henderson–Hasselbalch equation.

The unit used in the comparison of enzyme activities is the katal (abbreviation: kat). This is defined as the catalytic activity that will raise the rate of conversion of a specified substrate by one mole per second in a specified assay system. The katal replaces the former 'enzyme unit' (abbreviation: U). 1 kat $= 6 \times 10^7$ U.

Because enzyme assay using kinetic methods measures enzyme activity rather than the actual amount of the enzyme, the level of serum enzymes is sometimes measured by radioimmunoassay (see p. 77). In practice, the vast majority of clinical enzyme assays are based on catalytic activity because of ease of automation and low cost. Mass measurements have, however, become established in certain situations, notably:

- Isoenzyme measurements, where the differences in protein structure can be exploited by use of specific antisera (e.g. for CK-MB and LDH 1).
- Where the enzyme has naturally occurring inhibitors of activity (e.g. trypsin in serum).

Diagnostic enzymes

In diagnosis it is often useful to measure serum enzymes released as a result of tissue breakdown. In cases of acute viral hepatitis (illustrated in Fig. 6.19), there is a rapid rise in the level of serum aminotransferase (transaminase) activity; this occurs considerably earlier than the rise in the serum bilirubin level that occurs with jaundice.

In myocardial infarction, aspartate aminotransferase (AST) and creatine kinase (CK) levels rise about 6 h after the acute episode, whereas 2-hydroxybutyrate dehydrogenase (HBDH) and lactate dehydrogenase (LDH) levels rise much later. It should be noted that 2-hydroxybutyrate is not a normal metabolite, but is used as a preferred substrate for the heart LDH isoenzyme, which is thus referred to as HBDH. Because of this selectivity, this assay is a better late marker for myocardial infarction than an assay using lactate. Three isoenzymes of CK have been identified, with subunits denoted M (for muscle) or B (for brain). CK-MM is the predominant form in skeletal muscle, which also contains about 3% CK-MB; CK-BB is found in cerebral tissue. In heart muscle, more than 40% of the total CK activity is found as CK-MB; thus the level of this isoenzyme in plasma is often measured in cases of myocardial infarction as a more precise indicator of heart muscle damage. The time courses of changes in the levels of various serum enzymes after myocardial infarction are shown in Fig. 6.20.

There are other enzymes of diagnostic interest and these are all grouped in Table 6.1. The measurement of specific

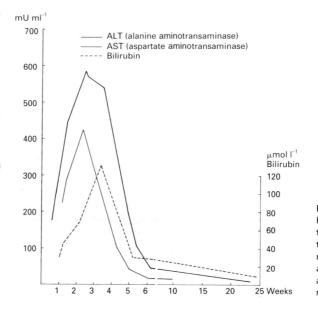

Fig. 6.19 Course of viral hepatitis. Alanine transaminase and aspartate transaminase are alternative names for alanine aminotransferase and aspartate aminotransferase, respectively.

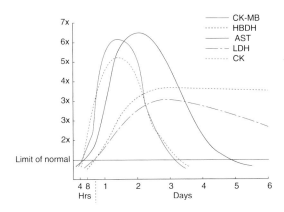

Fig. 6.20 Serum enzymes following cardiac infarction.

Table 6.1 Plasma markers and enzymes in diagnosis

Organ	Marker in serum (or urine where specified)
Brain	S100 protein (possible)
Heart	Creatine kinase (MB isoform), aspartate aminotransferase, lactate dehydrogenase, troponins
Kidney	Nitrogenous waste products in serum (creatinine, urea)
	Urinary enzymes, e.g. alkaline phosphatase, N-acetyl β-glucosaminidase, lysozyme
	Urinary protein – albumin is the protein measured. Small quantities are referred to as microalbuminuria, larger quantities (> 250 mg/day) as macroalbuminuria
Liver	Cellular alanine aminotransferase and aspartate aminotransferase, membranous alkaline phosphatase, γ-glutamyltransferase
	Classic liver function tests, e.g. bilirubin, decreased albumin and clotting factors
Pancreas	Amylase (P isoform), lipase
Skeletal muscle	Creatine kinase (MM form), aspartate aminotransferase, myoglobin, aldolase

proteins is also useful in diagnosis as was explained on p. 69 (Table 5.2).

γ-Glutamyltransferase catalyses the reaction:

Amino acid + glutathione = γ-glutamyl-amino acid + cysteinylglycine

This enzyme is involved in amino acid transport across membranes or in the salvage of glutathione. It is elevated in the blood of many alcohol drinkers, usually as a result of a combination of liver damage and enzyme induction. However, enzyme induction alone accounts for elevation in some patients with no other evidence of liver damage. Induction also accounts for its elevation in epileptics taking barbiturates. This is because consumption of alcohol or barbiturates causes considerable proliferation of the endoplasmic reticulum, inducing high levels of the enzyme.

The enzyme N-acetylglucosaminidase is found in increased amounts in the urine in cases of renal transplant rejection.

Markers for bone disease

The following enzymes, other proteins and small molecules can be measured in serum or urine to indicate the rate of bone formation or loss:

- Markers of bone formation (osteoblast activity): elevation in serum of osteocalcin, the bone isoform of alkaline phosphatase, procollagen type 1 C and N-terminal propeptides, and proline iminopeptidase can be used as indicators of bone formation.
- Markers of bone resorption (osteoclast activity): elevation in serum of tartrate-resistant acid phosphatase, N- and C-terminal type 1 collagen cross-link telopeptides (see p. 72), or the presence in urine of deoxypyridinoline,

pyridinoline, hydroxyproline and hydroxylysine can be used as indicators of increased bone resorption. (Deoxypyridinoline and pyridinoline are breakdown products of the crosslinks formed by lysine side chains of collagen.)

METABOLIC REGULATION AND CONTROL

FREE ENERGY AND CHEMICAL REACTIONS

All chemical reactions, including those catalysed by enzymes, are subject to the laws of thermodynamics. One of these laws defines a property known as free energy, which is associated with every chemical compound. This is sometimes referred to as the Gibbs free energy (after the American physical chemist Willard Gibbs) and is denoted by the symbol G. For a molecule in solution, free energy is concentration-dependent. The free energy of a particular component of a solution is equal to the free energy per mole times the number of moles of that component. The standard free energy, denoted by G^0, is equal to the free energy of the component at unit activity (in dilute solution this is approximately 1 mol l^{-1}). Thus, for the ith component of a solution:

$$G_i = G_i^0 + RT \ln a_i \qquad (3)$$

where R is the gas constant (8.134 J mol^{-1} K^{-1}), T the absolute temperature, and a_i the activity of the ith component (in dilute solution, activity approximates to concentration).

For a chemical reaction there is a quantity, ΔG, known as the free energy change of the reaction. This is the difference, *at any particular instant in time*, between the total of the free energies of the reactants and those of the products. ΔG is calculated as the free energies of the products minus those of the reactants, and will be negative if the sum of the free energies of the reactants exceeds the sum of those of the products. In other words, for a reaction:

$$A + B \rightarrow C + D$$

then, at any instant in time:

$$\Delta G = G_C + G_D - G_A - G_B$$

Using equation 3, and observing that $G_C^0 + G_D^0 - G_A^0 - G_B^0$ is termed the standard free energy change (ΔG^0) of the reaction, then:

$$\Delta G = \Delta G^0 + RT \ln \frac{[C]_C[D]_D}{[A]_A[B]_B} \quad (4)$$

where $[A]_A$, $[B]_B$, $[C]_C$ and $[D]_D$ are the concentrations pertaining at the moment for which ΔG is calculated.

All reactions proceed in a direction that tends to bring the free energies of the components on one side of the reaction equation to a value equal to those on the other. When the free energies on both sides are equal, equilibrium has been reached and the free energy change, ΔG, is now zero. If a reaction is written in such a way that ΔG is positive, ΔG for the reaction in the reverse direction will be negative, and the reaction will thus proceed in the reverse direction until equilibrium is reached.

As stated above, the standard free energy change, ΔG^0, is the free energy change when all components of a reaction are at unit activity (for practical purposes 1 mol l^{-1}). This is an important quantity that is used to compare free energy change between different reactions. It is a constant, at constant temperature. The fact that at equilibrium $\Delta G = 0$ offers a method for calculating ΔG^0. From equation 4 above, at equilibrium:

$$0 = \Delta G^0 + RT \ln \frac{[C]_E[D]_E}{[A]_E[B]_E}$$

or

$$\Delta G^0 = -RT \ln K_{eq}$$

where $[A]_E$, $[B]_E$, $[C]_E$ and $[D]_E$ are the equilibrium concentrations of A, B, C and D. Note that $\Delta G^{0'}$ is used to denote that one component, H$^+$, is not at unit activity when measurements are made at pH 7.0.

The fact that we can calculate standard free energy change in this way opens up the possibility of comparing biochemical reactions using these values, and allows us to study the influence that this will have on metabolic pathways. First, for a complex reaction, the free energy change is the sum of the free energy changes of the individual reactions (also called the partial reactions) that it comprises. Of special interest are certain reactions involved in the utilization and formation of ATP. The standard free energy change for the hydrolysis of ATP to ADP and P is negative, and is large compared with that for a phosphate ester such as glycerol -3-phosphate:

$$ATP^{4-} + H_2O \rightarrow ADP^{3-} + P + H^+$$

$$\Delta G^{0'} = -30.5 \text{ kJ mol}^{-1}$$

Glycerol-3-phosphate + $H_2O \rightarrow$ glycerol + P

$$\Delta G^{0'} = -9.2 \text{ kJ mol}^{-1}$$

In the past, the expression 'high energy compound' has been used in relation to ATP and other compounds that exhibit a similar large negative free energy change on hydrolysis. However, it is an expression that is useful only as a form of shorthand, and is an unnecessary and potentially misleading term that can be avoided by using the more correct terminology of free energy change.

Because of the large negative free energy change associated with the hydrolysis of ATP, complex reactions in which this is a partial reaction will often proceed in the direction that results in ATP conversion to ADP and P. However, in order that ATP concentrations can be maintained at a sufficiently high level, ADP must be phosphorylated to ATP. This can be achieved if the reaction is coupled to another reaction that exhibits a negative free energy change large enough to drive the phosphorylation, such as that occurring when NADH is oxidized by the respiratory chain, which can be coupled to oxidative phosphorylation (p. 139):

$$NADH + H^+ + O_2 \rightarrow NAD^+ + H_2O$$

$$\Delta G^{0'} = -222 \text{ kJ mol}^{-1}$$

ATP is also formed during glycolysis, a process known as substrate-level phosphorylation; for example:

Phosphoenolpyruvate + ADP $\rightarrow$ pyruvate + ATP

Thermodynamic laws therefore exercise a profound effect on metabolic pathways, and can never be contravened. They are often involved in a specific way: for example, when the ratio ATP to ADP, or NADH (NADPH) to NAD$^+$ (NADP$^+$) is altered. However, in addition to these, there are a number of other ways in which the activity of different pathways can be regulated. These are described in the sections below.

THE NEED FOR REGULATION

This section concerns primarily the biochemistry of higher animals. However, many of the mechanisms that will be described also apply, sometimes in modified form, to less complex assemblies of cells, or single cells. Metabolic events must meet the requirements for an organism to survive. These encompass sexual and reproductive activity, growth and development, mobility, the acquisition of energy-yielding foodstuffs and, in many animals, the need to store energy-yielding

materials in a form that can be readily metabolized in periods of fasting. In higher eukaryotes, metabolic activity is often controlled by the release of hormones and other messenger molecules, triggered by changes in the level of substances in the blood or by signals from the nervous system. In other cases, cellular activity might be controlled directly by changes in the cell environment. In addition, the processes involved in cell growth and development take place, not only during the embryonic and early postnatal periods but even in the adult animal, as the maintenance of tissue health involves a constant cycle of cell death and regeneration.

Major influences on the metabolism of a cell can originate either from the activation or repression of genes, or from processes at the plasma membrane that: (1) sense, through appropriate receptors, signals from the cell exterior originating from hormones and other messengers, or contact with other cells; or (2) take up, through specific transporter proteins, molecules in the environment that are of use to the cell. These activities at the plasma membrane in turn often result in gene activation or repression.

The different mechanisms that change enzymic activity in response to such stimuli include:

- changes in the rate of protein synthesis resulting from gene activation or repression
- changes in the rate of protein degradation
- phosphorylation or dephosphorylation of proteins
- activation of second messenger systems.

REGULATION BY GENES

Gene activation is often induced by signals from the cell exterior acting on receptors. This could result from contact with neighbouring cells, signalled through adhesion molecules (see p. 214); interaction of hormones, growth factors and other messengers with their receptors; or the uptake of nutrients through plasma membrane transporters. The principles of gene regulation are outlined in Chapter 3, and specific examples appear in other chapters, especially in relation to PEP carboxykinase (p. 181) and genes involved in lipoprotein metabolism (p. 182).

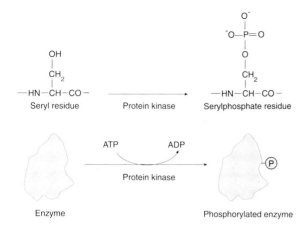

Fig. 6.21 Action of protein serine/threonine kinases.

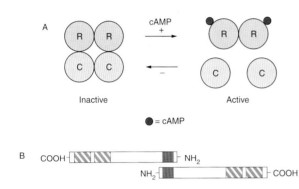

● = cAMP

Fig. 6.22 Protein kinase A dissociates in the formation of active enzyme. R indicates the regulatory subunit, C the catalytic subunit.

ENZYME PHOSPHORYLATION AND DEPHOSPHORYLATION

PROTEIN SERINE/THREONINE KINASES

Serine/threonine kinases catalyse the phosphorylation of protein serine or threonine residues (see Fig. 6.21). They are often known simply as S/T kinases. These kinases are associated most frequently with the regulation of intermediary metabolism. They are very often activated by second messengers (see p. 93) produced as a result of hormone action but they can also be activated during growth stimulation and a variety of other events. A number of serine/threonine kinases have wide specificity and are of major importance. Two of the most prominent are protein kinase A (indicating cyclic-AMP-stimulated) and protein kinase C (Ca²⁺-stimulated). The intervening letter has recently been allocated to another protein kinase, protein kinase B.

Protein kinase A (PKA) is activated by cyclic AMP (see Fig. 6.22). It is a protein kinase with broad specificity that mediates many of the actions of cyclic AMP, by phosphorylating serine or threonine residues on a number of other serine/threonine kinases (e.g. glycogen phosphorylase kinase; see p. 147). In the substrate protein, there is a characteristic sequence of amino acids that acts as a target motif for the active site of PKA. The consensus sequence is (R or K)–(R or K)–X–(S or T); for example, –RKXS–, where X is any amino acid. Before activation, PKA exists as a complex of catalytic and regulatory subunits. As shown in Fig. 6.22A, cyclic AMP binds to the regulatory subunits and thereby causes the regulatory and catalytic subunits to dissociate, and this activates the protein kinase. The regulatory subunit domain structure includes two cyclic AMP binding sites, shown in Fig. 6.22B as red hatched boxes, and a dimerization domain that binds two regulatory subunits together, thus creating a tetrameric inactive complex in the absence of cyclic AMP.

Protein kinase B (PKB) is a protein kinase that was originally discovered as the *akt* oncogene; this kinase is discussed in a later section (Chapter 16).

Protein kinase C (PKC) is activated by diacylglycerol and phospholipids and, in the case of some isoenzymes, also by Ca²⁺. Activation results from triggering of the phosphoinositide/Ca²⁺ second messenger system (see Chapter 15). PKC is a serine/threonine kinase that has a number of target protein substrates. Its activation is often associated with growth regulation, and it is activated by tumour promoters of the phorbol ester type that mimic diacylglycerol. Domains identified in PKC include the active site kinase domain, shown in black in Fig. 6.23, and two diacylglycerol/phospholipid binding sites, shown in red. Another domain, shown in pink, is thought to be a Ca²⁺-binding domain for the reasons given below. Identification of the function of these domains has been aided by the observation that limited proteolysis splits the protein into two peptides, one of which remains catalytic, the other binding diacylglycerol in a phospholipid-dependent manner. After this treatment, the liberated catalytic domain has constitutive activity; that is, it is active in the absence of the activator molecules diacylglycerol and Ca²⁺. This indicates that in the intact molecule the regulatory domain has an inhibitory function unless activator molecules are present, and that diacylglycerol and Ca²⁺ act to suppress this inhibition, possibly through conformational changes, as indicated in Fig. 6.23. The family of PKC enzymes has been found to embrace a number of isoenzymes, including those classified α–ζ. The domain structure of these is shown in Fig. 6.24. Domains C₁,

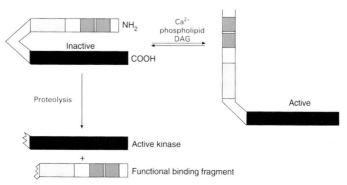

Fig. 6.23 The domains of protein kinase C.

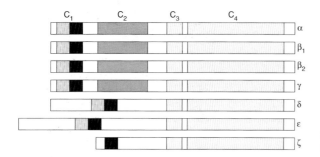

Fig. 6.24 The isoenzymes of protein kinase C.

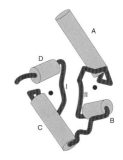

Fig. 6.26 The EF hand.

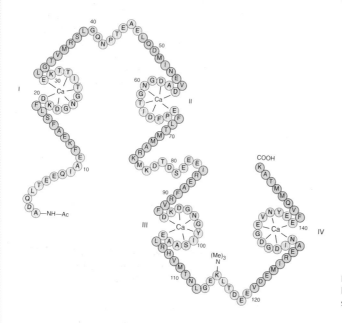

Fig. 6.25 Calmodulin has four Ca^{2+}-binding sites.

C_3 and C_4 are conserved in all subtypes. Domains $C_3 + C_4$ represent the catalytic C-terminal region. PKCs δ, ε and ζ do not have a C_2 domain, and as PKC ε (and also probably δ and ζ) is Ca^{2+}-independent, it might be that the C_2 domain confers Ca^{2+} dependence. The grey and black segments represent cysteine-rich domains, at least one of which is present in all PKCs. These overlap the diacylglycerol/phospholipid binding sites as shown in Fig. 6.23.

Ca^{2+}, CALMODULIN AND Ca^{2+}/CALMODULIN-DEPENDENT KINASE

Variation in the intracellular Ca^{2+} concentration is a major regulatory system in the control of cell function. Ca^{2+} can function as an independent molecule, but it also functions by binding to the protein calmodulin, the structure of which is shown in Fig. 6.25. This is a small, heat-stable protein, M_r 16 790, found in many eukaryotic cells. Its primary structure has been preserved almost perfectly throughout

evolution. As shown in Fig. 6.25, each calmodulin molecule binds four Ca^{2+}.

There is a structural relationship between calmodulin and other Ca^{2+}-binding proteins such as troponin C, which is a protein involved in muscle contraction (see p. 79), and parvalbumin, another muscle protein. This relationship extends to an arrangement of parts of the sequence, shown in red in Fig. 6.25, into a series of helices that form a structure known as an EF hand. This name derives from the fact that, in parvalbumin, the protein for which it was first proposed, two of the participating helices are known as E and F. The EF hand consists of a helix-loop-helix (HLH) domain, which forms a structure that can be likened to a human hand, in which the forefinger (represented by helix E) points forward, the second finger (represented by the loop) is curled back into the hand, with the thumb (represented by helix F) projecting out at a right-angle from it. An EF hand is illustrated in Fig. 6.26, where helix A represents the forefinger of an EF hand and helix B the

thumb, the Ca^{2+} being shown as a small red solid circle. Helices C and D form part of another EF hand. The loop, shown in grey in Fig. 6.25, holds a Ca^{2+}. This loop contains 6–8 oxygen atoms of Asp and Glu side-chains, which, together with the backbone carbonyls, bind the Ca^{2+} selectively even in the presence of 10^3-fold higher concentrations of Mg^{2+}. This HLH domain often occurs in pairs, calmodulin having two such pairs. When calmodulin binds Ca^{2+}, it acts as an activator of a number of serine/threonine protein kinases. These include myosin light chain kinase, glycogen-phosphorylase kinase and a group of protein kinases known collectively as Ca^{2+}-calmodulin (CAM) kinases.

PROTEIN TYROSINE KINASES

Tyrosine kinases catalyse phosphorylation of specific tyrosine residues in target proteins (Fig. 6.27). These kinases are associated with growth regulation, and many growth factor receptors possess this activity. Tyrosine kinases are of two major types. The first type consists of those that form part of the cytoplasmic domain of cell surface receptors and are thus integral membrane proteins (see Chapter 15). These include the growth factor receptors, which have kinase activity on their cytoplasmic domain. The second type is intracellular proteins. These mostly function downstream (i.e. at a subsequent stage of the activation process) of the plasma membrane receptors. The tyrosine kinases are described more fully later (see Chapter 15).

PROTEIN PHOSPHATASES

Any mechanism for regulation requires that the system be capable not only of being switched on, but also of being switched off. Thus protein kinase action must be balanced by the action of phosphatases,

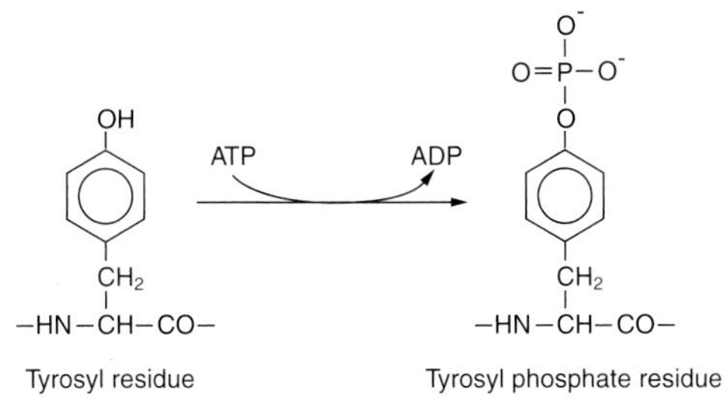

Fig. 6.27 The action of protein tyrosine kinases.

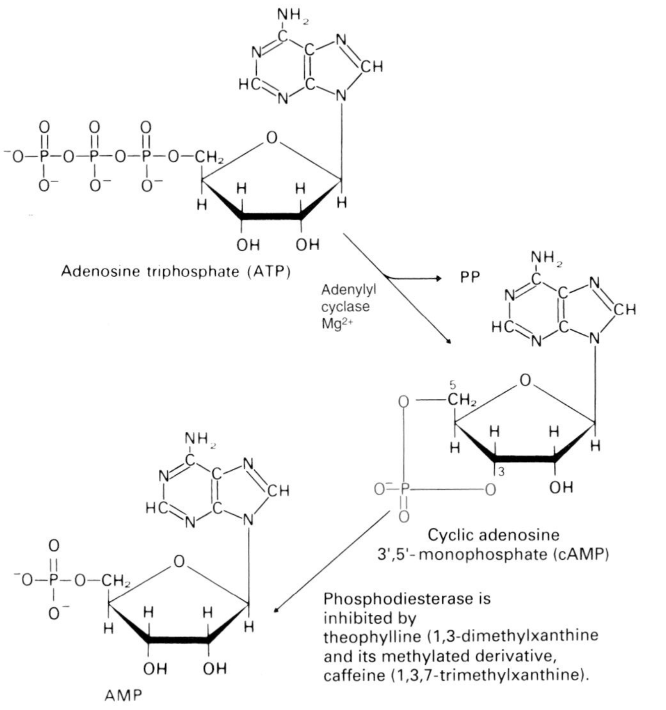

Adenosine triphosphate (ATP)

Adenylyl cyclase Mg^{2+}

PP

Cyclic adenosine 3',5'- monophosphate (cAMP)

AMP

Phosphodiesterase is inhibited by theophylline (1,3-dimethylxanthine) and its methylated derivative, caffeine (1,3,7-trimethylxanthine).

Fig. 6.28 The action of adenylyl cyclase and phosphodiesterase.

Table 6.2 Classification of Class I protein phosphatases

PP1	Dependent on ATP and Mg^{2+}, and acts mainly on phosphoproteins involved in glycogen metabolism, and in muscle contractility
PP2A	Stimulated by polycationic compounds such as histones or polylysine, and acts on phosphoproteins of glycolysis, gluconeogenesis, amino acid catabolism and fatty acid synthesis
PP2B	A calmodulin-binding Ca^{2+}-dependent enzyme and acts on protein kinases and proteins that have been phosphorylated by protein kinase A
PP2C	A Mg^{2+}-dependent enzyme, which acts on cyclic AMP-dependent protein kinase

Cyclic GMP is similarly synthesized by guanylyl cyclase from GTP, and functions as a second messenger in a number of systems, though not as widely as cyclic AMP.

CLINICAL IMPLICATIONS OF CYCLIC NUCLEOTIDES AND PROTEIN PHOSPHORYLATION

Diarrhea remains the number one killer of children less than 5 years of age throughout the world, often as a result of cholera (there have been six pandemics of cholera in recent memory). It is known that the *Vibrio cholerae* exotoxin induces intestinal secretion of Cl$^-$ ions; electrical neutrality is then maintained by secretion of Na$^+$ ions, and the accumulated salts lead to withdrawal of water from the circulation resulting in an iso-osmotic fluid diarrhea. This action of the toxin arises from persistent activation of adenylyl cyclase (see p. 206). Exotoxins of other bacteria, such as *E. coli*, activate guanylate cyclase and the resultant elevated cyclic GMP levels also induce secretion. The more severe consequences of the disease can be readily prevented by the oral administration of glucose and NaCl, as glucose uptake involves the simultaneous uptake of Na$^+$ (see Fig. 15.48).

Inhibition of phosphodiesterase by theophylline is considered to account for the bronchodilator action of the drug.

Sildenafil citrate (Viagra) selectively inhibits phosphodiesterase type V, which acts on cyclic guanosine monophosphate (cGMP). cGMP is the mediator of signalling by nitric oxide (see p. 208),

which remove the phosphate groups by a simple hydrolytic mechanism. Protein phosphatases have been grouped into classes according to their mechanism of action (Table 6.2). Class I protein phosphatases consist mainly of enzymes specific for serine/threonine phosphates. Within this class, there are phosphatases 1 and 2 (PP1 and PP2), characterized as described in Table 6.2.

Class II protein phosphatases comprise various enzymes that hydrolyse protein tyrosine phosphates. Enzymes having protein tyrosine phosphatase (PTPase) activity may be transmembrane or intracellular proteins.

SECOND MESSENGERS

CYCLIC AMP AND CYCLIC GMP

Cyclic AMP was the first compound to be discovered and described as a second messenger, molecules such as hormones being regarded as first messengers. The role and structure of cyclic AMP were discovered in the search for a heat-stable activator of the glycogen phosphorylase system. The membrane-bound enzyme, adenylyl cyclase, catalyses the formation of cyclic AMP from ATP, as shown in Fig. 6.28, and the enzyme phosphodiesterase hydrolyses the bond between the phosphate and the 3'-hydroxyl of the ribose. Between them, therefore, adenylyl cyclase and phosphodiesterase regulate the concentration of cyclic AMP. The actions of adenylyl cyclase are described more fully in Chapter 15. In addition to its effects on intermediary metabolism, cyclic AMP has a profound effect in many cellular events, including growth stimulation, cell differentiation and development. It mediates the action of many hormones on genes, acting through the cyclic AMP response element, CRE. The associated transcription factor is CREB (see p. 180).

93

which is an important vasodilator. The clinical effect of Viagra, which increases cGMP concentrations, thus results from the consequent relaxation of the smooth muscle in the corpus cavernosum.

Protein kinases and protein phosphatases are potential targets for drugs. One of the first of these is Glivec, a tyrosine kinase inhibitor (see Chapter 16).

Ca²⁺ AND PHOSPHOINOSITIDES

Another second messenger system of importance depends on enzymes that cleave phosphoinositides, leading to release of Ca^{2+} as well as yielding products that function in their own right. This system is described in Chapter 15.

ALLOSTERIC PROPERTIES OF ENZYMES

STRUCTURAL ASPECTS

The rate of an enzyme reaction can be affected by the presence of a compound that combines with the enzyme at a site other than the active site. Such a compound is known as an allosteric modulator, allosteric modifier or allosteric effector, and its binding site is known as an allosteric site. Such enzymes characteristically yield sigmoid plots when rate is plotted against substrate concentration (Fig. 6.29), indicating that there is cooperativity in the binding of substrate molecules, similar to that found in the binding of oxygen to hemoglobin. If the ligands bringing about the allosteric behaviour are the same (e.g. as for hemoglobin), the effect is known as homotropic. If they differ from each other, it is heterotropic.

The behaviour of an allosteric molecule can be analysed by a model, named the Monod–Wyman–Changeux model after its originators; this is summarized in Fig. 6.30. The model envisages the binding of substrate to one of two different states: the T (tense) state and the R (relaxed) state (compare hemoglobin; see p. 63). The R state predominates when an allosteric modifier is bound, otherwise the T state is the predominant form. Cooperativity is exhibited only by the T state. If a molecule is entirely in the R state as a result of binding an allosteric activator, non-sigmoid (i.e. Michaelis–Menten) kinetics result. Intermediate states can be thought of as involving hybrid forms, in which some subunits with substrate bound might be in the R state, whereas other subunits are in the T state. Other models that include

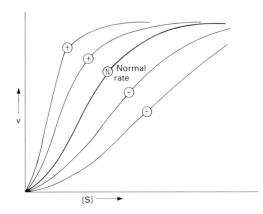

Fig. 6.29 Allosteric enzymes exhibit sigmoid kinetics. Modulators can influence the substrate-velocity curve positively (+) or negatively (-); in each case two different concentrations of modulator are shown, the effect increasing with increase in modulator concentration.

many more of the possible combinations have been described, but lead to more complex analyses.

ANALYSIS OF COOPERATIVE PHENOMENA: THE HILL EQUATION

The Hill equation is used to analyse binding situations where cooperativity is manifested; that is, where binding sites exist for more than one ligand and the binding of each ligand facilitates binding of successive ligands. The simplifying assumption is made that the ligand fully occupies all possible sites simultaneously, so that only fully occupied or empty protein molecules are present. The Hill equation is derived in Box 6.2.

BOX 6.2

DERIVATION OF THE HILL EQUATION

An equilibrium expression can be written as:

$$K = [R][L]^n/[RL_n]$$

where $[RL_n]$ is the concentration of receptor with n ligands bound
In such a case:

$$y = [RL_n]/[R_{Tot}]$$
Since
$$[RLn] = [R_{Tot}] - [R]$$
then
$$1 - y = [R]/[R_{Tot}]$$

and we can obtain the equation:

$$y/(1 - y) = [RL_n]/[R]$$
But
$$[RL_n] = [R][L]^n/K$$
and so
$$y/(1 - y) = [L]^n/K$$
giving
$$\log [y/(1 - y)] = n \log[L] - \log K$$

This is the Hill equation. n is known as the Hill coefficient; y is the fractional saturation.

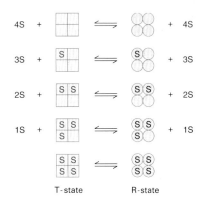

Fig. 6.30 The Monod–Wyman–Changeux model.

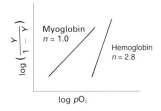

Fig. 6.31 The Hill plot for myoglobin and hemoglobin.

In the derivation of the Hill equation, a number of assumptions are made about the binding of ligand to protein that will not be fulfilled in practice. However, the Hill coefficient can be used as a convenient, although oversimplified, indication of the nature of the ligand-binding interaction. If $n = 1$, there is no cooperativity, as in the case of myoglobin (see Fig. 6.31). If $n > 1$, positive cooperative activity is present; the nearer n approaches the number of binding sites, the higher the cooperativity. If $n < 1$, negative cooperativity is occurring.

THREE-DIMENSIONAL STRUCTURE OF ALLOSTERIC ENZYMES

Most allosteric enzymes are oligomeric proteins and, as outlined above, this is one basis for explaining the sigmoid kinetics curve. A notable exception is hexokinase D, a monomeric protein that exhibits cooperative behaviour with its substrate, glucose (see p. 97). Three-dimensional structures have been obtained for a number of allosteric enzymes. One example of such an allosterically regulated enzyme is phosphofructokinase (PFK), an enzyme of the glycolytic pathway (see p. 134). There are three isoforms, which are encoded by separate genes and are differentially expressed in specific tissues. They are designated A, B and C, the tissues in which they are most abundant being muscle, liver and brain, respectively. PFK is inhibited by one of its own substrates (ATP) and by citrate. It is activated by AMP/ADP and fructose 2,6-bisphosphate (see p. 178). Rabbit muscle PFK is tetrameric, each subunit consisting of two pear-shaped domains linked by a helical region. The four subunits pack together as shown in Fig. 6.32. Such a tetramer carries four active sites and a number of allosteric sites. The active site is in a cleft on each subunit as indicated by B in the figure. The allosteric sites lie in clefts formed between subunits, as shown by C′ at the bottom of the molecule and A and A′ at the top.

The more detailed structure shown in Fig. 6.33 indicates more clearly the structure of the active site and that of the activator allosteric site for AMP/ADP lying between the subunits. The protein shown is the PFK from *Bacillus stearothermophilus*, which is smaller than the rabbit muscle enzyme. Its subunits are smaller, each of the monomers of the rabbit enzyme corresponding to a dimer of the bacterial enzyme. The bacterial enzyme exists as a tetramer, but only two of the subunits are shown in Fig. 6.33. β Strands are represented by arrows A–K, and α helices by cylinders 1–13. The substrates ATP and fructose 6-phosphate are shown in the active site, and the activator ADP in the effector site.

CONFORMATIONAL CHANGES ACCOMPANYING T TO R TRANSITION

It is known that the three-dimensional structure of an allosteric enzyme undergoes conformational change on transition from the T to the R state. These changes have been determined for hemoglobin, and also for phosphorylase, the enzyme that degrades glycogen. Figure 6.34 indicates some of the changes that occur in phosphorylase. The active enzyme exists as dimers. In the upper part of the figure, a

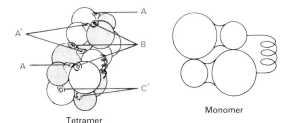

Fig. 6.32 Subunit composition of phosphofructokinase. The different sites indicated are for binding substrates and effectors as follows: A, fructose 6-phosphate; A′, fructose 2,6-bisphosphate; C′, ATP inhibitor; B, ATP substrate.

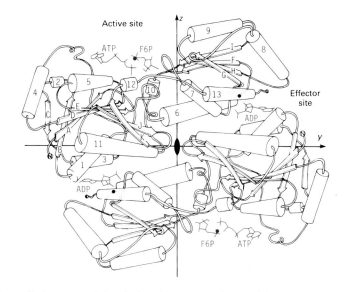

Fig. 6.33 Detailed structure of phosphofructokinase. Two subunits of the PFK tetramer are viewed along the *x*-axis. β Strands are represented by arrows (A–K) and α helices by cylinders (1–13). Each subunit consists of two domains: domain 1 is on the left in the upper subunit. The substrates ATP and fructose 6-phosphate (F6P) are shown in the active site, and the activator ADP in the effector site.

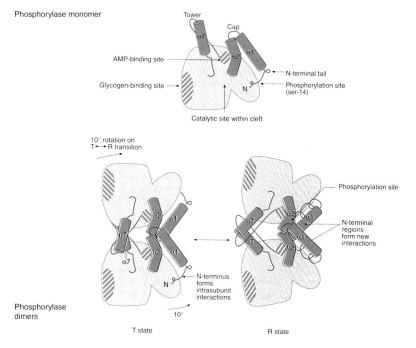

Fig. 6.34 Structural changes in T ↔ R interconversion of phosphorylase.

monomer is represented to show some of the main features of the molecule. Three of the helices of the molecule ($\alpha 1$, $\alpha 2$ and $\alpha 7$) are picked out for study; the rest of the molecule is represented by the outline shape, various binding sites being indicated by red hatching. $\alpha 7$ is referred to as the tower helix. Residues 40–45 lying between $\alpha 1$ and $\alpha 2$ are referred to as the 'cap'. Dimers are shown in the lower part of the figure, indicating the changes that occur as a result of the T to R transition. As indicated, the monomers rotate $10°$ in relation to the vertical axis, and the three helices shown change their orientation, especially in the case of the tower helix. Movement of this helix indirectly leads to movement of an arginine into the catalytic site, displacing an aspartate. When Ser-14 is phosphorylated, the 20 N-terminal residues form an ordered helical conformation, which is also found in the dephosphorylated R state.

METABOLIC CONTROL ANALYSIS

HISTORICAL BACKGROUND

The rate at which metabolic pathways function is known as flux. It is obvious that a cell faces a constantly changing external environment, and to respond to these changes it must regulate the flux in a variety of pathways. The study of the methods by which it does this is known as metabolic control analysis and, over the years, many attempts have been made to analyse these mechanisms. The hypotheses that have been put forward for the most part lead into mathematical treatments that are beyond the scope of this book. However, one concept, that of feedback regulation, is relatively well established.

FEEDBACK REGULATION

It has long been recognized that the end-product of certain pathways can inhibit the passage of substrates down the pathway. For example, if isoleucine is added to a culture of *E. coli*, the de novo synthesis of isoleucine by the bacterium is strongly inhibited. There is a close correlation between the concept of feedback inhibition and the allosteric property of enzymes. Indeed, allosteric effects in enzyme action were first recognized during investigations of feedback inhibition in the 1950s. Simple feedback inhibition is illustrated in Fig. 6.35, in which product S_3 is shown inhibiting enzyme 1. Such an inhibition will normally be allosteric, as the

Simple feedback inhibition

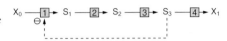

Fig. 6.35 Simple feedback inhibition.

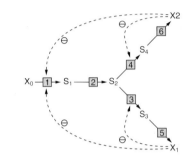

Fig. 6.36 Nested feedback inhibition.

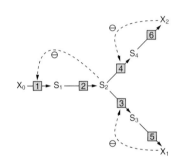

Fig. 6.37 Sequential feedback inhibition.

structure of S_3 will seldom be similar to the structure of X_0, so competitive inhibition is an unlikely candidate. Various types of more complex networks of feedback inhibition are known, two of which, nested inhibition and sequential inhibition, are shown in Figs 6.36 and 6.37, respectively.

The mechanism by which feedback inhibition is exerted might well often involve a single enzyme. Such enzymes are regulatory enzymes, with allosteric properties. Other enzymes of the pathway will then be involved in adjusting the concentration of metabolites in the remaining steps of the pathway (known as homeostatic control), so the levels of these metabolites remain within limits such that other pathways in which they may be intermediates are not perturbed.

GENETIC DIVERSITY OF ENZYMES

VARIANT FORMS OF ENZYMES

As is the case with all proteins (see, for example, the section on protein families,

p. 58), considerable diversity of primary structure is found between enzymes that nevertheless have the same or very similar functions. Modification of even a single amino acid residue might have a profound influence on function. By contrast, it might be found that other differences are associated with minor or even negligible changes in function. The following sections illustrate some of this diversity, and other examples will be found in subsequent chapters. In general, the term isoenzyme (sometimes contracted to isozyme) is applied to enzymes that have different structures but which catalyse the same reaction. It is now almost misleading to refer to 'an enzyme' because so many different structures can fulfil a particular function. In many cases, these structures have been grouped into families that carry out particular, or related, enzyme activities. Despite this, it is still common to refer to 'an enzyme' as referring to the proteins associated with a particular activity, but always bearing in mind the provisos outlined above. Variations between enzyme structures can arise in different ways, some of which are listed in Table 6.3.

VARIANTS OF HEXOKINASE

Hexokinase, an enzyme that carries out the reaction:

$$\text{Glucose} + \text{ATP} \rightarrow \text{glucose 6-phosphate} + \text{ADP}$$

can exist in several genetically distinct forms. These enzymes illustrate the way in which the existence of genetically independent proteins having related enzymic activities must be taken into account in analysing metabolic activity.

Four distinct isoenzymes of hexokinase have been identified in mammalian tissues, designated hexokinase A, B, C and D, or alternatively hexokinase I, II, III and IV, respectively. These isoenzymes are related in structure but a major structural difference is that hexokinase D is a protein of about 50 kDa, whereas the remainder have a molecular mass of approximately 100 kDa. The larger proteins might possibly have evolved by duplication and fusion of a gene encoding an ancestral 50-kDa hexokinase resembling hexokinase D, having two halves showing extensive amino acid sequence similarities to each other, and to hexokinase D. These are known as the N-terminal and C-terminal halves, both of them, in hexokinase B, having a site that is catalytically active. By contrast, in hexokinases A and C only the C-terminal half is active. Figure 6.38

Table 6.3 Variant forms of enzymes

Group	Reason for multiplicity	Example
1	Genetically independent proteins*	Malate dehydrogenase in cytosol and mitochondria
2	Heteropolymers (hybrids) of two or more polypeptide chains, non-covalently bound*	Hybrid forms of lactate dehydrogenase
3	Genetic variants (allelozymes)*	Glucose-6-phosphate dehydrogenase in man
4	Conjugated or derived proteins: (a) Proteins conjugated with other groups (e.g. phosphate) (b) Proteins derived from single polypeptide chains	Phosphorylase a, glycogen synthase D The family of chymotrypsins arising from chymotrypsinogen
5	Polymers of a single subunit	Glutamate dehydrogenase of M_r 1 000 000 and 250 000
6	Conformationally different forms	All allosteric modifications

* These classes fall into the category of isoenzymes

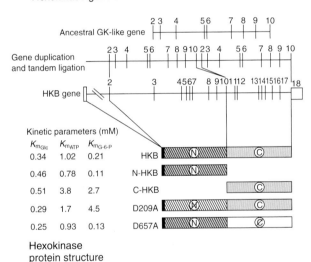

Fig. 6.38 Gene evolution of hexokinase B (HKB). GK, glucokinase.

illustrates a possible model of gene evolution of hexokinase B, in which an ancestral gene undergoes duplication and tandem ligation (i.e. the duplicate genes are ligated nose to tail), leading to the mammalian hexokinase B. Exon 1 codes for the first 21 amino acids, and exons 2–10 and 10–18 code for the N-terminal and C-terminal halves, respectively, each corresponding to the ancestral gene exons 2–10. Figure 6.38 also shows the kinetic parameters of the wild-type, the N-terminal and C-terminal halves expressed separately, and two mutations, in which Asp-209 or Asp-657 is mutated to Ala, that abolish activity of the N-terminal and C-terminal halves, respectively. An important distinguishing property of the hexokinases is their degree of inhibition

by glucose 6-phosphate, which these experiments indicate has a higher K_m in the case of hexokinase B with the C-terminal half.

Why should an animal require four different isoenzymes? A number of clues indicate possible reasons. First, the isoenzymes have different cellular locations, substantial amounts (up to 80% in some tissues) of hexokinase A being associated with mitochondria, hexokinase B also to some extent binding to mitochondria and hexokinase C being localized at the periphery of the nucleus. Much attention has been paid to their different kinetic parameters. These differ considerably. Hexokinase C is inhibited by high concentrations of glucose, and hexokinase D is active only at concentrations of

glucose above 1 mmol l^{-1}, and shows cooperative behaviour at concentrations above this, which correspond to those in blood. For this reason, hexokinase D has received special attention as possibly having a distinct physiological role, as explained below.

HEXOKINASE D

Some years ago, it was suggested that, because hexokinase D has a lower affinity for glucose than other hexokinases, and becomes active only in the range of blood glucose concentrations, it could play a special role after a meal in the metabolism of glucose in the liver, in which it is the predominant form. It was also pointed out that it was more specific for glucose than fructose at low concentrations than the other isoenzymes, and has therefore often been referred to by the name glucokinase, a convention we also adopt. However, its specificity for fructose or glucose is dependent on the concentrations of the two substrates, and the name glucokinase is something of a misnomer. It is relatively insensitive to inhibition by glucose 6-phosphate in comparison to the other three isoenzymes. Apart from this, and its low affinity for glucose, hexokinase D has a highly typical tissue distribution, the gene being expressed only in hepatocytes and the insulin-secreting pancreatic β cells.

The gene has two promoters. Transcription in islet β cells is initiated exclusively at the upstream promoter and in liver cells exclusively at the downstream promoter. The exon–intron organization of the human gene is shown in Fig. 6.39, filled boxes representing the exons, the arrows the sites of transcription initiation. Lines I and II show how differential splicing of the primary transcripts results in a different exon 1 in islet cells (exon 1β) and liver (exon 1L). Exons 2–10 are the same in the two tissues. The gene in liver is hormonally regulated by insulin, hepatic glucokinase activity falling during fasting and being restored by glucose refeeding. Similar changes are not found for the β cell enzyme. Cyclic AMP (the level of which is increased in liver by glucagon) exerts dominant negative control over glucokinase gene expression. Thus there are reasons for believing that hexokinase D plays a distinct role in glucose metabolism.

HETEROPOLYMERS

Lactate dehydrogenase (LDH), which interconverts lactate and pyruvate (see, for

Exon structure of hexokinase D

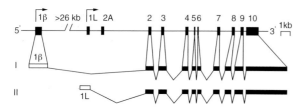

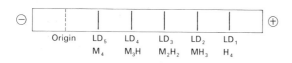

Fig. 6.39 Hexokinase D gene structure in liver and β cells.

Fig. 6.40 Electrophoresis of lactate dehydrogenase reveals isoenzymes.

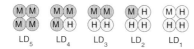

Fig. 6.41 Lactate dehydrogenase forms five isoenzymes from two subunits.

example, p. 135), is a good example of the formation of isoenzymes through the formation of heteropolymers. After electrophoresis of a tissue extract, several protein bands possessing LDH activity are detected, as shown in Fig. 6.40. This arises because two different types of subunit, of different charge, are present in the cell, termed H for heart and M for muscle. These are so called because heart muscle contains substantial amounts of a tetramer of four H subunits and skeletal muscle contains substantial amounts of a tetramer with four M subunits. The different forms, termed LD_1–LD_5, arise from heterotetramers of differing content of these two types of subunit, as shown in Fig. 6.41.

ALLELIC VARIANTS OF ENZYMES

In eukaryotes, every individual has at least two genes encoding a particular protein: one allele inherited from the male parent and the other from the female parent. However, each of these might be one of a number of allelic forms, as occurs in the case of hemoglobins. The possession of different allelic forms can have a variety of consequences for the individual if the allelic forms have different kinetic properties. An example of this can be found in the case of different alcohol dehydrogenases and their role in the metabolism of ethanol.

CLINICAL IMPLICATIONS – THE METABOLISM OF ETHANOL

Ethanol metabolism is mediated by three distinct pathways. The major pathway, which accounts for some 80%, is via alcohol dehydrogenase as described below. The second is mediated by a member (CYP2E1) of the cytochrome P450 family of proteins, the so-called microsomal ethanol oxidizing system (MEOS), located in the smooth endoplasmic reticulum of the liver. This enzyme system has a higher K_m for ethanol and thus functions preferentially at high concentrations of ethanol in the blood. It is also – like other cytochrome P450s – inducible, particularly by ingestion of ethanol. This explains why chronic alcoholics, in the absence of serious liver disease, metabolize ethanol at about twice the rate of normal subjects. The third, minor pathway, involves the peroxisomal enzyme, catalase.

Primary alcohols serve as substrates for liver alcohol dehydrogenase (ADH) but the enzyme is much more active with ethanol than with methanol. Methanol is highly toxic, being oxidized systematically (hepatic) and locally (neurones, retinal cells) to formaldehyde. Methanol toxicity is associated with paralysis, loss of consciousness and irreversible blindness. However, alcohol dehydrogenase has a much higher affinity for ethanol than methanol and thus acute methanol poisoning can be treated by infusion of ethanol and by the administration of 4–methyl pyrazole, a potent inhibitor of alcohol dehydrogenase. ADH also acts on ethylene glycol, which might be ingested accidentally, and thus initiates its conversion to toxic oxalic acid. In such cases, ethanol is given to compete with the harmful substrate and prevent its oxidation

by ADH. ADH forms acetaldehyde from ethanol in the cytosol:

$$CH_3CH_2OH + NAD^+ \rightarrow CH_3CHO + NADH + H^+$$

Mitochondrial acetaldehyde dehydrogenase (ALDH) predominantly converts the acetaldehyde to acetate:

$$CH_3CHO + H_2O + NAD^+ \rightarrow CH_3COOH + NADH + H^+$$

Acetate is then converted to acetyl CoA for further metabolism. Acetaldehyde is a highly reactive substance and is thus probably responsible for many of the toxic effects of ethanol, including the addictive and dependency phenomena of chronic alcoholics. Human ADH is a dimer and is polygenic, being formed from three different subunits classed α, β and γ, each of which has several subclasses. The way in which ADH is classified is shown in Table 6.4.

The different subunits are distributed throughout several populations as shown in Table 6.5, and give rise to isoenzymes with quite marked differences in kinetic parameters (Table 6.6).

Each individual possesses a number of these different isoenzymes, as seen in Fig. 6.42, which shows characteristic distributions found on starch gel electrophoresis for a typical Caucasian and a typical Oriental. The different kinetic properties of the $\beta_1\beta_1$ and $\beta_2\beta_2$ enzymes lead to markedly different activities at physiological pH, as shown in Table 6.6; the $\beta_2\beta_2$ enzyme is much more active than the $\beta_1\beta_1$ enzyme and hence acetaldehyde is formed more rapidly.

Caucasians have two principal isoenzymes for the oxidation of acetaldehyde, ALDH-1 and ALDH-2, whereas about 40% of Orientals have only ALDH-1. Because ALDH-2, the mitochondrial enzyme, has a high affinity for its substrate, its absence will markedly

Table 6.4 Classification of alcohol dehydrogenases (ADH)

Gene	Allele	Polypeptide
ADH1	ADH_1	α
ADH2	ADH_2^1	β_1
	ADH_2^2	β_2
	ADH_2^3	β_3
ADH3	ADH_3^1	γ_1
	ADH_3^2	γ_2
ADH4	ADH_4	π
ADH5	ADH_5	χ
ADH6	ADH_6	δ, ε

Table 6.5 Racial variation in allele frequency of alcohol dehydrogenases (ADH)

	β_1 ADH$_2^1$	β_2 ADH$_2^2$	β_3 ADH$_2^3$	γ_1 ADH$_3^1$	γ_2 ADH$_3^2$
White American	>95	>5	<5	50	50
White European	90	10	<5	60	40
Japanese	35	65	<5	95	5
Blacks	85	<5	15	85	15

Table 6.6 Kinetic properties of different alcohol dehydrogenase class I isoenzymes

Kinetic constraint	Isoenzyme					
	$\alpha\alpha$	$\beta_1\beta_1$	$\beta_2\beta_2$	$\beta_3\beta_3$	$\gamma_1\gamma_1$	$\gamma_2\gamma_2$
K_m ethanol (mM)	42	0.05	0.94	36	1.0	0.5
V_{max} (U mg^{-1})	0.6	0.23	10.0	7.0	2.2	0.87

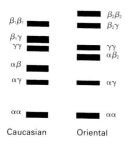

Caucasian   Oriental

Fig. 6.42 Electrophoresis of alcohol dehydrogenase isoenzymes.

increase the concentration of acetaldehyde in atypical subjects. The inactive ALDH-2 is probably the main cause of an undesirable effect of alcohol consumption by Orientals, who might flush and experience nausea and palpitations in response to ingesting even low amounts of ethanol. It will be noted that both reactions involved in ethanol metabolism generate NADH. The liver has to dispose of the increased NADH by the electron transport chain but with difficulty. Many enzymes are sensitive to product inhibition by NADH, but particularly lactate dehydrogenase, causing a reduction of the production of pyruvate from lactate. Thus hypoglycemia and accumulation of hepatic triacylglycerols are consequences of ethanol ingestion. The effects are particularly pronounced after food deprivation. It is claimed that the altered redox (NADH/NAD) during ethanol metabolism is responsible for most of the toxic and metabolic effects of ethanol ingestion.

A number of ALDH inhibitors have been devised, of which disulfiram (Antabuse) is the best known (structure in Fig. 6.43); these compounds have been used to prevent flushing in those patients on aversion therapy.

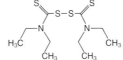

Fig. 6.43 Structure of disulfiram.

PRIMARY STRUCTURE OF ENZYMES

The primary structure of cytochrome c, an enzyme of the respiratory chain (see p. 139), is known for more than 60 different species spanning the evolutionary tree from primitive organisms to higher primates. It is assumed that these sequences

reveal the way that changes have occurred as evolution has progressed. They show that the structure of the protein has essentially been conserved over many millions of years of evolution, but that changes of amino acid residues have occurred at many positions in the protein, without altering its main function. Some residues are identical throughout all species, i.e. they have been conserved throughout evolution. There are 26 such invariant residues; they are shown in Fig. 6.44. Invariant residues are those that are underlined. The residues with side-chains packed against the heme have black dots, those with side-chains completely buried in the protein interior are shown as full red circles, and those that are half-buried are indicated by half-red circles. Most of the invariant amino acids are buried in the heme pocket, including the histidine and methionine involved in coordinating the Fe^{2+}. It is therefore thought that these have a unique function, and that any mutations that might have occurred to change them proved seriously disadvantageous to the animal and the mutation thus did not survive.

ENZYME PRIMARY STRUCTURE AND CONVERGENT EVOLUTION: NICOTINAMIDE NUCLEOTIDE BINDING SITES

The nicotinamide nucleotide binding site in many dehydrogenases has a characteristic structure of a series of β strands. A similar

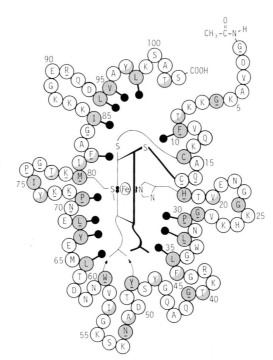

Fig. 6.44 Cytochrome c has 26 invariant residues. See text for further explanation.

arrangement of β strands is found in many enzymes that bind the nicotinamide nucleotides, even though these proteins otherwise show little sequence similarity. The presence of this common domain (see p. 58) in proteins that originated from widely separate points in the evolutionary tree has given rise to the concept of convergent evolution, i.e. that proteins of very different initial structure gradually evolved domains that converged towards a similar type of structure.

CLINICAL IMPLICATIONS – GENETIC ENZYME DEFECTS AND POLYMORPHISM

Inborn errors of metabolism

Many thousands of diseases resulting from inborn errors of metabolism, historically mainly involving enzymes but now known to include many non-enzymic proteins, have been recognized. In these diseases, a genetic variation – often the result of a point mutation – leads to expression of a protein that functions differently from the protein having the normal function, leading to overt disease symptoms. However, there will be other variants within a human population that do not lead to overt symptoms, the expressed protein functioning within normal limits. Changes that do not give rise to overt symptoms are known as silent mutations. Heterozygotes will often be symptomless, because the defective gene is fully compensated by the normal gene. Genetic diseases include sickle-cell hemoglobin (p. 63), phenylketonuria (p. 123) and galactosemia (p. 113).

Polymorphism and disease

While for a long time it has been known that a single gene defect can lead to clinically recognized disease, e.g. the inborn errors of metabolism, the many studies of gene structure now available have revealed that individual genes can exhibit many variations in structure – polymorphisms – and that the effect of these polymorphisms can be widespread and fundamental. Moreover, such polymorphisms are found in all regions of DNA, including those that appear not to code for protein or nucleic acid.

Single nucleotide polymorphisms

Many polymorphisms involve a change in just one nucleotide and hence are known as single nucleotide polymorphisms (SNPs).

Polymorphisms and alleles

The different forms of a gene are known as alleles. Such alleles can be grouped according to their presence and effect on a population:

1. Alleles that are so embedded in a population that they are distributed in clearly defined subpopulations with characteristic allelic genotypes. An example is found in the different alcohol dehydrogenases described in a previous section of this chapter (p. 99). In many cases, these subpopulations appear not to be linked in any way with disease, whereas in others they might be. For example, apolipoprotein E has 5 alleles – E_1 to E_5 – some genotypes of which are linked to Alzheimer's disease.
2. Other alleles that have not penetrated a population so widely, such as those that underlie genetic diseases (e.g. phenylketonuria). Such polymorphisms are not necessarily harmful and might even be beneficial, as with the apoAI(Milano) mutation, which protects against heart disease (p. 172).

The search for SNPs related to disease

Although many SNPs have no obvious connection with disease, it is now recognized that a connection, hitherto undetected, might exist. Such a connection might be due to linkage with more than one SNP. Linkage with SNPs in non-coding regions may lead to identification of nearby genes that are responsible for disease. The search is therefore now on to find linkage between SNPs and disease. A prime candidate is diabetes type 2, although investigations of SNPs and other diseases (e.g. asthma) have also been reported. This work will be greatly assisted by automated methods of gene structure analysis now becoming available. These include so-called SNP chips ('snipchips'), which are essentially glass slides to which are bound nucleotide sequences complementary to SNPs that are under investigation. Each spot on the slide has a complementary sequence of an individual SNP of interest. The slide is then washed with a clinical sample containing the genes under investigation, which will bind to the plate, eliciting a signal wherever a gene binds and the chip can then be read and positives recorded. This is known as a microarray.

The gene copy number and copy number polymorphism (CNP)

The number of copies of a gene in the human genome can vary from individual to individual. Extensive stretches of DNA might be subject to duplication or deletion. These large-scale copy number polymorphisms (CNPs) are a significant source of human genetic diversity. In one study, two individuals differed by 11 CNPs of average length 465 kilobases, determined by microarray analysis, of germline origin. Gene dosage variation has been suggested to be involved in neurological disease and cancer.

What is normal?

The question arises – not for the first time for clinical biochemists – 'what is normal?' Determination of the primary structure of a protein leads to a consensus sequence that reflects the composition of the majority of the samples used in the analysis. The increasing ease of sequencing genes and proteins will permit more accurate estimates of the extent of microheterogeneity in protein structure.

Nomenclature for protein polymorphisms

The convention for denoting replacement of an amino acid is based on the single letter code. Thus for apoAI(Milano), R173C indicates that cysteine replaces arginine at position 173. A deletion is denoted by Δ, e.g. Δ508, the residue 508 being lost.

COENZYMES AND WATER-SOLUBLE VITAMINS

THE ROLE OF COENZYMES

Early attempts to purify enzymes led to the discovery that dialysis caused a loss of activity that in many cases could be traced to the fact that some components were lost when the mixture containing the enzyme was dialysed, i.e. the mixture was enclosed within a semipermeable membrane that allowed only small molecules to pass through it, the outside of the membrane being bathed in buffer so that the small molecules escaped into the surrounding buffer. It was obvious that these small molecules were essential for enzyme activity, and they thus became known as coenzymes. The term cofactor includes such compounds, but is also used to describe other molecules, such as metal ions, that might be necessary for enzyme activity, whereas coenzyme is a term generally reserved for organic molecules that are necessary for enzyme function. Some coenzymes, such as the nicotinamide nucleotides, are included in the written reaction, appearing in their transformed form as products. Kinetically, such molecules are treated as a substrate in their own right, whereas others, such as pyridoxal phosphate (p. 106), are regarded as functioning essentially in the enzyme mechanism and are not normally regarded as substrates. In some cases, the coenzyme remains tightly bound to the enzyme, as in the case of flavin nucleotides (p. 103), which are oxidized or reduced while bound to the enzyme protein.

After the discovery and identification of vitamins, many were found to exert their action by functioning as coenzymes. This is especially true of the water-soluble vitamins such as B_1 and B_6. Other vitamins were found to be necessary for the synthesis of coenzymes, such as the function of riboflavin in the synthesis of the flavin nucleotides. Often, several compounds can function to satisfy a vitamin requirement. Equivalent forms of a vitamin are known as vitamers.

NICOTINAMIDE NUCLEOTIDES

Many biochemical reactions involve oxidation and reduction. This often takes the form of the removal of hydrogen atoms (usually two) from a molecule in the case of oxidation, or addition of hydrogen atoms in the case of reduction. Removal of one hydrogen atom from a molecule leaves an unpaired electron, and thus it is usual that two are removed so that the two unpaired electrons can then pair, as for example in the formation of a double bond. One of the most important coenzymes used in the transfer of hydrogen atoms is nicotinamide adenine dinucleotide (NAD^+), the structure of which is shown in Fig. 6.45; others are FAD and FMN. NAD^+ normally functions to remove two hydrogen atoms from a compound that it oxidizes, but only one hydrogen atom is transferred intact to NAD^+, to position 4 of the nicotinamide ring. In the case of the other hydrogen atom, its electron is transferred to NAD^+, neutralizing the positive charge on position 1 of the nicotinamide ring, and the proton that is left goes into solution.

The general form of reactions involving NAD^+ is:

$$RH_2 + NAD^+ \rightarrow R + NADH + H^+$$

For convenience, when writing metabolic pathways the H^+ is often omitted. However, it is important to appreciate that it is always involved in the reaction. The same applies to $NADP^+$ and its reduced form.

Nicotinamide adenine dinucleotide phosphate ($NADP^+$) is the oxidized form of a related coenzyme, in which the hydroxyl at C-2 of the ribose attached to the nicotinamide is esterified to phosphate. Reduction of the nicotinamide ring of $NADP^+$ occurs in a manner exactly analogous to that for NAD^+. These coenzymes are water soluble and are usually free to diffuse away from the enzyme after reaction. Nicotinamide nucleotides can also be tightly bound to enzymes, having a role in maintaining enzyme structure.

A useful property of these coenzymes is that the absorption spectra of the oxidized and reduced forms differ, in that the reduced form absorbs light much more strongly in the region of the spectrum near 340 nm (Fig. 6.46). Thus many dehydrogenase reactions can be followed by measuring the change in absorbance at 340 nm.

ADENINE NUCLEOTIDE COENZYMES

Adenosine 5′-triphosphate (ATP), the structure of which is shown in Fig. 6.47, is formed during tissue respiration from adenosine 5′-diphosphate (ADP). This function of respiration has profound significance, because ATP is involved in many reactions, not only in phosphoryl group transfer, but in others in which it is split to ADP and orthophosphate. The large negative free energy change associated with hydrolysis of ATP (p. 90) ensures that many of these reactions proceed in the direction in which ATP is hydrolysed. Thus this partial reaction often has the function of driving an overall reaction in a particular direction. The three compounds ATP, ADP and AMP are part of a system that regulates the flow of certain pathways, as evidenced by a number of examples discussed in the following pages. The

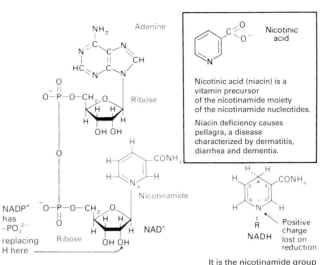

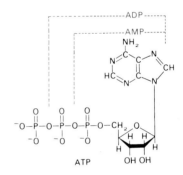

Fig. 6.47 Adenine nucleotide structures.

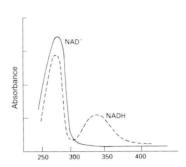

Fig. 6.46 Increased absorbance at 340 nm can be used to measure NADH.

Fig. 6.45 The structures of nicotinamide nucleotides.

enzyme adenylate kinase is one factor in regulating the relative amounts of the adenine nucleotides. It catalyses the reaction:

$$ATP + AMP \leftrightarrow 2\,ADP$$

Another major influence on the extent of ATP biosynthesis is the overall state of cell metabolism and the corresponding greater or lesser requirement for the utilization of ATP in the performance of work. The respiratory chain is regulated by the relative proportions of ADP and ATP, as discussed on p. 141. A quantity known as the energy charge is defined by the expression:

$$\frac{[ADP] + \frac{1}{2}[ADP]}{[ATP] + [ADP] + [AMP]}$$

ATP, ADP and AMP are important allosteric modifiers of a number of reactions, such as the reaction catalysed by phosphofructokinase (p. 178).

NUCLEOTIDE COENZYME SYSTEMS IN METABOLIC REGULATION

The regulation of pathways is a function of the ATP/ADP/AMP system, and also of the NAD$^+$/NADH and NADP$^+$/NADPH systems. The cell has the capacity to regulate the ratios of these compounds one to another within a particular system. Over short time intervals, the components of each of the coenzyme systems:

1. ATP + ADP + AMP
2. NADH + NAD$^+$
3. NADPH + NADP$^+$

sum to a constant total in any given cell compartment. If one component of any of these three systems increases, it does so at the expense of the other component(s) of the system, i.e. if NADH increases, NAD$^+$ decreases, or if ATP levels change, those of ADP or AMP (or both, in certain situations) will undergo compensatory change. Of course, over longer time intervals, the total amounts of these compounds can change, due to biosynthesis or degradation, if the physiological situation demands. The relative concentrations of the components of each of these systems is often a parameter in determining their allosteric effects on regulatory enzymes.

The relative concentrations of these coenzymes differ in different cell compartments (Fig. 6.48); this has a directive effect on metabolic pathways within those compartments. Thus, in the cytosol, the tendency is for reactions involving NAD$^+$ to proceed towards

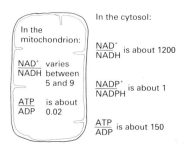

Fig. 6.48 Cell compartments differ in ratios of nucleotide coenzymes.

NADH (oxidation of the substrate). Because of this, NADPH is often the coenzyme used for reduction in the cytosol (note the NADP$^+$/NADPH ratio in Fig. 6.48), the more favourable ratio facilitating reduction.

THIAMINE DIPHOSPHATE

Thiamine (vitamin B$_1$) is the precursor of thiamine diphosphate (older name thiamine pyrophosphate), which is a coenzyme for some important oxidative decarboxylation reactions. In oxidative decarboxylation, loss of CO_2 from an α-keto acid is accompanied by oxidation of the resulting aldehyde to an acid. Such reactions include those catalysed by pyruvate dehydrogenase and oxoglutarate dehydrogenase. Thiamine diphosphate is

also a coenzyme for transketolase. The way in which it functions in the mechanism of the pyruvate dehydrogenase complex is shown in Fig. 6.49. This complex consists of three enzyme activities, which involve NAD$^+$, thiamine diphosphate and lipoate as shown in the figure. The enzyme activities are carried out by three subunits of the complex, denoted E$_1$, E$_2$ and E$_3$. Reaction 1 involves decarboxylation of pyruvate and catalyses attachment of an hydroxyethyl group to thiamine diphosphate, from which it is transferred (reaction 2) to oxidized lipoate, a step that achieves conversion of the hydroxyethyl group to an acetyl thioester attached to the lipoate. Reactions 1 and 2 are catalysed by E$_1$. E$_2$ catalyses the formation of acetyl CoA by exchange of the acetyl group from lipoamide onto the free sulfhydryl group of coenzyme A (reaction 3), and the lipoate is then reoxidized by E$_3$ with NAD$^+$ as coenzyme (reaction 4). The overall reaction is:

$$Pyruvate + CoA + NAD^+ \rightarrow$$
$$acetyl\ CoA + CO_2 + NADH$$

α-KETO ACID DEHYDROGENASE COMPLEXES

The pyruvate dehydrogenase complex (PDC) is one of a family of α-keto acid dehydrogenase complexes that share a

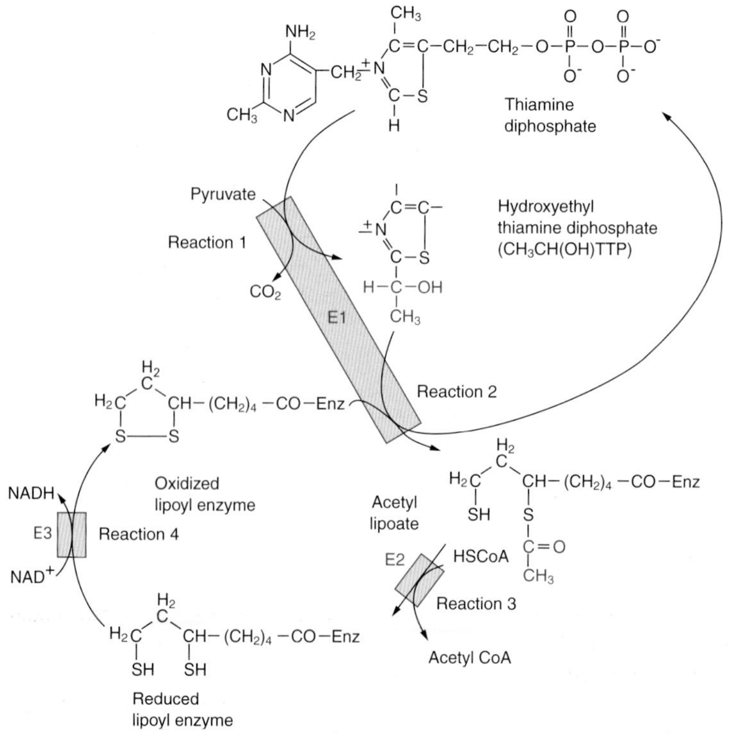

Fig. 6.49 Reactions of the pyruvate dehydrogenase complex.

common mechanism. The family includes those of α-ketoglutarate dehydrogenase and branched chain α-keto acid dehydrogenase (involved in the breakdown of the carbon chains of the branched chain amino acids leucine, isoleucine and valine). All these complexes consist of three catalytic components E_1, E_2 and E_3. Specific genes for E_1 and E_2 exist for each complex, whereas the E_3 component, which catalyses the same reaction for all three complexes, is encoded by a single gene. In pyruvate dehydrogenase, the E_1 component is a heterotetramer of two each of α and β subunits. A kinase involved in regulation of the enzyme (see p. 91) phosphorylates three specific serines on the $E_1\alpha$ subunit. Regulation of gene expression is important during embryogenesis and differentiation, but also in the adult for adjusting amounts of enzyme in different physiological conditions. For example, feeding diets high in glucose to rats results in increases in the amounts of component proteins. Some of the promoter-regulatory regions of PDC-$E_1\alpha$ are shown in Fig. 13.17. Altogether, seven distinct nuclear-protein binding domains are known, together with *cis*-acting elements.

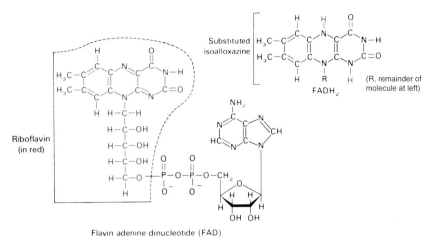

Fig. 6.50 Flavin nucleotide structures.

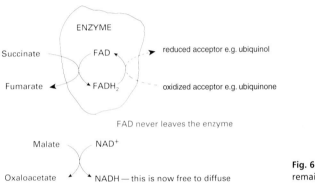

Fig. 6.51 Flavin nucleotides remain bound to the enzyme.

CLINICAL IMPLICATION – THIAMINE DEFICIENCY DISEASE

Thiamine was originally discovered as the vitamin deficient in the diet of those suffering from beri-beri, a disease found in Asian populations dependent on rice diets. If the rice is polished, the thiamine is removed. The disease is associated with neuropathy and cardiomyopathy. An experimental deficiency can be induced in laboratory animals and is associated with neurological symptoms. For example, pigeons show a characteristic reaction in not being able to hold their heads erect, which can readily be reversed by administering the vitamin. In Western countries, thiamine deficiency can be associated with alcohol abuse, including heavy binge drinking, especially when this is accompanied by a poor diet.

FLAVIN NUCLEOTIDES

Flavin adenine dinucleotide (FAD) and flavin mononucleotide (FMN) are coenzymes of a class of dehydrogenases known as flavoproteins. The structure of FAD is shown in Fig. 6.50. It consists of a substituted isoalloxazine linked to ribitol phosphate, which is in anhydride linkage with AMP. FMN is riboflavin phosphate,

i.e. FAD without the adenosine monophosphate moiety. FAD and FMN function as hydrogen atom acceptors, and are normally tightly bound to the protein of a flavin dehydrogenase. The hydrogen atoms are accepted at the positions on the isoalloxazine ring shown in red in Fig. 6.50. These then have to be passed on to an acceptor for the coenzyme to be reoxidized. The situation is summarized in Fig. 6.51. Flavin coenzymes remain tightly bound to the apoenzyme throughout the reaction, unlike nicotinamide coenzymes, which behave as soluble substrates for the dehydrogenase.

CLINICAL IMPLICATION – RIBOFLAVIN DEFICIENCY DISEASE

Riboflavin (vitamin B_2) was isolated in the course of investigations into a B vitamin fraction that prevented a skin condition in rats. Human deficiency, however, rarely occurs nowadays. It can result from eating a diet that consists largely of corn (maize). Where it does occur, it can cause skin lesions resembling sebborrhoea.

COENZYME A

As shown in Fig. 6.52, coenzyme A (CoA) is a complex molecule containing a phosphorylated derivative of ADP linked to pantothenic acid (which itself is a combination of pantoic acid and β-alanine), which is then linked to the decarboxylation product of cysteine. One of the most important derivatives of CoA results from linkage of its thiol group to an acetyl group to form acetyl CoA. CoA functions as an activating group in many acyl group transfer reactions, in β-oxidation and in reactions involving acetyl CoA. Its free sulfhydryl (–SH) group reacts with a carboxyl group to form a thioester, which is in some ways analogous to the ester formed between an alcohol and a carboxyl group. The thioester group has special properties that result from the chemistry of the sulfur atom. This induces electron displacements that make the carbonyl carbon susceptible to attack (e.g. by nucleophilic groups, leading to acyl transfer). In other reactions, the methyl carbon is activated. One of the

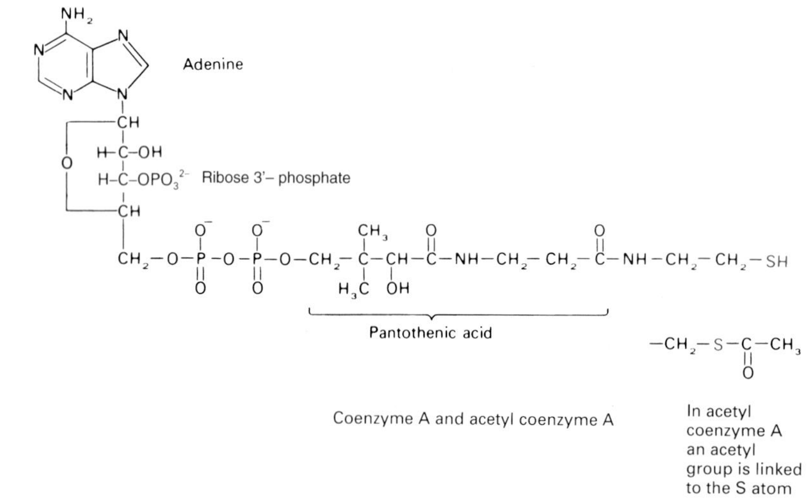

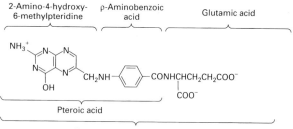

Fig. 6.52 The structure of coenzyme A.

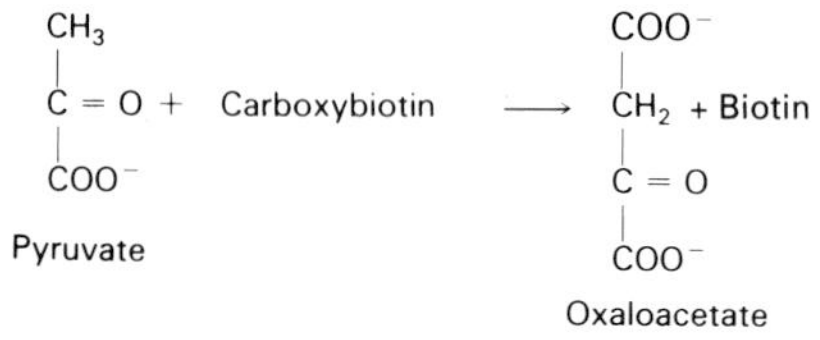

Fig. 6.53 The pyruvate carboxylase reaction requires biotin.

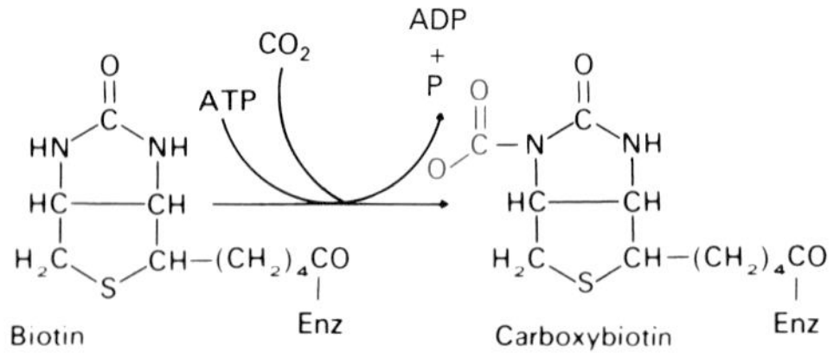

Fig. 6.54 The formation of carboxybiotin.

Fig. 6.55 Components of folic acid. Folate is pteroylglutamate.

components of CoA, pantothenic acid, is a water-soluble vitamin.

BIOTIN

Biotin is a water-soluble vitamin and is a prosthetic group of certain carboxylation enzymes, including pyruvate carboxylase (Fig. 6.53) and acetyl-CoA carboxylase. These enzymes utilize ATP in the modification of biotin-enzyme to N-carboxybiotin-enzyme by the addition of CO_2, which is then transferred to the substrate. Biotin is covalently bound through its carboxyl group to a lysyl side-chain of the enzyme (Fig. 6.54).

CLINICAL IMPLICATIONS – BIOTIN DEPENDENCY

Although nutritional biotin deficiency is virtually unknown, the binding of biotin to the protein lysyl groups is carried out by the enzyme holocarboxylase synthetase. During normal breakdown of enzyme protein, lysyl biotin is released and degraded by the enzyme biotinidase, and the biotin that is released is recycled. Deficiency of holocarboxylase synthetase results in failure to utilize biotin. Clinical features characteristically include feeding problems, acidosis, and an acute progressive encephalopathy during infancy. Deficiency of biotinidase will cause failure to utilize or recycle biotin. Features include alopecia, skin rash, developmental delay, hypotonia, seizures, acidemia, aciduria, hearing problems, and vision problems, which develop during childhood. Both conditions typically respond to biotin therapy.

FOLATE COENZYMES

The transfer of a methylene or methyl group often involves folic acid, a water-soluble vitamin, in its tetrahydrofolate form. In this form, positions 5, 6, 7 and 8 of the pteridine ring are reduced. The various components of the folic acid molecule are shown in Fig. 6.55. The predominant form in portal plasma is tetrahydrofolate, which is converted in the liver to 5-methyltetrahydrofolate, in which form it normally circulates. Although it has a single glutamate in plasma, intracellular folates are attached to a chain of several glutamates, a conjugation necessary for retention within cells. 5-Methyltetrahydrofolate is converted to tetrahydrofolate by reaction with cobalamin to form methylcobalamin, which then reacts with homocysteine to form methionine and regenerate cobalamin (note that this does not constitute net synthesis of methionine, which must be provided in the diet as a precursor for homocysteine). Dihydrofolate is formed in this reaction, which is then converted to tetrahydrofolate by dihydrofolate reductase.

Tetrahydrofolate reacts either with serine, to form 5,10-methylenetetrahydrofolate, in which a methylene bridge is formed between C-5 and C-10, or alternatively with formiminoglutamate, a metabolite of histidine (p. 126), to form 5-formiminotetrahydrofolate, in which the formimino group –CH=NH is transferred to C-5 (see Fig. 6.56). These can be converted to other forms, as shown in the figure. Figure 6.57 indicates the pathways in which individual tetrahydrofolate derivatives function as methyl donors. The importance of folates in the biosynthesis of purines and pyrimidines is responsible for defective cell division in folate deficiency.

CLINICAL IMPLICATIONS – FOLATES IN MEDICINE

These pathways are defective in vitamin B_{12} deficiency (see below) and cellular depletion of folate coenzymes eventually ensues, resulting in reduction in purine and thymidylate biosynthesis. Epidemiological studies have demonstrated a correlation between a folate-poor diet and neural tube defects such as spina bifida. Intervention trials have shown that dietary

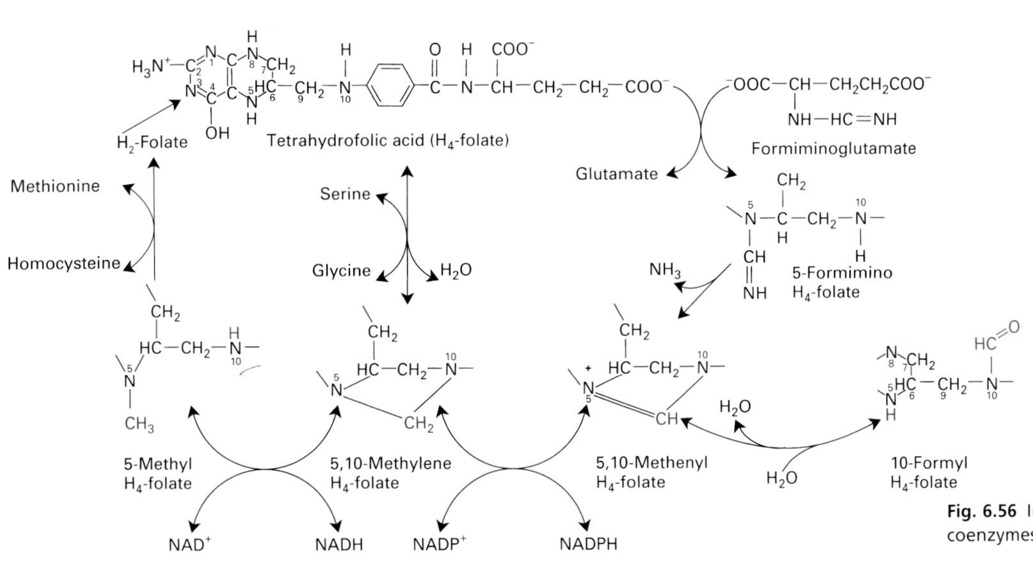

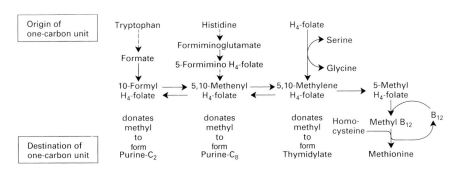

Fig. 6.56 Interconversions of folate coenzymes.

Fig. 6.57 Donation of methyl groups by folate coenzymes. Methyl B_{12}, methylcobalamin (see p. 106).

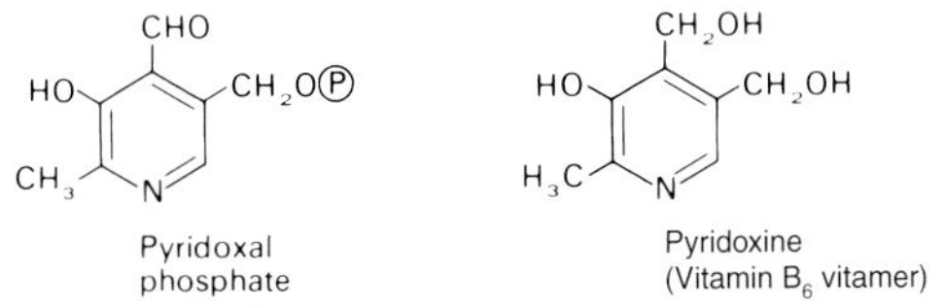

Fig. 6.58 Structures of pyridoxal phosphate (the active form of vitamin B_6) and pyridoxine.

supplementation with folates in women seeking to become pregnant, continued through the early stages of any ensuing pregnancy, can greatly decrease the occurrence of these defects.

Because folate metabolism is an essential component of the pathways for the synthesis of purines and pyrimidines for DNA synthesis, intervention in these pathways is a strategy in cancer chemotherapy. Thus in the synthesis of thymidylate from uridylate by thymidylate synthase 5,10-methylenetetrahydrofolate is converted to dihydrofolate, and for this to re-enter the folate cycle it must be converted to tetrahydrofolate by dihydrofolate reductase, an enzyme that is inhibited by methotrexate and other drugs (see p. 26).

Elevated homocysteine levels in plasma have been suggested as a risk factor for coronary heart disease. A common polymorphism, C677T, exists for the gene that encodes methylenetetrahydrofolate reductase, which converts 5,10-methylenetetrahydrofolate to 5-methyltetrahydrofolate needed for conversion of homocysteine to methionine. This C to T substitution reduces enzyme activity and increases homocysteine levels. Dietary folate supplementation can reduce the level of plasma homocysteine, and could have value in reducing the risk of heart disease.

PYRIDOXAL PHOSPHATE

Pyridoxal phosphate is a derivative of the water-soluble vitamin B_6. Pyridoxine, pyridoxamine and pyridoxal (see Fig. 6.58) are all vitamers of B_6. Pyridoxal phosphate acts as a coenzyme in transamination, and in some amino acid decarboxylation reactions such as the decarboxylation of glutamate to γ-aminobutyric acid (GABA), as described on p. 126. It is also involved in some reactions that catalyse racemization of isomers. In a transamination reaction, as shown in Fig. 6.59, the aldehyde group of pyridoxal phosphate first reacts with the amino group of the amino acid, with loss of water, to form a type of compound known as a Schiff base. By a rearrangement of bonds and addition of water, a keto acid and pyridoxamine phosphate are formed. The pyridoxamine phosphate then transfers its amino group to another keto acid, to form an amino acid and pyridoxal phosphate, as shown in the Fig. 6.59.

CLINICAL IMPLICATIONS OF VITAMIN B_6

Vitamin B_6 deficiency is rare in humans because the vitamin is widely distributed in common foodstuffs and, in addition, is synthesized in appreciable quantities by intestinal bacteria. There have been claims

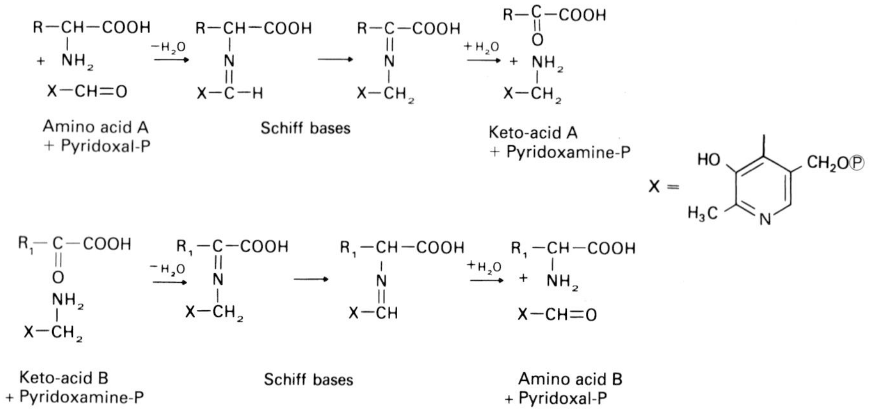

Fig. 6.59 Schiff base formation is involved in the mechanism of transamination.

that increased B_6 intake can be beneficial, but these are not well substantiated, and, if taken in large excess, it can have harmful effects. The main abnormality seen in B_6 deficiency is a photosensitive dermatitis, which is readily cured by administration of the vitamin. Laboratory animals made B_6-deficient can be susceptible to spontaneous epileptiform convulsions, and are more susceptible to convulsive drugs which act as GABA antagonists.

VITAMIN B_{12}

Vitamin B_{12} was first isolated in the cyanocobalamin form, and identified as the factor in raw liver that alleviates the symptoms of pernicious anemia. Four pyrrole rings form a porphyrin-like structure around a cobalt atom. This cobalt atom has coordinate bonds that link it with other groups in the molecule. Cobalamin is the name given to the structure shown in Fig. 6.60 in black. This structure shows in red a 5′-deoxyadenosyl group linked to the sixth coordination position of the cobalt atom. The sixth coordination position is occupied by the cyano group in cyanocobalamin in place of the 5′-deoxyadenosyl group, and by a methyl group in methylcobalamin. Methylcobalamin acts as a coenzyme in the methylation of homocysteine (see p. 122), and 5′-deoxyadenosylcobalamin is the coenzyme in a reaction in which methylmalonyl-CoA is converted to succinyl-CoA.

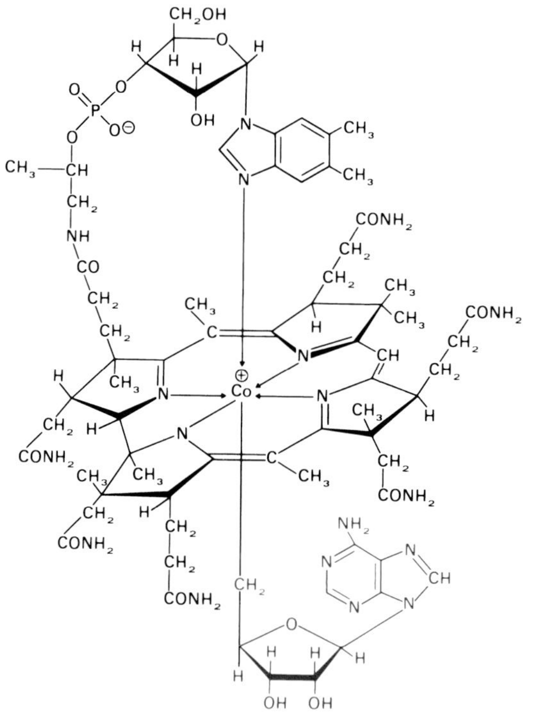

CLINICAL IMPLICATIONS – VITAMIN B_{12} AND PERNICIOUS ANEMIA

Vitamin B_{12} is present only in foods of animal origin, especially liver, fish and eggs.

Fig. 6.60 5′-Deoxyadenosylcobalamin is one form of vitamin B_{12}.

Deficiency rarely occurs, but is precipitated by lack of intrinsic factor, a protein secreted by the gastric mucosa and required for efficient absorption of the vitamin. Lack of intrinsic factor leads to pernicious anemia, which can be treated by parenteral vitamin B_{12}.

VITAMIN C (ASCORBIC ACID) AND ITS CLINICAL IMPLICATIONS

Ascorbic acid was identified as the component in fresh vegetables and fruit that prevented the onset of scurvy, a disease characterized by defective connective tissue resulting in bleeding gums and loss of teeth. Its action in the prevention of scurvy may be explained by its involvement in the hydroxylation of proline (see below). The structure of ascorbic acid, and of its ionized form ascorbate, are shown in Fig. 6.61. Ascorbic acid can act as a reducing agent, being oxidized to dehydroascorbic acid. It has an important role in collagen synthesis. Proline is oxidized to hydroxyproline after it has been incorporated into collagen precursor peptides (p. 72). The reaction involves oxoglutarate and dioxygen (O_2) as shown in the reaction equation:

-Pro-Gly- + 2-oxoglutarate + O_2 →
-Hypro-Gly- + CO_2 + succinate + H_2O

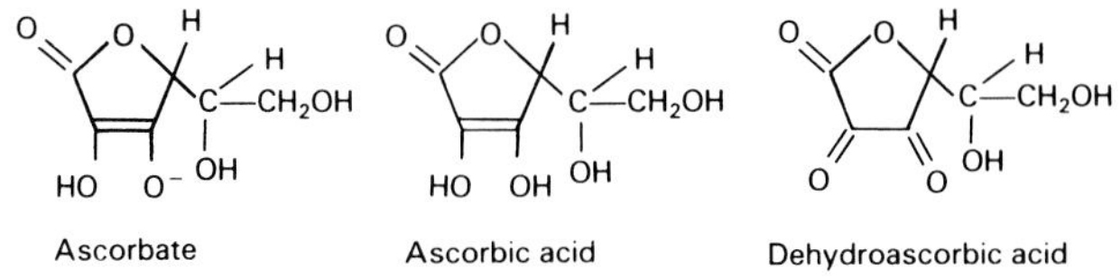

Fig. 6.61 Structures of ascorbic acid and its ionized (ascorbate) and oxidized (dehydroascorbic acid) forms.

Ascorbate   Ascorbic acid   Dehydroascorbic acid

Fe^{3+} and ascorbic acid are required in this reaction, in the absence of which abnormal collagen is formed.

Ascorbic acid also plays a role in the detoxification of reactive oxygen species (see p. 142). It is important in the uptake of iron, as discussed on p. 71. Humans are among the few higher animals that are unable to synthesize L-ascorbic acid, owing to a deficiency of the enzyme L-gulonolactone oxidase, the enzyme catalysing the terminal step in the synthesis of the vitamin.

Carbohydrates: structures and interconversions

7

Carbohydrates, sometimes referred to as sugars, consist of monosaccharides and their derivatives. Polymers are known as oligosaccharides or polysaccharides, depending on length. Carbohydrates can be considered as having two distinct and vital functions: first, as substrates, the oxidation of which provides energy for biosynthetic reactions and work, and second, as structural components.

Glucose is of special importance as an energy source. It is derived from the energy-storage polymers starch (in plants) and glycogen (in animals). Glucose acts as a substrate for glycolysis, one of the main energy-yielding oxidative pathways.

Various sugars, including mannose, galactose and fucose and their amino and sulfated derivatives, are present in complex polysaccharides, which have structural roles and play an important part in recognition functions and adhesion (see later chapters).

Monosaccharides form groups of isomeric molecules distinguished from each other by the configuration of their hydroxyl groups and the position of the carbonyl group. Hexoses have six carbon atoms and pentoses have five. The aldoses have the carbonyl group on a terminal carbon (i.e. they are aldehydes) and the ketoses on an internal carbon (i.e. they are ketones).

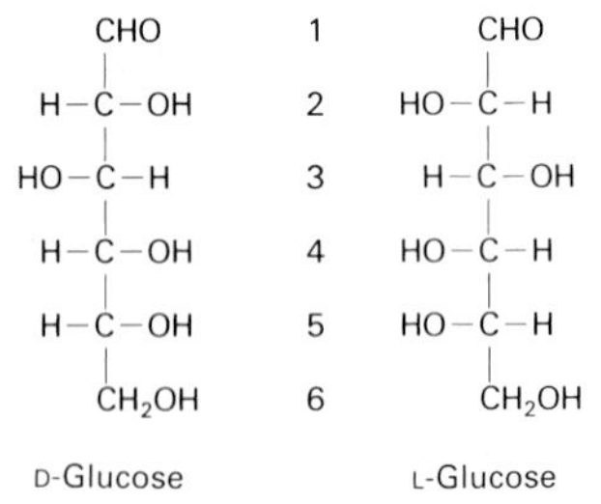

Fig. 7.1 Glucose exists as optical isomers. D-Glucose is sometimes called dextrose.

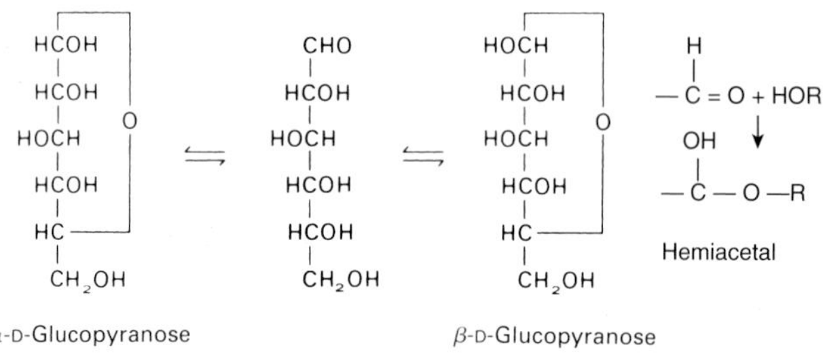

Fig. 7.2 α and β forms of sugars equilibrate spontaneously.

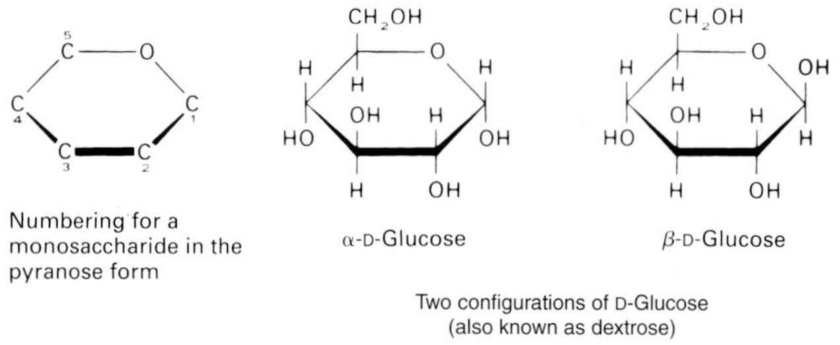

Numbering for a monosaccharide in the pyranose form

α-D-Glucose

β-D-Glucose

Two configurations of D-Glucose (also known as dextrose)

Fig. 7.3 The monosaccharide ring structure and its numbering.

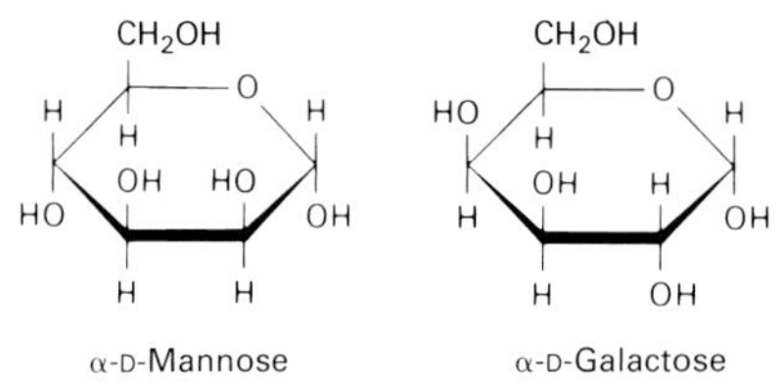

α-D-Mannose

α-D-Galactose

Isomers of this type are termed *epimers*, and enzymes that change the configuration on one hydroxyl group to convert one sugar into another are termed *epimerases*.

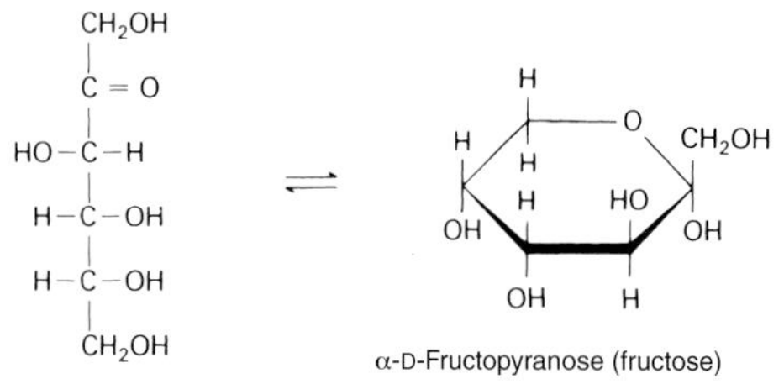

α-D-Fructopyranose (fructose)

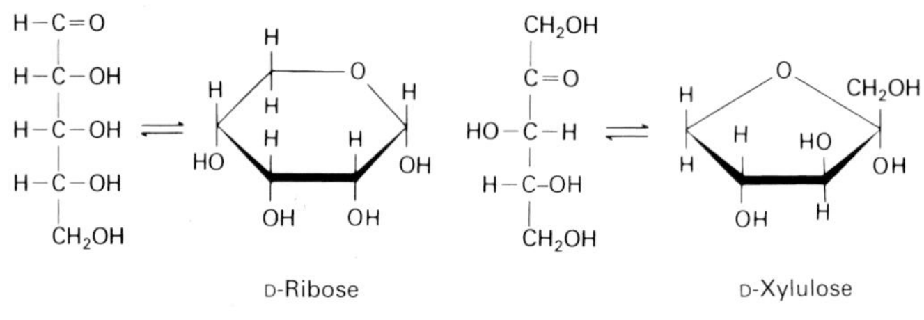

D-Ribose

D-Xylulose

Fig. 7.4 The structures of other mono-saccharides.

MONOSACCHARIDES AND DISACCHARIDES

MONOSACCHARIDE STRUCTURES

Carbohydrates (also loosely known as sugars) are found as monosaccharides or as polymers containing monosaccharide units. Monosaccharides consist of polyhydric alcohols, from three to ten or more carbons in length, and contain either an aldehyde group (when they are called aldoses) or a ketone group (in the case of ketoses). They contain centres of asymmetry, and are thus chiral molecules (see p. 9). For example, glucose, which is widely distributed as a monosaccharide or as a component of larger molecules, exists in two forms, D-glucose and L-glucose (see Fig. 7.1). The configuration on carbon 5 (denoted C-5) determines whether the molecule is designated D or L, and is related to the configuration of D- or L-glyceraldehyde. The two glucose molecules are mirror images, and the configuration of all the other hydroxyls is similarly reversed between the two molecules in the Fischer projection used in the figure. The Fischer projection is a two-dimensional representation of a three-dimensional shape, and has the convention that bonds shown horizontally are regarded as projecting to the back of the paper, and those shown vertically as coming up out of the paper (each carbon being considered separately). The configuration at each carbon can be denoted R or S (see p. 9), a notation that applies to individual carbons, not whole molecules. In mammalian carbohydrates, the D-forms predominate. A monosaccharide with six carbons is known as a hexose, one with five carbons as a pentose.

The open chain form of a monosaccharide is in equilibrium with a ring form, as shown in Fig. 7.2 for D-glucose, through the formation of a hemiacetal bond between the carbonyl group and a hydroxyl group (in an acetal, two alcohols are linked to the carbonyl group; hence hemiacetal when only one is

involved). The ring closure can occur to give either of two configurations, an α or a β form, as shown in the figure. These ring forms can be represented as in Fig. 7.3. The α and the β forms are in equilibrium with each other, interconverting via the open chain form. Sugars that differ only in the configuration at the hemiacetal bond are known as anomers, and the carbon bearing the hydroxyl group involved is known as the anomeric carbon. Note that, in the α configuration, the anomeric hydroxyl always projects to the opposite face of the

ring from C-6, whereas in the β configuration it projects to the same face as C-6. Depending on the size of the ring formed, the structure is designated pyranose, if a six-membered ring, or furanose, if a five-membered ring. Monosaccharides that differ only in the configuration of one of the carbons other than the anomeric carbon are known as epimers; the structures of galactose and mannose, two epimers of glucose, are shown in Fig. 7.4. The structures of two pentoses are also shown in this figure, as well as the structure of an important ketose, fructose, shown in the pyranose configuration.

The hemiacetal group reacts readily with certain oxidizing agents, such as Fehling's solution. This reaction forms the basis of the well-known 'reducing test' for sugars, such as glucose or mannose, that have a free hemiacetal group, i.e. they reduce Fehling's solution. Some disaccharides (see below) possess a free hemiacetal group. An important exception is sucrose (see Fig. 7.9), in which the constituent monosaccharides are linked through their anomeric carbons, which as a result are not oxidizable and do not give a positive reducing test.

A six-membered ring structure can adopt either a chair or boat conformation, as shown in Fig. 7.5 for cyclohexane. Bonds perpendicular to the plane of the molecule are termed axial, those in the plane of the molecule being equatorial. The six-membered ring of D-glucose adopts a chair conformation (Fig. 7.6).

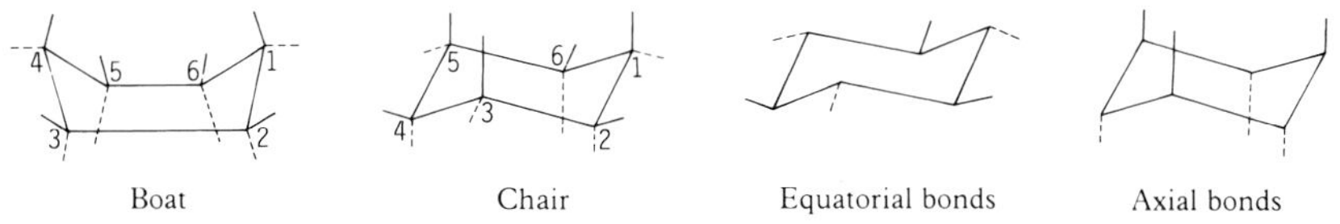

GLYCOSIDES

Monosaccharides can form a number of derivatives. One of the most common is formed by reaction of an alcohol with the hemiacetal group, the resulting compound being known as a glycoside. This is illustrated in Fig. 7.7 for the reaction of D-glucose with methanol. The more specific names, glucoside, mannoside or galactoside, can be used to specify the sugar involved. A glycoside will be of either the α or β configuration, according to the specificity of the enzyme that forms it, and there is no spontaneous interconversion between α and β forms once the glycosidic link has been formed. Enzymes known as glycosidases hydrolyse glycosides; they are specific for either the α or the β form.

AMINO SUGARS AND SULFATED DERIVATIVES

One of the hydroxyls of a monosaccharide, most often that at C-2, can be replaced by an amino group, which is often acetylated as shown in Fig. 7.8. These amino sugars are found in the complex polysaccharides in glycoproteins and proteoglycans, in which hydroxyl groups can also be sulfated (see, for example, p. 113). Sulfated sugars are also found in glycolipids (p. 195).

DISACCHARIDES

A disaccharide consists of two monosaccharides linked by a glycosidic

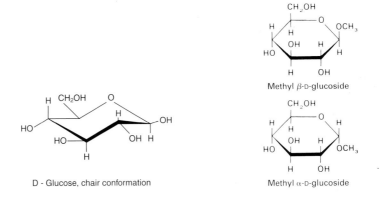

Fig. 7.5 Boat and chair conformations.

Fig. 7.6 The chair conformation of D-glucose.

Fig. 7.7 Methylglycosides of D-glucose.

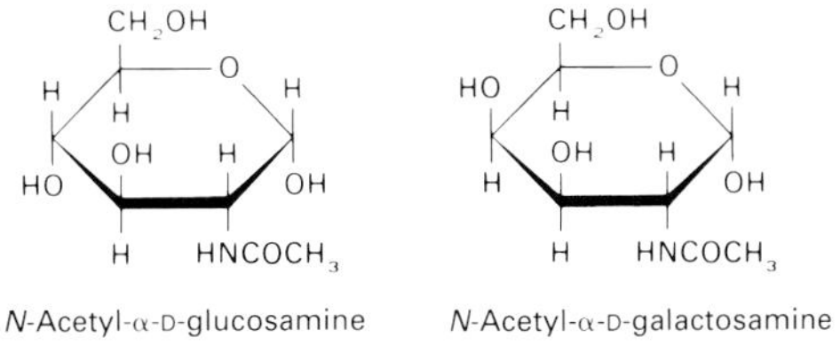

Fig. 7.8 N-Acetylated amino sugars.

bond. The structures of some important disaccharides are shown in Fig. 7.9. Lactose is the sugar found in milk, and consists of a molecule of galactose in glycosidic linkage with the hydroxyl on C-4 of glucose. The galactose is in the β configuration, and the linkage is referred to as a β1-4 link. Maltose is a disaccharide that often results from hydrolysis of polymers of glucose, such as starch. Sucrose, the sweetening agent obtained from sugar cane or beet, is unusual in that it is formed by a bond between the two hemiacetal linkages of the constituent monosaccharides, and thus has no free hemiacetal group.

POLYSACCHARIDES

STRUCTURE OF POLYSACCHARIDES

Polysaccharides are polymers of monosaccharide units. Where the number of monosaccharide units is in the range 1–10, the term oligosaccharide is used rather than polysaccharide. Some polysaccharides function as storage compounds, the prime examples being glycogen (p. 146) and starch (which consists of a mixture of amylose and amylopectin) (p. 112). Other polysaccharides function as structural carbohydrates, which are highly diverse in structure and sometimes referred to as complex carbohydrates. The main chains of glycogen, amylopectin and amylose are linked by α1-4 bonds, supplemented in glycogen and amylopectin by occasional α1-6 bonds, which have the effect of creating branches in the chains (p. 146). A great variety of linkages is found in the structural polysaccharides. Most of these linkages involve a glycosidic bond, the differences between one linkage and another resulting from the various hydroxyl groups to which the hemiacetal is linked, and whether the bond is α or β. Glycan is another term used to denote polysaccharide. Where the glycan is composed of a single type of monosaccharide, it can be more specifically named by replacing the ending 'ose' of the sugar by the suffix 'an'; hence starch, which contains only glucose, is termed a glucan.

111

The structures of amylose and cellulose (an important constituent of plant cell walls) are shown in Fig. 7.10. Humans cannot digest cellulose because they cannot hydrolyse its β1–4 links. However, it is degraded by bacteria in the stomach of ruminants, who can therefore utilize cellulose as a nutrient.

GLYCOPROTEINS AND PROTEOGLYCANS

Carbohydrate is found attached to many globular proteins, which are therefore classed as glycoproteins. The term proteoglycan is used to describe certain complexes of carbohydrate and protein typically found in the glycocalyx that surrounds cells, in the synovial fluid of joints, as well as in the basement membrane. Figure 7.11 shows an electron micrograph, together with a key to the structure, of such a molecule. The carbohydrates are attached to core proteins which are held on a central strand of hyaluronic acid through link proteins. Figure 7.12 shows the repeating disaccharide units of which the carbohydrates frequently found in such substances are composed. These molecules usually contain amino sugars and sulfated hydroxyl groups, and are often referred to as glycosaminoglycans. Such molecules bear negative charges, arising partly from the sulfate groups but also from carboxyl groups of the glucuronic acid units that some of them contain. Figure 7.13 shows the structure of glucuronic acid, together with the structure of gluconic acid for comparison. Glucuronic acid results from oxidation at C–6 of glucose, while gluconic acid is the product of oxidation at C–1. Glucuronic acid plays an important role in glucuronides, as explained on p. 114.

INTERCONVERSIONS OF MONOSACCHARIDES

THE IMPORTANCE OF NUCLEOTIDE–SUGAR INTERMEDIATES

Certain compounds in which monosaccharides are linked to a nucleoside diphosphate are important in carbohydrate metabolism. One of these is uridine diphosphoglucose (UDPG), shown in Fig. 7.14. It is formed enzymically by reaction between UTP and glucose 1-phosphate. Similar compounds such as uridine diphosphogalactose, guanosine diphosphomannose and guanosine diphosphofucose are formed by reaction

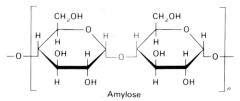

(Glucose) — Maltose — (Glucose)

(α-D-Glucosyl-(1 → 4)-α-D-glucose)

(Glucose) — Sucrose — (Fructose)

(β-D-Fructosyl-α-D-glucose)

(Galactose) — Lactose — (Glucose)

(β-D-Galactosyl(1→4)-β-D-glucose)

Fig. 7.9 The structures of maltose, sucrose and lactose.

Amylose

(-α-D-glucosyl-(1 → 4)-α-D-glucosyl-)

Cellulose

Fig. 7.10 The structures of amylose and cellulose.

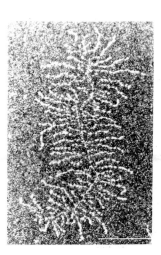

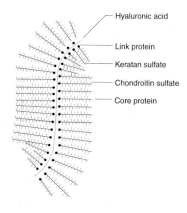

- Hyaluronic acid
- Link protein
- Keratan sulfate
- Chondroitin sulfate
- Core protein

Fig. 7.11 The structure of a proteoglycan isolated from bovine cartilage.

The anticoagulant heparin binds antithrombin. The complex inhibits enzymes of the bloodclotting cascade.

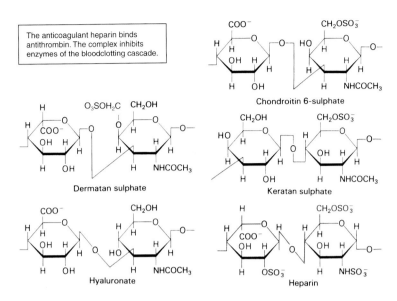

Chondroitin 6-sulphate

Dermatan sulphate

Keratan sulphate

Hyaluronate

Heparin

Fig. 7.12 The structures of some complex polysaccharides.

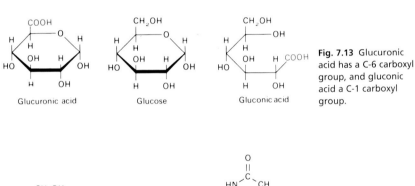

Glucuronic acid

Glucose

Gluconic acid

Fig. 7.13 Glucuronic acid has a C-6 carboxyl group, and gluconic acid a C-1 carboxyl group.

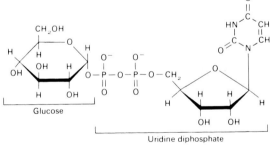

Glucose

Uridine diphosphate

Fig. 7.14 Uridine diphosphoglucose is an intermediate in many reactions of glucose.

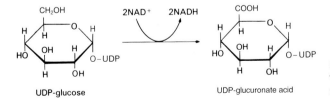

UDP-glucose

UDP-glucuronate acid

Fig. 7.15 UDP-glucose is the precursor of UDP-glucuronate.

between the appropriate nucleoside triphosphate and the sugar 1-phosphate. UDP-glucuronic acid is formed from UDP-glucose by oxidation of the C-6 hydroxyl group to a carboxyl group (Fig. 7.15).

GALACTOSE METABOLISM

Galactose is a component of the oligosaccharide chains of glycoproteins, proteoglycans and glycolipids. It is also a component of lactose, the sugar of milk.

The initial step in its metabolism is the formation by a specific kinase, galactokinase, of galactose 1-phosphate, which then reacts with UTP to form UDP-galactose (Fig. 7.16). An epimerase interconverts UDP-galactose and UDP-glucose (Fig. 7.17). UDP-galactose can also be formed by the enzyme UDP-glucose-hexose 1-phosphate uridylyltransferase (uridyltransferase), which catalyses the reaction of galactose 1-phosphate with UDP-glucose, resulting in the reversible cycle shown in Fig. 7.18.

CLINICAL IMPLICATIONS – GALACTOSEMIA

In galactosemia, an inborn error of metabolism, the infant fails to thrive and, if untreated, could develop liver disease, mental disease, cataracts and renal tubular damage due to the elevated levels of galactose or galactose 1-phosphate, or both, in tissues. In this condition, galactokinase might be deficient, giving a mild form of the disease, or most commonly, a deficiency of uridyltransferase. In the absence of this enzyme in infancy there is no route for the conversion of galactose 1-phosphate to UDP-galactose, because the enzyme shown in Fig. 7.16 forming UDP-galactose is not expressed until later in life.

In adults, the toxicity of galactose is less severe due to the metabolism of galactose 1-phosphate by UDP-glucose pyrophosphorylase which can accept galactose 1-phosphate in place of glucose 1-phosphate. Galactosemia is treated by the exclusion of galactose from the diet.

MANNOSE METABOLISM

Mannose can be phosphorylated by hexokinase to mannose 6-phosphate, which can be converted to or formed from fructose 6-phosphate (see Fig. 7.19). Mannose 6-phosphate can be converted to mannose 1-phosphate, from which GDP-mannose can be formed, and this can be converted to GDP-fucose. GDP-mannose and GDP-fucose are intermediates in the formation of complex carbohydrates.

THE FORMATION OF N-ACETYLNEURAMINIC ACID (SIALIC ACID)

Sialic acid (see p. 195) is an important constituent of many complex carbohydrates, especially gangliosides. It is synthesized via N-acetylmannosamine 6-phosphate, extra carbons being added from

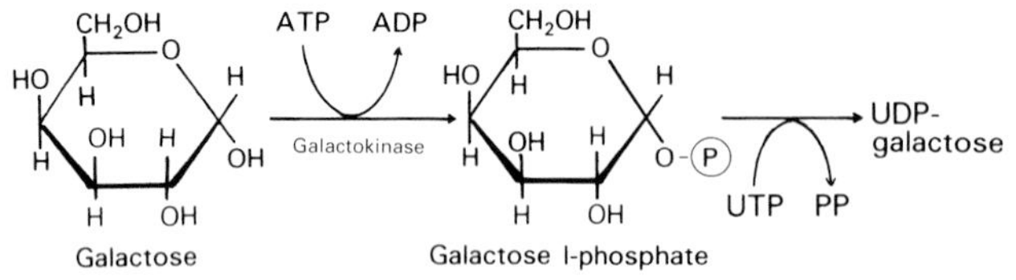

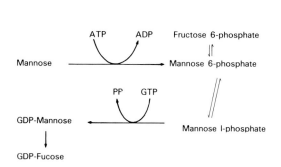

Fig. 7.16 Galactose is converted to UDP-galactose.

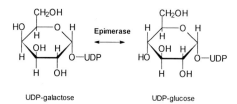

Fig. 7.17 UDP-galactose and UDP-glucose can epimerize.

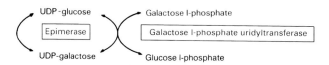

Fig. 7.18 Galactose 1-phosphate uridyltransferase interconverts galactose 1-phosphate and glucose 1-phosphate and their UDP derivatives.

Fig. 7.19 Mannose metabolism.

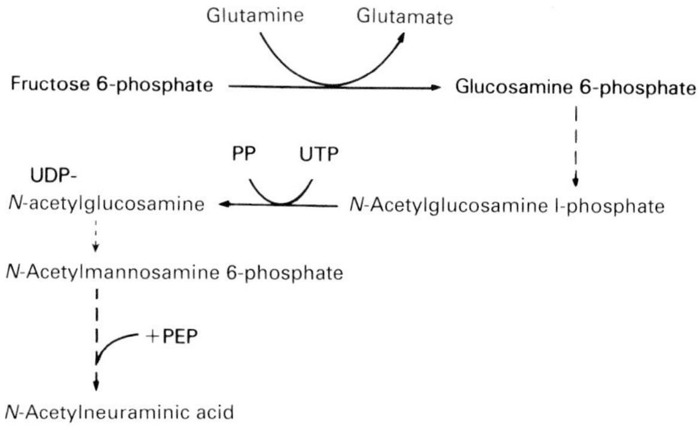

Fig. 7.20 Formation of *N*-acetylneuraminic acid from fructose 6-phosphate. PEP, Phosphoenohpyrurale

phosphoenolpyruvate in a reaction pathway of several steps. *N*-Acetylmannosamine 6-phosphate is synthesized from fructose 6-phosphate in the series of reactions outlined in Fig. 7.20.

DETOXIFICATION MECHANISMS

THE FORMATION OF GLUCURONIDES

Compounds that are not very soluble in water are not easily excreted but they can be rendered more soluble by metabolism. One such mechanism involves the addition of glucuronic acid by formation of a glycosidic link between the glucuronic acid and a compound having a hydroxyl group, as shown in Fig. 7.21. In some cases, the hydroxyl group might have been introduced into an aromatic ring by enzymes known as monooxygenases, which catalyse the reaction:

$$RH + O_2 + NADPH + H^+ \rightarrow ROH + H_2O + NADP^+$$

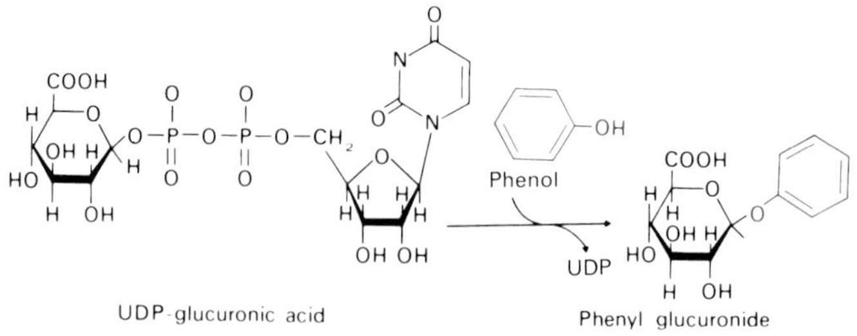

Fig. 7.21 The formation of glucuronides.

Enzymes of this type are found in the smooth-surfaced endoplasmic reticulum and other membranes and are members of a large family of monooxygenases, the cytochrome P450 family, different members of which are specific for particular substrates. Only one of the oxygen atoms of the dioxygen molecule is incorporated into the aromatic ring, the other reacting to form water with two hydrogen atoms arising from NADPH oxidation. Phenobarbital causes a proliferation of the endoplasmic reticulum of liver; thus one of the results of administering the drug is to increase the

amount of cytochrome P450 enzymes. These enzymes derive their name from their absorption of light at about 450 nm in the presence of reducing agent. They act on lipid-soluble substrates such as steroids, fatty acids and xenobiotics. The gene is designated *CYP* and this can be used in naming the enzymes. Thus, cholesterol side-chain cleavage enzyme is P450 11A1 or CYPXIAI.

Enzymes that hydrolyse the glycosidic bond of glucuronides are, in common with other glycosidases, specific for the α or β configuration of the bond, being known as β-glucuronidases and α-glucuronidases.

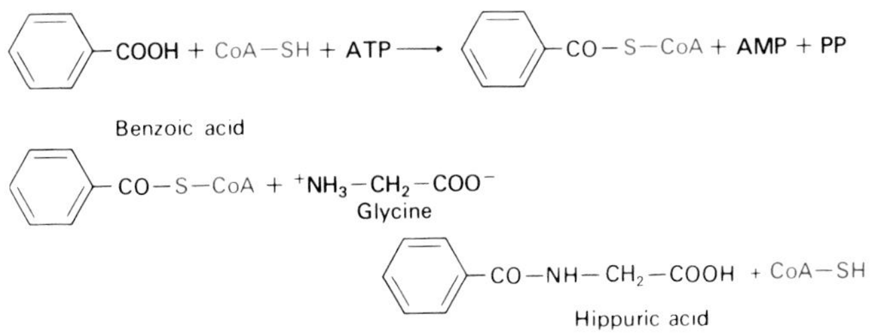

Fig. 7.22 The formation of hippuric acid.

OTHER ROUTES FOR DETOXIFICATION

The formation of glucuronides is not the only route by which potentially toxic molecules can be detoxified. Compounds such as acids are conjugated with glycine, as shown in Fig. 7.22; the resulting glycine conjugates are excreted more readily than the unreacted compound. Other compounds are conjugated with the sulfhydryl group of glutathione, to form conjugates known as mercapturic acids.

Nitrogen metabolism

8

Body protein is in a constant state of turnover through the activity of biosynthetic and degradative pathways. The first step in the breakdown of an amino acid involves removal of the amino group by one or other of the aminotransferases. Activity of the urea cycle leads to the excretion of the amino nitrogen as urea. Pathways exist for the breakdown of the residual carbon chains.

Some amino acids can be synthesized in animals by transfer of an amino group to a readily available keto acid. Amino acids that can be made in this way are non-essential; those that cannot, must be obtained from the diet and are known as essential amino acids.

The biosynthesis of biologically important compounds such as thyroxine, histamine and adrenaline and the synthesis of heme are described, together with a description of the porphyrias. The role of creatine in energy provision in muscle is a specialized use for an amino acid derivative.

PROTEIN BREAKDOWN AND EXCRETION OF NITROGEN

TRANSAMINATION

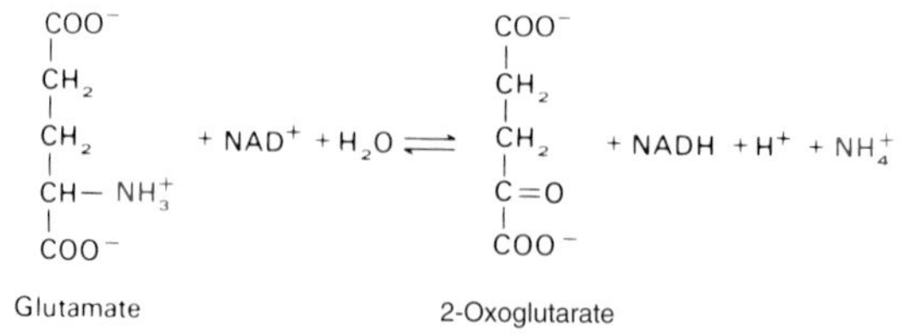

In the total breakdown of a protein, one of the most important tasks is the removal and excretion of the nitrogen atoms. This occurs after hydrolysis of the protein by peptidases to its constituent amino acids. If total excretion of nitrogen exceeds intake over any measured period, the animal is said to be in negative nitrogen balance. If the reverse is the case, as in a growing animal, a state of positive nitrogen balance exists, whilst a perfect balance between the two processes is referred to as nitrogen equilibrium.

In cases where the bodily requirement for amino acids is already fully satisfied, excess amino nitrogen is excreted as urea. The amino groups are transferred to the amino acids aspartate and glutamate, which, as explained below, act as substrates of reactions leading to incorporation of the amino nitrogen into urea. The transfer of an amino group from an amino acid to an α-keto acid to form a different amino acid is known as transamination, and is catalysed by enzymes known as aminotransferases (formerly transaminases). In the case of glutamate, the amino group can be directly removed by the action of glutamate dehydrogenase, which catalyses an oxidative deamination (Fig. 8.1).

A generalized transamination is shown in Fig. 8.2. The mechanism involves pyridoxal phosphate and has been described on p. 106. Individual aminotransferases exist for all the common amino acids, but there are two keto acids, oxoglutarate and pyruvate, that are of particular importance as acceptors of the amino group. The terminology 'oxo' is used in chemical names to denote a keto group, but 'keto acid' is used to denote the class of compound. On transamination oxoglutarate and pyruvate yield glutamate and alanine, respectively. There is an important aminotransferase for which glutamate or alanine can act as substrate, their keto acids acting as the other substrate as appropriate, as shown in Fig. 8.3. The route for the excretion of amino groups requires the formation of urea by the urea cycle, which is described below. The nitrogen enters the cycle either as ammonia or by transfer from aspartate. (The term 'ammonia' is used to indicate the sum of NH_4^+ and NH_3. Either ammonium ion or free ammonia is used to denote each specifically.) Transamination related to urea formation therefore channels

the amino group towards ammonia or aspartate. Many aminotransferases transfer the amino group from individual amino acids to oxoglutarate either directly (Fig. 8.4) or indirectly via alanine aminotransferase, as in Fig. 8.5.

Aminotransferases also exist that transfer amino groups directly to oxaloacetate from individual amino acids (Fig. 8.6) to form aspartate. In addition, aspartate aminotransferase transfers the glutamate amino group to oxaloacetate to form aspartate (Fig. 8.7). Thus, cooperation between these various enzymes channels the amino group into the urea cycle, as summarized in Fig. 8.7. This figure also shows that ammonia is formed from amines. This results from the action of monoamine oxidase (see Fig. 8.8), which is an enzyme with an important role in the degradation of compounds such as

adrenaline, noradrenaline and serotonin (see Fig. 8.23). Monoamine oxidase inhibitors (e.g. phenelzine and isocarboxazid) are sometimes used as antidepressant drugs based on their action in increasing the concentration of noradrenaline and serotonin in the synaptic gap and exerting an increased postsynaptic effect. The cyclopropylamines are better antidepressants (e.g. trimipramine, dothiepin). They act by preventing the

Fig. 8.1 The glutamate dehydrogenase reaction.

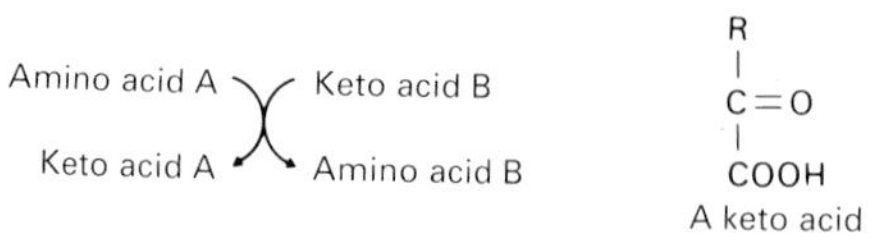

Fig. 8.2 The transamination reaction.

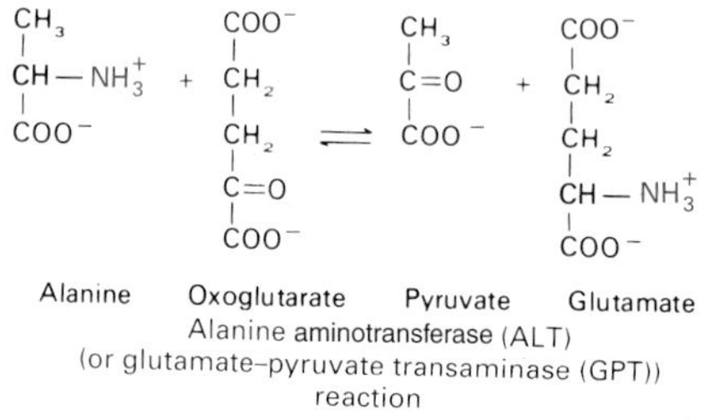

Fig. 8.3 The reaction of alanine aminotransferase.

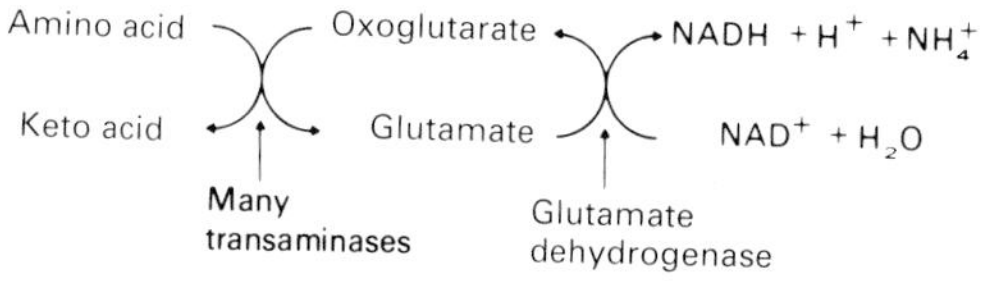

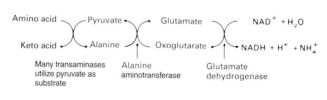

Fig. 8.4 The role of glutamate dehydrogenase.

Fig. 8.5 Many aminotransferases utilize pyruvate as substrate.

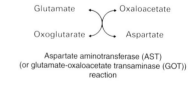

Aspartate aminotransferase (AST) (or glutamate-oxaloacetate transaminase (GOT)) reaction

Fig. 8.6 The aspartate–oxoglutarate aminotransferase reaction.

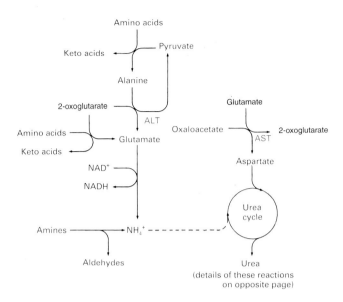

Fig. 8.7 General scheme for transfer of amino groups to urea.

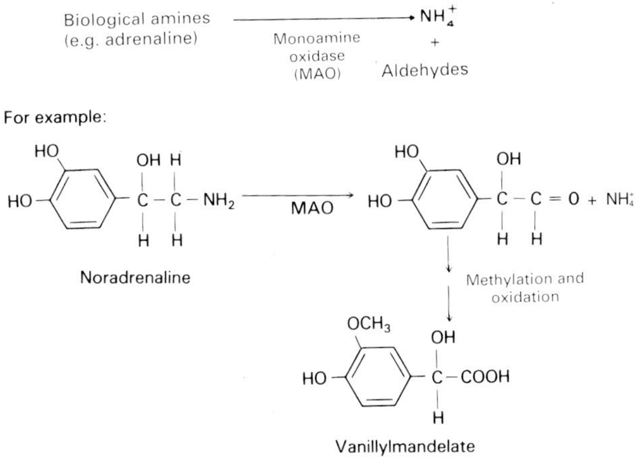

(details of these reactions on opposite page)

Biological amines (e.g. adrenaline) →[Monoamine oxidase (MAO)] NH_4^+ + Aldehydes

For example:

Noradrenaline →[MAO]→ ... + NH_4^+

Methylation and oxidation

Vanillylmandelate

Fig. 8.8 The monoamine oxidase reaction.

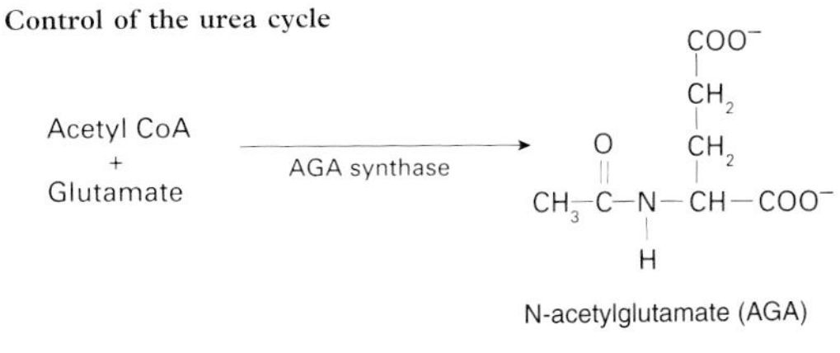

Control of the urea cycle

Acetyl CoA + Glutamate →[AGA synthase]→ N-acetylglutamate (AGA)

Fig. 8.9 The synthesis of N-acetylglutamate.

CPS II, which is involved in pyrimidine biosynthesis, differs in that it utilizes glutamine as substrate, is a cytosolic enzyme and is not activated by N-acetylglutamate; instead, it is activated by PRPP (phosphoribosylpyrophosphate; see p. 26) and inhibited by UTP.

GLUTAMINE BIOSYNTHESIS

A widespread reaction that also converts ammonia to a non-toxic form is the synthesis of glutamine by the reaction:

Glutamate + NH_3 + ATP → glutamine + ADP + P

This acts to detoxify ammonia in many tissues, and to act as a vehicle for its transport. The glutamine thus formed can be used in synthetic reactions, as for the biosynthesis of purines and pyrimidines, or can be transported to the liver for conversion to urea. Most urea is synthesized from ammonia that has been released from glutamine by the enzyme glutaminase, which hydrolyses glutamine to glutamate and ammonia. In the liver, glutamine synthase is localized to hepatocytes surrounding the central vein of liver lobules, while the enzymes of the urea cycle are expressed in hepatocytes in the periportal regions of the lobules. The influence of liver morphology on metabolism in the liver is discussed in a later section (p. 179). It seems likely from its distribution that another function of glutamine synthase might be to scavenge any ammonia that is not dealt with by the urea cycle enzymes. Glutamine synthesized in this way is secreted by the liver into the blood and can be hydrolysed in the kidney with the release of ammonia into the urine.

THE UREA CYCLE

The enzyme pathway that catalyses the formation of urea is known as the urea cycle. It is noteworthy that it was the first of the cyclical pathways to be discovered by Hans Krebs (the other being the citric acid cycle), and it is therefore often referred to as the Krebs urea cycle. The reactions of the cycle are shown in Fig. 8.11. The start of the cycle can be regarded as the reaction between the amino acid ornithine and carbamoyl phosphate, to form citrulline. This then reacts with aspartate to form argininosuccinate, from which fumarate is then removed to yield arginine, which is hydrolysed by arginase to yield urea and regenerate ornithine for the next turn of

active reuptake into cellular stores of released noradrenaline.

CARBAMOYLPHOSPHATE SYNTHASE

Ammonia at concentrations above $50\,\mu M$ is toxic for the central nervous system, and it is thus essential that its concentration be kept low. Degradation of the residual carbon chains of amino acids releases large amounts of carbon dioxide, which also must be disposed of. Carbamoylphosphate synthase I (CPS I) plays a major role in removing both of these metabolites. This form of the enzyme is the most abundant

protein in the mitochondrial matrix, and links free ammonia (K_m $38\,\mu M$) with CO_2 utilizing two molecules of ATP to form carbamoyl phosphate, one of the molecules of ATP donating the phosphoryl group and the other being hydrolysed to ADP and P, which results in a negative free energy change for the reaction. The enzyme has an absolute requirement for N-acetylglutamate (AGA), which is synthesized from acetyl CoA and glutamate (Fig. 8.9). Because AGA synthase is activated by arginine, this amino acid has a stimulatory effect on urea synthesis (see Fig. 8.10). Another form of the enzyme,

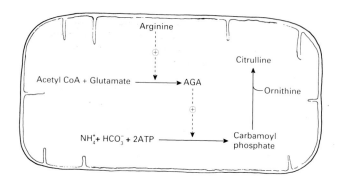

Fig. 8.10 *N*-acetylglutamate activates carbamoylphosphate synthetase.

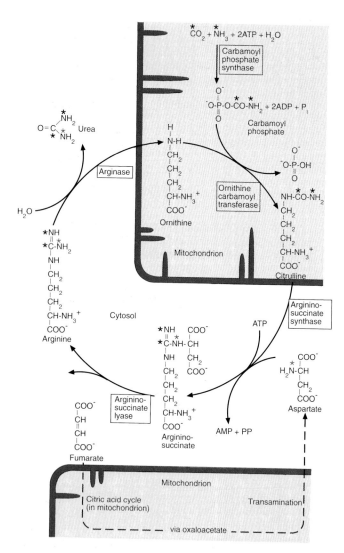

Fig. 8.11 The urea cycle.

summarized in Table 8.1. The prognosis varies with the severity of the disease. For example, a neonatal form of carbamoylphosphate synthase deficiency is associated with complete or almost complete absence of the enzyme, and normally results in death in the neonatal period. However, partial deficiency of the enzyme also occurs, with correspondingly longer survival to early adulthood or later.

THE SUPPLY OF AMINO ACIDS

ESSENTIAL AND NON-ESSENTIAL AMINO ACIDS

Higher animals are able to synthesize only some of the amino acids required for protein synthesis. The amino acids that cannot be made must be obtained from dietary sources, and are known as the essential, or indispensable, amino acids. Plants and bacteria are able to synthesize all the amino acids needed for their protein synthesis, and many unusual ones besides. Those that can be synthesized in animals are referred to as non-essential, or dispensable, amino acids. Tables 8.2–8.4 list the amino acids in these different categories. Dietary proteins can be segregated into those that provide a good balance of the essential amino acids and those that do not. Some animal proteins, such as collagen and gelatin (which is derived from it), have poor nutritional value because of their unusual amino acid composition. Vegetable proteins often lack certain amino acids; wheat gluten, for example, is relatively poor in lysine and some rice protein is deficient in lysine and threonine. Because the deficiency is not the same in all vegetable proteins, however, mixtures of proteins provide adequate nutrition.

SYNTHESIS OF NON-ESSENTIAL AMINO ACIDS

The non-essential amino acids can be synthesized from carbohydrate precursors, provided a source of amino nitrogen is available. Pyruvate, oxaloacetate and oxoglutarate are all intermediates of carbohydrate metabolism (see, for example, the citric acid cycle, p. 136). They are the keto acids of alanine, aspartate and glutamate, respectively, and the amino acids can thus be formed from them by transamination. Serine is synthesized from 3-phosphoglyceric acid, an intermediate in the glycolytic pathway (p. 134). The

the cycle. This regeneration of the starting material is an important characteristic of cyclical pathways. The formation of carbamoyl phosphate and citrulline takes place in the mitochondria, the remaining reactions being cytoplasmic.

The urea cycle is activated by glucocorticoids and glucagon, both of which activate the gene encoding CPS I, glucocorticoids acting through the glucocorticoid receptor and glucagon acting through cyclic AMP and CREB

(CRE binding protein, see p. 180). In combination with other factors, these form complexes that interact with the promoter region of the gene.

CLINICAL IMPLICATIONS – INHERITED DEFECTS OF UREA CYCLE ENZYMES

Several inherited diseases that are due to deficiency of one or other of the urea cycle enzymes are known; these are

Table 8.1 Inherited abnormalities of the urea cycle enzymes

Deficient enzyme	Disease	Type of inheritance	Characteristic features
Carbamoylphosphate synthase	Hyperammonemia	Autosomal recessive	Hyperammonemia and aminoacidemia without orotic aciduria
Ornithine carbamoyltransferase	Hyperammonemia	X-linked dominant	Hyperammonemia and aminoacidemia with orotic aciduria
Argininosuccinate lyase	Argininosuccinic-aciduria	Autosomal recessive	Mild argininosuccinic acidemia with argininosuccinic aciduria
Arginase	Argininemia	Autosomal recessive	Argininemia (variable with dietary load) and argininuria
Argininosuccinate synthetase	Citrullinemia	Autosomal recessive	Citrullinemia and hyperammonemia with orotic aciduria

Table 8.2 Non-essential amino acids synthesized directly by transamination from metabolites readily available from major pathways

Amino acid	Metabolite from which synthesized
Alanine	Pyruvate
Aspartate	Oxaloacetate
Glutamate	Oxoglutarate

Table 8.3 Non-essential amino acids synthesized by special pathways

Amino acid	Metabolite from which synthesized
Proline	Ornithine via glutamic semialdehyde
Glycine	Serine
Serine	3-Phosphoglycerate
Cysteine	S-Adenosylmethionine and serine
Tyrosine	Phenylalanine
Arginine	Ornithine*

*Arginine may be needed in the diet for adequate growth rates in the young.

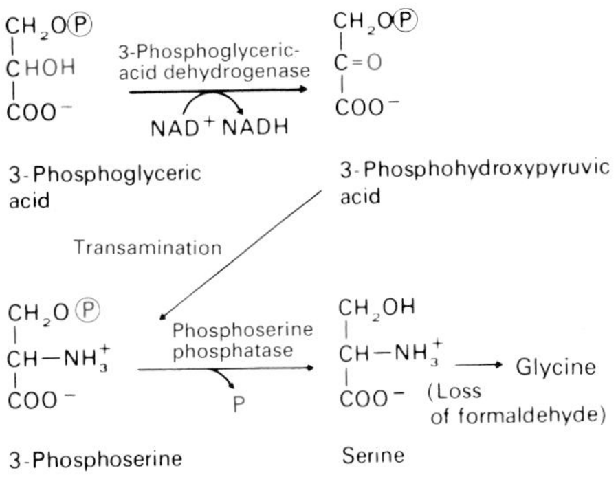

Fig. 8.12 Serine is synthesized from 3-phosphoglycerate.

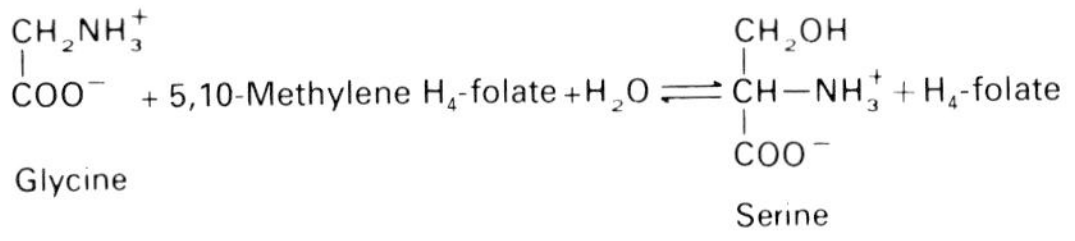

Fig. 8.13 Glycine and serine are interconverted.

Table 8.4 Essential amino acids in man

- Histidine
- Isoleucine
- Leucine
- Lysine
- Methionine
- Phenylalanine
- Threonine
- Tryptophan
- Valine

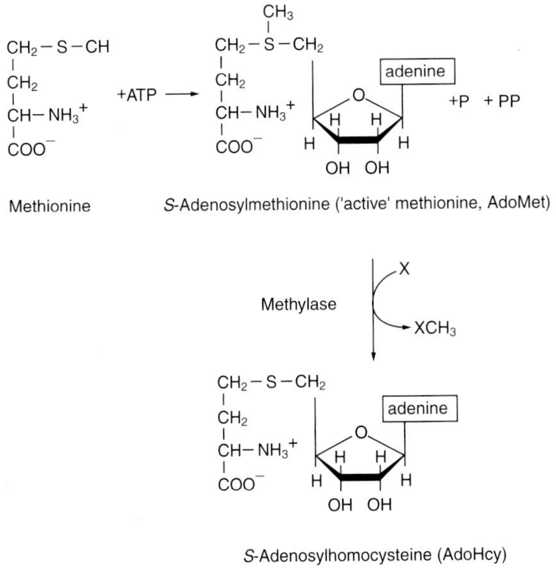

Fig. 8.14 S-Adenosylmethionine is formed from methionine and ATP.

pathway for the biosynthesis of serine is shown in Fig. 8.12. Glycine and serine are interconverted by the reaction shown in Fig. 8.13, which is also required for the de novo synthesis of glycine.

S-Adenosylmethionine (AdoMet), which acts as a methyl donor in a number of reactions (see, for example, the biosynthetic pathway for adrenaline, p. 125), is formed from methionine and ATP (Fig. 8.14). A generalized reaction for methyl transfer is shown in Fig. 8.15. The first two steps in the pathway for the formation of cysteine involve conversion of S-adenosylmethionine to S-adenosylhomocysteine, by transfer of the methyl group to an acceptor such as

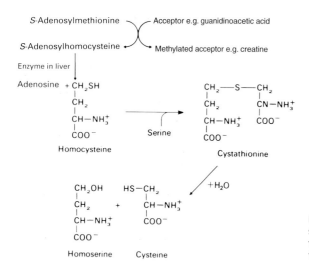

Fig. 8.15 Cysteine is synthesized from serine with the sulfhydryl group derived from methionine.

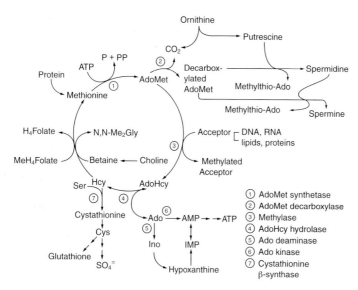

Fig. 8.16 S-Adenosylmethionine is a methyl group donor in many pathways.

1. AdoMet synthetase
2. AdoMet decarboxylase
3. Methylase
4. AdoHcy hydrolase
5. Ado deaminase
6. Ado kinase
7. Cystathionine β-synthase

CATABOLISM OF ESSENTIAL AMINO ACIDS AND THE FORMATION OF ADRENALINE, HISTAMINE, THYROXINE AND SEROTONIN

CATABOLISM OF PHENYLALANINE AND TYROSINE

Phenylalanine can be transaminated to phenylpyruvic acid by a normally minor pathway that is brought into play in the inherited disease phenylketonuria (see below). The normal pathway of phenylalanine degradation is by conversion to tyrosine. The first step in tyrosine degradation is its transamination to 4-hydroxyphenylpyruvate (Fig. 8.18). This undergoes an oxidative decarboxylation, catalysed by 4-hydroxyphenylpyruvate dioxygenase, in which an additional hydroxyl group is introduced into the benzene ring, forming homogentisate. The reaction is complex, involving ascorbate as coenzyme. Further oxidation by homogentisate dioxygenase leads to ring opening and the formation of maleylacetoacetate, which is further degraded to fumarate and acetoacetate as shown in Fig. 8.18.

CLINICAL IMPLICATIONS – THE FIRST INHERITED DISEASES TO BE DESCRIBED

The reactions shown in Fig. 8.18 are noteworthy in that several of the enzymes, if deficient, lead to diseases that were among the first ever to be described as genetic in origin by Archibald Garrod at the beginning of the twentieth century. Among these are alcaptonuria, which results from a deficiency of homogentisate dioxygenase, in which homogentisate accumulates and is excreted in the urine, which can turn black on standing, and albinism, a condition in which there is a lack of pigmentation (e.g. of the skin and hair), which is due to a deficiency of enzymes that form melanin from tyrosine. Another

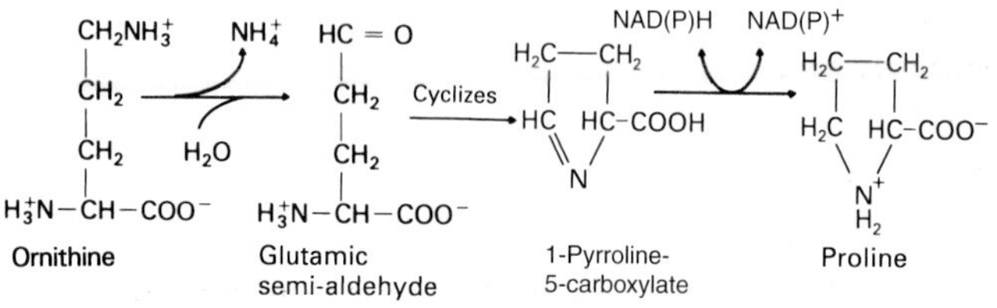

guanidinoacetic acid to form creatine. S-Adenosylhomocysteine (AdoHcy) is then cleaved to adenosine and homocysteine. The homocysteine then reacts with serine, which supplies the carbons and amino group of cysteine, cystathionine being formed, which is then cleaved to homoserine and cysteine.

S-Adenosylmethionine participates in a number of other reactions as shown in Fig. 8.16. Thus, after decarboxylation, it can yield propylamine ($CH_3CH_2CH_2NH_3^+$), which is involved in the biosynthesis of spermine and spermidine, (polyamines important in nucleic acid metabolism). Betaine and methyltetrahydrofolate function as alternative methyl donors in the conversion of homocysteine (Hcy) to methionine. However, in folate deficiency, homocysteine tends to accumulate (see p. 105). Blood levels of homocysteine can be used as an indication of folate status.

Proline is formed from ornithine after removal of the amino group by transamination to form glutamic semi-aldehyde, which cyclizes to 1-pyrroline-5-carboxylate (see Fig. 8.17). This is then reduced by NADH to proline.

Tyrosine is formed from phenylalanine by the action of phenylalanine hydroxylase; this reaction is discussed in the following section.

Fig. 8.17 Proline is synthesized from ornithine.

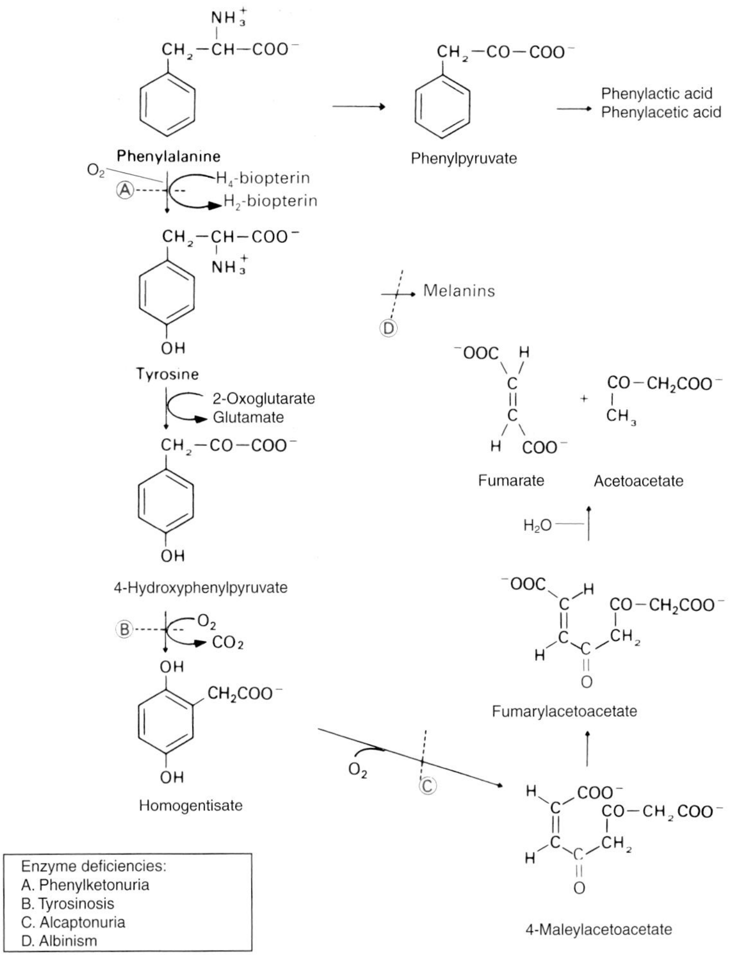

Fig. 8.18 The catabolism of phenylalanine and tyrosine.

Enzyme deficiencies:
A. Phenylketonuria
B. Tyrosinosis
C. Alcaptonuria
D. Albinism

CLINICAL IMPLICATIONS – PHENYLKETONURIA

The inherited disease, phenylketonuria, arises from mutations in the phenylalanine hydroxylase gene. Deficiency of the enzyme results in inability to catabolize phenylalanine, which accumulates in the liver, as a result of which a minor pathway is brought into play transaminating the phenylalanine to phenylpyruvate. If the condition is untreated, severe, irreversible mental retardation results. Phenylketonuria can be diagnosed by detecting phenylpyruvate in the urine of infants. A better way is to use a microbiological test to detect the elevated blood levels of phenylalanine; this is known as the Guthrie test, and permits even earlier detection. The condition is treated by giving a diet low in phenylalanine, using modified protein hydrolysates; this is successful to a considerable extent. Phenylketonuria was the first genetic disease for which a successful therapy was devised. Variants of the disease result from deficiency in synthesis of tetrahydrobiopterin or reduction of dihydrobiopterin. In these cases, administration of 5-hydroxytryptophan, the precursor of serotonin, and DOPA (3,4-dihydroxyphenylalanine), the precursor of catecholamines, prevents a serious deficiency of these neurotransmitters. The sweetening agent, aspartame, is the methyl ester of

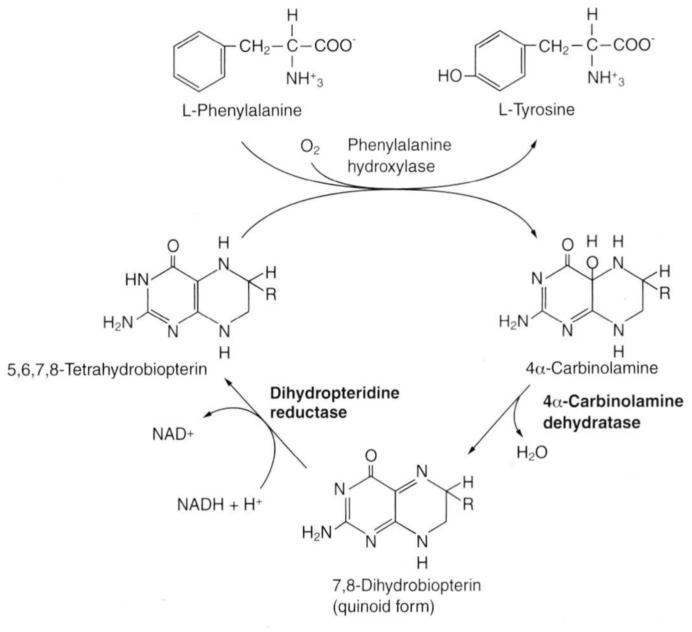

genetic disease associated with this pathway is tyrosinosis, due to a deficiency of 4-hydroxyphenylpyruvate dioxygenase, in which 4-hydroxyphenylpyruvate and tyrosine accumulate in the urine.

PHENYLALANINE HYDROXYLASE

Phenylalanine hydroxylase is one of a family of aromatic amino acid hydroxylases that introduce a hydroxyl group into an aromatic ring; related enzymes are tyrosine hydroxylase and tryptophan hydroxylase. These enzymes share many physical, structural and catalytic characteristics. They are monooxygenases, utilizing molecular oxygen and a pteridine coenzyme, that reduce one oxygen atom to H_2O via 4a-carbinolamine, the other oxygen atom providing the hydroxyl oxygen. In the case of the aromatic amino acid hydroxylases, the coenzyme is tetrahydrobiopterin, which is oxidized to dihydrobiopterin in the course of the reaction. It is then reduced back to tetrahydrobiopterin by dihydropteridine reductase using NADH as coenzyme (see Fig. 8.19).

Fig. 8.19 The phenylalanine hydroxylase reaction.

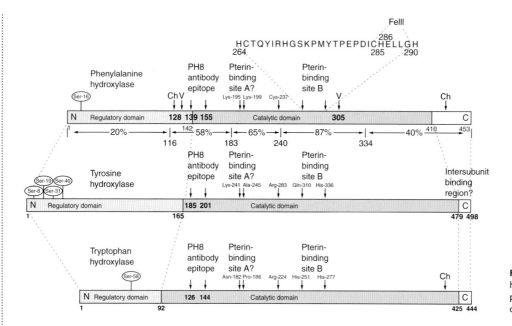

Fig. 8.20 The aromatic amino acid hydroxylases. Ch and V indicate points of cleavage by chymotrypsin and V8 protease.

N-aspartylphenylalanine, and is broken down to phenylalanine by gut bacteria. It should therefore be excluded from diets for patients with phenylketonuria.

The gene encoding phenylalanine hydroxylase is expressed only in liver and is the product of a single locus. About 200 mutations are known. The gene is 65 kb in length with multiple introns; about 10% of mutations are in the introns and affect proper splicing (see Chapter 3). Prenatal diagnosis in families with a history of the disease can be achieved by techniques of molecular genetics to identify the family's specific mutation. Figure 8.20 shows some structure–function relationships among the three aromatic amino acid hydroxylases, which indicate that the genes probably have a common evolutionary origin.

THE FORMATION OF THYROID HORMONES

The synthesis of thyroxine (T$_4$) and triiodothyronine (T$_3$) involves the iodination of tyrosine residues of thyroglobulin, a protein contained in the follicle within the thyroid gland. The reactions are summarized in Fig. 8.21. Within the follicle, colloid that contains thyroglobulin is taken into vesicles in which it is degraded. As outlined in Fig. 8.22, vesicles containing the colloid are taken from the main colloid reserve by a process of phagocytosis, at step (i) in Fig. 8.22. Step (ii) involves the transfer of hydrolytic enzymes from dense granules (g), and this is followed (iii) by digestion of the colloid, a process that can be followed histochemically using a periodic

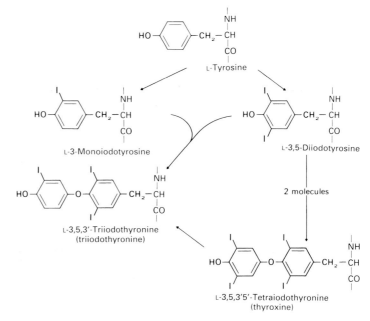

Fig. 8.21 The biosynthesis of thyroxine and triiodothyronine.

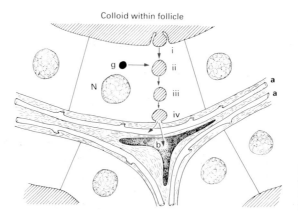

Fig. 8.22 Ultrastructural features of thyroxine biosynthesis. N, cell nucleus. See text for further details.

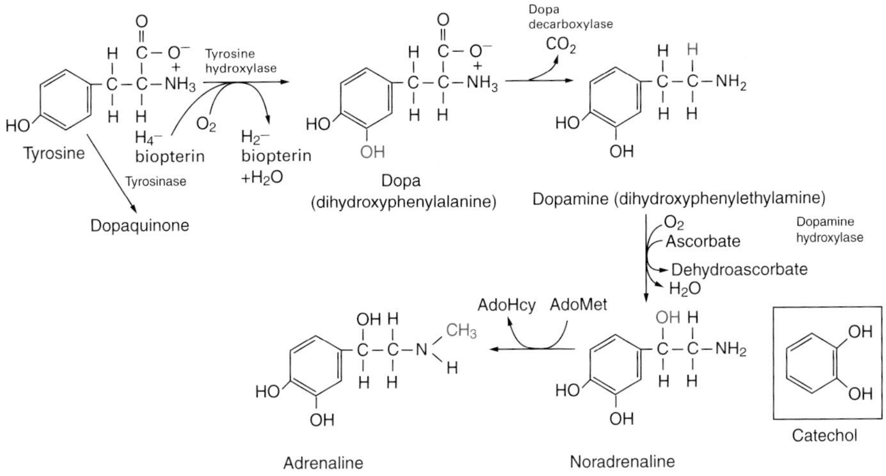

Fig. 8.23 The biosynthesis of adrenaline and noradrenaline from tyrosine.

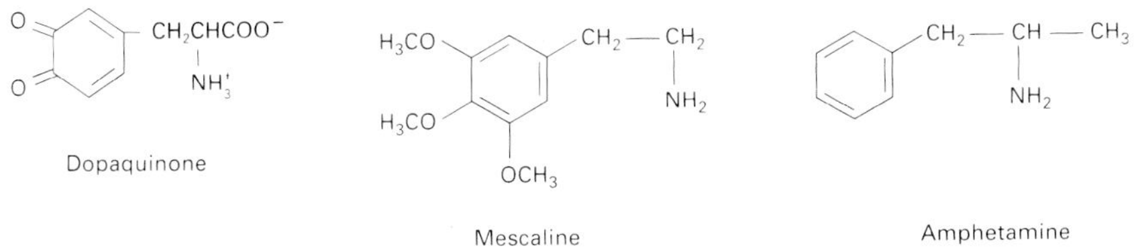

Fig. 8.24 Structures of some catecholamine-related drugs.

acid Schiff reaction, which is specific for carbohydrates. A decrease in staining indicates the breakdown of glycoproteins of the colloid. Extrusion of iodothyronines occurs into the thyroid blood capillary (a) or lymphatic capillary (b) at step (iv). T_4 is the major component secreted and is present in blood at concentrations 20–50-fold higher than those of T_3. However, T_4 is converted in tissues to T_3, which is the component thought to bind to the receptors in the nucleus, leading to an increase in mRNA and protein synthesis.

THE FORMATION OF ADRENALINE (EPINEPHRINE) AND NORADRENALINE (NOREPINEPHRINE)

Adrenaline and noradrenaline are hormones secreted by the adrenal medulla. Both function as neurotransmitters – adrenaline for some brainstem neurons and noradrenaline in the sympathetic and central nervous systems. They are formed by the biosynthetic pathway shown in Fig. 8.23, and are known as catecholamines because they are catechols (aromatic o-diols) and also contain an amino group. The name also embraces any of their derivatives with these structural characteristics.

The biosynthetic pathway from tyrosine begins with the introduction of a second hydroxyl group into the tyrosine ring by tyrosine 3-monooxygenase (tyrosine

hydroxylase), an enzyme that catalyses a similar type of reaction to that of phenylalanine hydroxylase (p. 123). This is followed by a decarboxylation step to form dopamine. Noradrenaline is formed from dopamine by another hydroxylation, this time introducing an aliphatic hydroxyl at the β position of the dopamine side-chain; the reaction is catalysed by the enzyme dopamine β-monooxygenase, which utilizes ascorbate as a coenzyme to donate hydrogen atoms. Biosynthesis of adrenaline then results from a methylation utilizing S-adenosylmethionine.

Related in structure to dopamine are mescaline, a hallucinogenic drug extracted from the mescal buttons of the spineless peyote cactus, and amphetamine, a synthetic drug that produces a feeling of mental alertness and well-being (see Fig. 8.24).

CLINICAL IMPLICATIONS – PARKINSON'S DISEASE

Dopamine is also involved in neurotransmission. It is particularly important in the substantia nigra, a part of the midbrain so called because of its content of the black pigment, melanin, of which dopaquinone is a precursor, formed from tyrosine by tyrosinase. The substantia nigra is important in mediating motor activity of the brain. Destruction of the nigrostriatal cells in the substantia nigra

causes Parkinson's disease. Symptoms of the disease, such as tremor, can be alleviated by administration of L-DOPA, which crosses the blood–brain barrier and is converted to dopamine, which does not cross the blood–brain barrier and so is not effective when administered directly.

THE FORMATION OF HISTAMINE AND CATABOLISM OF HISTIDINE

Histamine is an important autacoid, i.e. a compound secreted by one cell to act on another, and is formed by histidine carboxylase (see Fig. 8.25). It is acted upon by monoamine oxidase, which inactivates it; the product, imidazolyl aldehyde, is oxidized to imidazolyl acetate, in which form it is excreted in the urine. The other pathway for the degradation of histidine is shown in Fig. 8.26. Formiminoglutamate (FIGLU) is required for the formation of one of the folate coenzymes, formiminotetrahydrofolate (see p. 105). FIGLU accumulates and is excreted in the urine in formiminotransferase deficiency and in folate or vitamin B_{12} deficiency.

THE FORMATION OF SEROTONIN AND THE METABOLISM OF TRYPTOPHAN

Tryptophan serves as the precursor of two important compounds, serotonin and nicotinamide. Serotonin

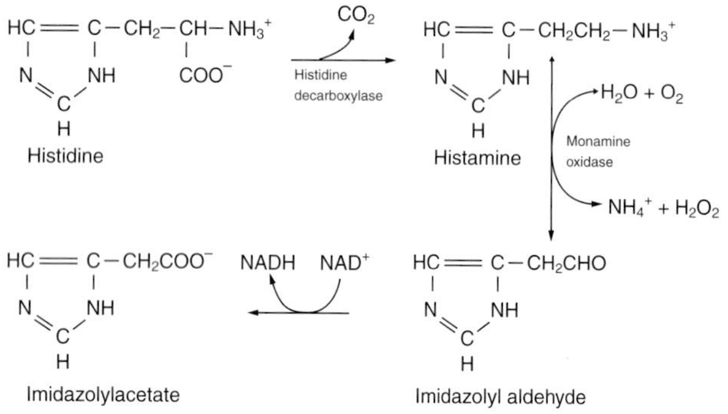

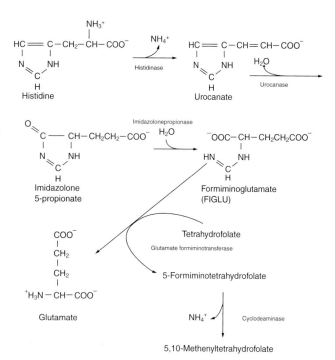

Fig. 8.25 The biosynthesis and catabolism of histamine.

Fig. 8.26 The metabolism of histidine.

Phosphocreatine and creatine can be metabolized to creatinine. This breakdown is fairly constant over a 24-hour period, and urinary creatinine is often used as a reference substance in assessing metabolite excretion in urine.

γ-AMINOBUTYRIC ACID

γ-Aminobutyric acid, $NH_2CH_2CH_2CH_2COOH$, normally referred to by its abbreviation, GABA, is formed by glutamate decarboxylase, which removes the α-carboxyl group of glutamate. It acts as an inhibitory neurotransmitter in the brain, as does glycine. Other amino acids or their derivatives that have neurotransmitter function include glutamate, adrenaline, noradrenaline, dopamine, histamine and serotonin (5-hydroxytryptamine), the formation of all of which has been described. Their action in the brain is independent of the blood concentration, where some of these circulate as hormones. The neurotransmitter function of GABA is involved in some of the effects of vitamin B_6 deficiency.

THE BIOSYNTHESIS AND METABOLISM OF HEME

BIOSYNTHESIS OF HEME

As a component of hemoglobin, cytochromes, myoglobin and various heme-containing enzymes, heme is of central importance. Its biosynthesis in erythroid and non-erythroid tissues is finely but distinctly regulated by feedback inhibition – by heme – of 5-aminolevulinate (ALA) synthase (ALAS), the initial and rate-limiting step in heme biosynthesis (Fig. 8.29). Heme biosynthesis begins with the formation of ALA from succinyl CoA and glycine by the pyridoxine-dependent ALA synthase. Two molecules of ALA condense to form porphobilinogen (PBG), the reaction being catalysed by the thiol-dependent enzyme ALA dehydratase (ALAD). This enzyme is inhibited by Pb^{2+} and thus chronic lead poisoning leads to a secondary porphyria with anemia, abdominal pain and neurological symptoms as found in certain porphyrias (see below). Four molecules of PBG condense to form the transient intermediate hydroxymethylbilane (HMB) catalysed by the enzyme

(5-hydroxytryptamine) is formed by hydroxylation of tryptophan by tryptophan monooxygenase followed by decarboxylation. Serotonin is a neurotransmitter with varied and widespread effects. The pathway by which it is degraded is shown in Fig. 8.27. Some types of mood changes and depression are associated with the levels of serotonin in the brain. The action of some antidepressant drugs, e.g. Prozac and Seroxat, is related to their ability to inhibit serotonin reuptake into the presynaptic neuron.

Also shown in Fig. 8.27, a pathway exists in animals, including humans, for the biosynthesis of nicotinamide adenine dinucleotide (NAD) from tryptophan. However, if tryptophan levels in the diet are low, this pathway might not be sufficiently active to form adequate amounts of nicotinamide, and deficiency symptoms, leading to pellagra, may occur.

PHOSPHOCREATINE

Some reactions of nitrogen metabolism that are important in muscle involve creatine, a guanidinium compound derived from arginine, as shown in Fig. 8.28. The guanidinium group can be phosphorylated by the enzyme creatine kinase, using ATP as phosphorylating agent, and the product, phosphocreatine can react with ADP to form ATP and creatine. During muscular contraction, a sudden drop in ATP levels leads to the formation of ATP by creatine kinase. This provides ATP to sustain contraction in the interval before glycolysis is activated.

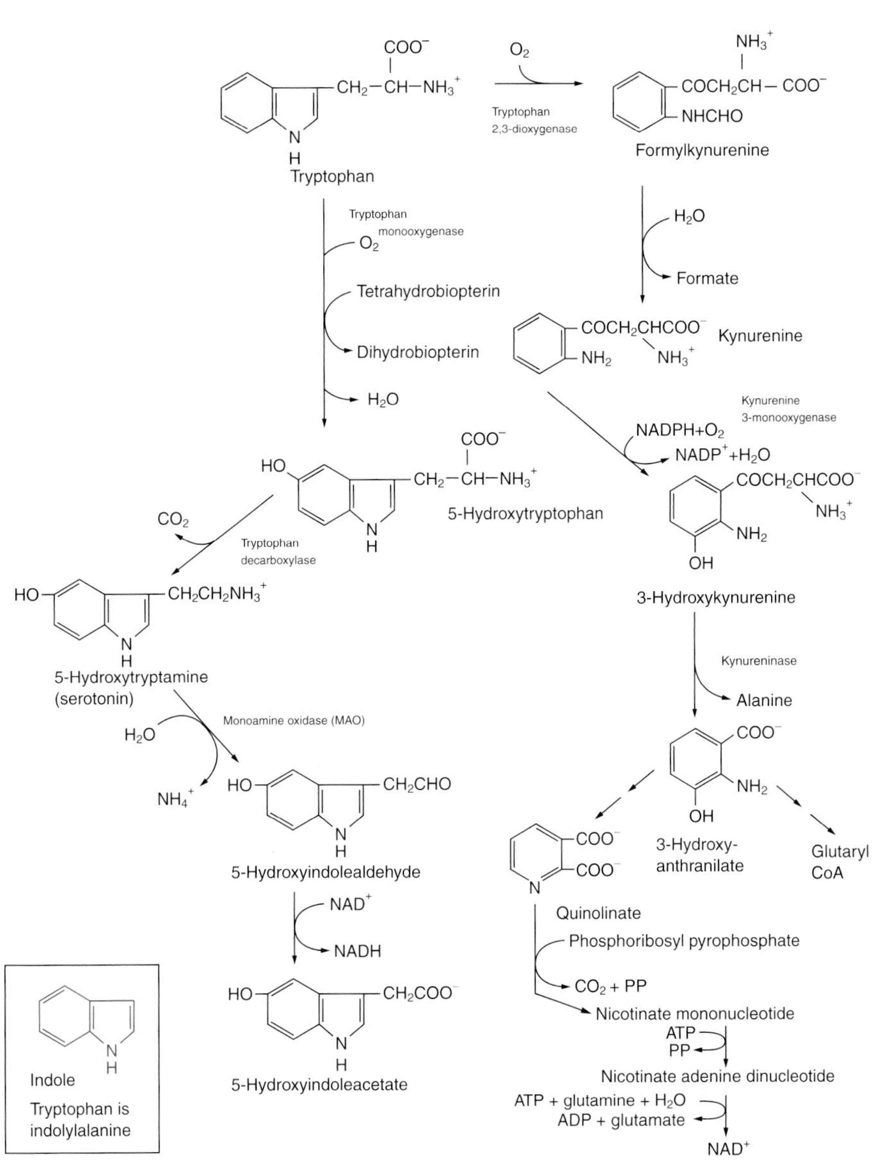

Fig. 8.27 The catabolism of tryptophan.

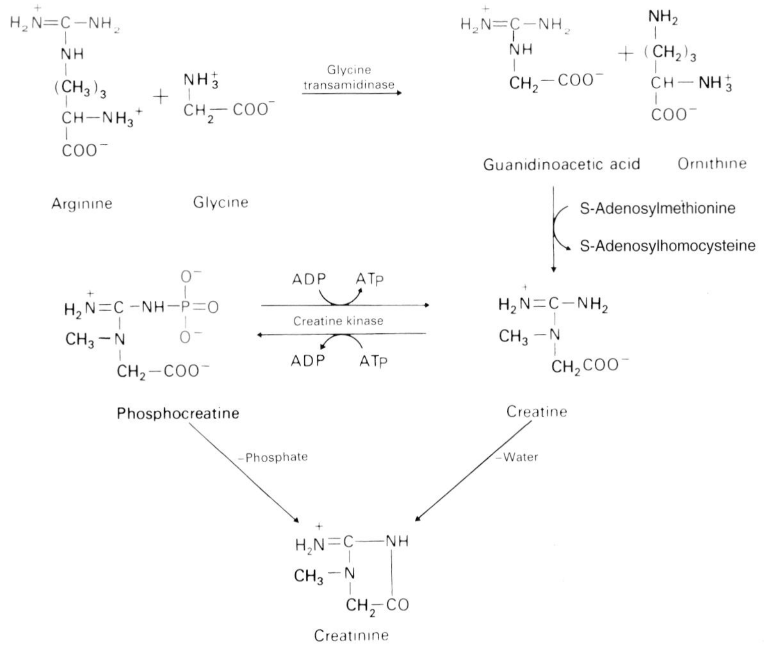

Fig. 8.28 The biosynthesis of creatine and creatinine from arginine and glycine.

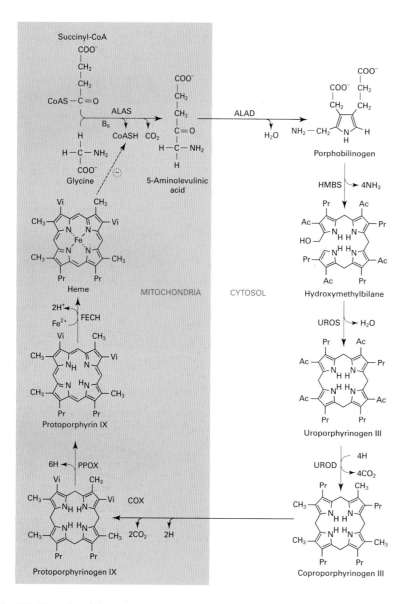

only the latter can be further oxidized to form protoporphyrin IX and thus lead to heme synthesis. These latter three enzymes coproporphyrinogen oxidase (COX), protoporphyrinogen oxidase (PPOX) and ferrochelatase (FECH) are mitochondrial enzymes and deliver heme in to the proximity of ALA synthase, also a mitochondrial enzyme. The other enzymes are cytosolic and thus are found in high concentrations in erythrocytes and may be readily assayed for diagnostic purposes. Ferrochelatase specifically requires Fe^{2+}, and free fatty acids facilitate the enzyme activity. The pathway is regulated by feedback inhibition by heme of ALA synthase (see Fig. 8.30).

CLINICAL IMPLICATIONS – THE PORPHYRIAS

The genes for the eight enzymes of heme biosynthesis have been fully characterized and a wide variety of mutations give rise to the genetic porphyrias (Table 8.5). Broadly, they are classified into the acute neuropsychiatric (hepatic), cutaneous or mixed porphyrias.

Acute porphyrias

The acute porphyrias are characterized by recurrent attacks of abdominal pain accompanied by vomiting, constipation, muscle pains and weakness with variable psychological consequences. Untreated, there might be progressive paralysis, epileptic seizures, severe metabolic disturbances and death. The currently proposed pathogenic mechanisms involve neurotoxicity due to excess ALA levels, but heme deficiency and free-radical-mediated cytotoxicity have also been suggested.

Fig. 8.29 The pathway for the biosynthesis of heme. Ac, acetic $-CH_2COO^-$; ALAD, ALA dehydratase; ALAS, ALA synthase; COX, coproporphyrinogen oxidase; FECH, ferrochelatase; HMBS, HMB synthase; PPOX, protoporphyrinogen oxidase; Pr, propionic $-CH_2CH_2COO^-$; UROD, uroporphyrinogen decarboxylase; UROS, uroporphyrinogen III synthase; Vi, vinyl $-CH{:}CH_2$.

hydroxymethylbilane synthase (HMBS, formerly known as PBG deaminase). Dipyrrole intermediates are formed during its synthesis by the second most rate-limiting enzyme in the pathway. HMB can cyclize non-enzymatically to form uroporphyrinogen I, whereas uroporphyrinogen III synthase (UROIIIS) catalyses the biologically active III isomer. Uroporphyrinogen I and III differ only in that the order of the carboxymethyl, or acetic (Ac) and carboxyethyl or propionic (Pr) side-chains are reversed on one of the pyrrole rings. Although both can be decarboxylated by uroporphyrinogen decarboxylase (UROD) to form, respectively, coproporphyrinogen I and III,

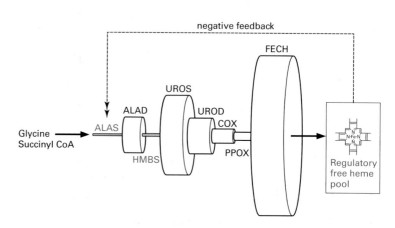

Fig. 8.30 Hepatic heme biosynthesis as a metabolic pipeline. Abbreviations as for Fig. 8.29. Regulatory enzymes are shown in red. ALAS is the primary regulatory enzyme, HMBS is considered a secondary regulator, as coproporphyrinogen and protoporphyrinogen are selective inhibitors of HMBS (see text for mixed porphyrias).

Table 8.5 The genetic porphyrias

Pathway	Enzyme deficiency	Disease	Clinical features	Diagnostic tests
Succinyl CoA + Glycine ↓ δ-Aminolevulinic acid (ALA) ↓	ALA synthase	Not reported	–	–
	ALA dehydratase	Doss porphyria (AR)	Abdominal pain	Raised urinary ALA and coproporphyrinogen III
Porphobilinogen (PBG) ↓	HMB synthase	Acute intermittent porphyria (AD)	Abdominal pain Gastrointestinal disturbance Motor and autonomic neuropathy	Raised urinary ALA, PBG and porphyrins
Hydroxymethylbilane (HMB) ↓	Uroporphyrinogen III synthase	Congenital erythropoietic porphyria (AR)	Severe skin lesions Hemolytic anemia	Normal urinary ALA and PBG Raised urinary and fecal porphyrins Raised erythrocyte protoporphyrins
Uroporphyrinogen III ↓	Uroporphyrinogen decarboxylase	Porphyria cutanea tarda (AD)[a]	Marked skin lesions	Normal urinary ALA and PBG Increased urinary and fecal porphyrins
Coproporphyrinogen ↓	Coproporphyrinogen oxidase	Hereditary coproporphyria (AD)	Neuropsychiatric features ± skin lesion	Raised urinary ALA and PBG Increased urinary and fecal coproporphyrinogen III
Protoporphyrinogen ↓	Protoporphyrinogen oxidase	Variegate (S African) porphyria (AD)	Neuropsychiatric features ± skin lesion	Characteristic plasma fluorescence Raised fecal porphyrins
Protoporphyrin IX ↓ Heme	Ferrochelatase	Erythropoietic protoporphyria (AD)[b]	Acute photosensitivity Mild anemia	Increased erythrocyte and fecal protoporphyrins

AR, autosomal recessive; AD, autosomal dormant.
(AD)[a] 15% of patients with porphyria cutanea tarda are hereditary; the majority are due to liver damage in susceptible individuals.
(AD)[b] Co-inheritance of a ferrochelatase expression allele and severe ferrochelatase defect required for clinical expression.

Therapy aims to reduce ALA synthase activity by raising intracellular free heme with infusions of heme salts, high-carbohydrate feeding and administering heme oxygenase inhibitors. Approximately 75% of acute attacks involve a precipitating cause, including:

- administration of porphyrinogenic drugs, most of which act by inducing hepatic cytochrome P450 enzymes
- altered sex hormone status resulting from either exogenously administered hormones or premenstrual/pregnancy alterations
- infections, malignant disease or undue stress.

Avoidance of precipitating agents is an important strategy of patient care. It is believed that the raised levels of PBG, ALA and circulating porphyrins are produced in the liver, hence their classification as acute hepatic porphyrias. Liver transplantation has proved highly effective in a patient with persistent recurrent attacks of acute intermittent porphyria.

Cutaneous porphyrias

Cutaneous porphyrias are characterized by marked photosensitivity with or without severe tissue destruction. UV photoactivation of the high levels of porphyrin intermediates in cutaneous tissues leads to cellular damage. Treatment involves avoidance of sunlight, use of UV-blocking creams, avoidance or removal of hepatotoxic agents, use of β-carotene as a cytoprotective antioxidant and in certain forms of porphyria, use of chloroquine as a porphyrin complexing agent facilitating their urinary excretion.

Mixed porphyrias

Both cutaneous and acute neuropsychiatric symptoms occur in mixed porphyria. The pathogenesis of the acute attacks in patients with mixed porphyria, i.e. variegate porphyria and hereditary coproporphyria is of interest. There is evidence that accumulating coproporphyrinogen and protoporphyrinogen are selective inhibitors of HMBS, effectively mimicking acute intermittent porphyria with raised levels of ALA and PBG.

CLINICAL IMPLICATIONS – METABOLISM OF HEME

Heme is oxidized progressively to methemoglobin, biliverdin and bilirubin (Fig. 8.31) with conjugation to form bilirubin mono- and di-glucuronide (Fig. 8.32). This is catalysed by the inducible cytochrome P450 enzyme heme oxygenase, followed by biliverdin reductase. Conjugation of bilirubin is by hepatic bilirubin UDP glucuronyl transferase, genetic deficiency of which leads to accumulation of the lipophilic unconjugated bilirubin (Crigler–Najjar

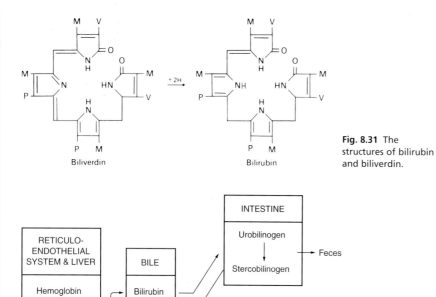

Fig. 8.31 The structures of bilirubin and biliverdin.

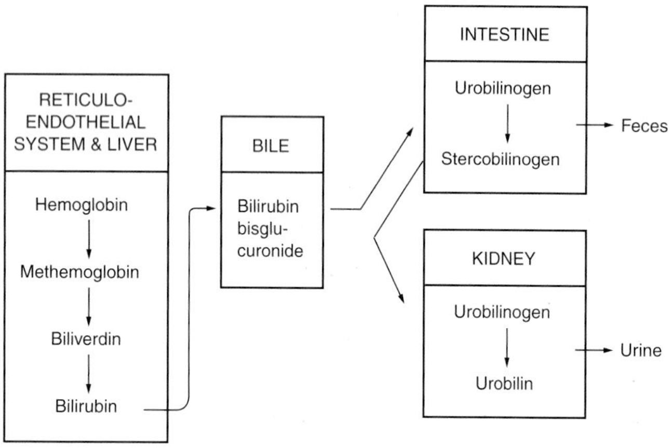

Fig. 8.32 The metabolic fate and excretion of biliverdin and bilirubin.

syndrome). Presenting at birth the neurotoxic free bilirubin causes serious CNS damage, particularly of the basal ganglia, resulting in kernicterus. Administration of heme oxygenase inhibitors limits bilirubin formation. Use of exchange blood transfusions, exposure to UV light to catalyse the photoisomerization of bilirubins to non-toxic forms and administration of phenobarbitone, which induces conjugases, are other therapeutic strategies.

Note that conjugated bilirubin glucuronide is water soluble and excreted in both bile and urine. Biliary obstruction either within the liver, in the bile duct or gall bladder leads to jaundice with pale stools and dark urine. Jaundice due to impaired conjugation as a result of excess red cell breakdown (hemolysis) or genetic or acquired defects in conjugation due to hepatic damage leads to jaundice with increased urinary bilirubin excretion.

9

Oxidative catabolism of glucose and fatty acids

This chapter describes the forces driving metabolic reactions, together with the mechanisms by which cells achieve energetically unfavourable reactions. A sequence of chemical reactions follows the same rules as single reactions and proceeds in a direction that exhibits a negative free energy change. As complex molecules in general have high molar free energy, their biosynthesis must occur in a series of partial reactions linked to other reactions releasing energy to 'drive' the coupled reaction. This often involves reactions in which ATP is a substrate, because the partial reaction resulting in the hydrolysis of its phosphate anhydride bond exhibits a large negative free energy change. A continual regeneration of ATP to drive synthetic processes is achieved by coupling the formation of ATP with the oxidation of glucose (glycolysis) or fatty acids (β-oxidation); both of these catabolic processes are exergonic. The products of glycolysis and β-oxidation are further oxidized to CO_2 and H_2O by the citric acid cycle and electron transport chain of heme-containing cytochromes, with further formation of ATP (oxidative phosphorylation).

β-OXIDATION AND GLYCOLYSIS

FORCES DRIVING METABOLIC PROCESSES

It has been explained (p. 89) that chemical reactions proceed in a direction that results in negative free energy change. The sequences of reactions that form metabolic pathways are governed by the same set of thermodynamic rules as individual reactions, i.e. they proceed in a direction such that the products, at any instant in time, are of lower free energy than the reactants. In general, the degradation of large molecules to smaller molecules is a process associated with a negative free energy change, because oxidation processes are exothermic. The synthesis of large molecules from smaller molecules is a process leading to an increase in free energy of the molecules synthesized, so reactions of synthetic pathways include partial reactions having a negative free energy change that drive the pathway in the direction of synthesis. Remember that the overall free energy change of a reaction is the sum of the free energy changes of the partial reactions of which it is composed. Thus, as explained on p. 90, the inclusion of the partial reaction ATP → ADP + P, which has a large negative free energy change, can be linked to a biosynthetic partial reaction with a positive, but smaller, free energy change, so that the reaction proceeds in the direction of biosynthesis.

Ultimately, all life depends on the utilization of energy emitted by the sun. The process of photosynthesis uses photons to drive the formation of carbohydrates from carbon dioxide and water, and all animal life depends on the nutrients produced by this process (Fig. 9.1). The strategy employed by living organisms to provide the energy required for organized existence is thus to obtain nutrients that can be subjected to oxidation, and thereby provide components such as ATP that can react in synthetic pathways to ensure those pathways exhibit an overall negative free energy change. The concentration of the reactants contributes to the free energy change of a reaction. Thus, if the concentration of NADPH is much greater than that of NADP⁺ then, in a particular cell compartment, reactions utilizing NADPH will proceed in the direction resulting in reduction of any cosubstrate. This is another device used for driving pathways of synthetic reactions. These concepts are summarized in Fig. 9.2.

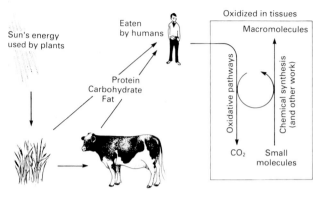

Fig. 9.1 Metabolic energy is derived ultimately from the sun.

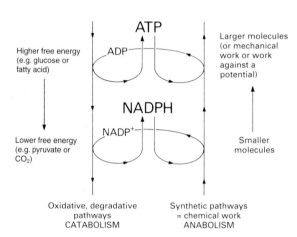

Fig. 9.2 Nicotinamide and adenine nucleotides link catabolic and anabolic pathways.

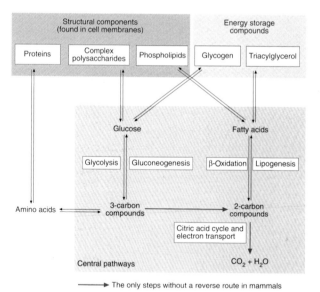

Fig. 9.3 Map of the major routes of metabolism.

The end-products of biosynthesis are of two types: structural components and energy-storage compounds. As shown in Fig. 9.3, there is a continual synthesis and degradation of all these components, the major intermediates being amino acids, glucose and fatty acids. An important step, indicated by the red arrow in Fig. 9.3, has fundamental implications for the interaction of carbohydrate and lipid metabolism, in that once the three-carbon compound pyruvate has been converted to the two-carbon acetyl radical (acetyl CoA) it is not possible for this to be utilized for net synthesis of carbohydrate.

THE MAJOR OXIDATIVE PATHWAYS OF THE CELL

The pathways, summarized in Fig. 9.4, that generate the major part of the ATP and NADH formed in the cell are:

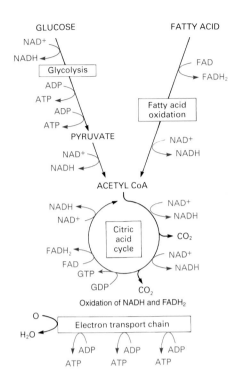

Fig. 9.4 Outline of pathways oxidizing glucose and fatty acid.

- glycolysis
- fatty acid oxidation
- the citric acid cycle
- electron transport coupled to oxidative phosphorylation.

Of the two initial substrates for these two pathways, fatty acid is in a considerably more reduced state than glucose (see Fig. 9.5) because most of its carbons are fully reduced, whereas all the carbons of glucose already bear one oxygen atom. On total combustion, the heat produced from fat is 37 kJ g^{-1}, whereas the amount for carbohydrate is 16 kJ g^{-1} (Fig. 9.6). Thus fat provides a more condensed form of energy for storage than carbohydrate, and the energy reserves of a well-fed animal consist mainly of its adipose tissue.

THE β-OXIDATION PATHWAY OF FATTY ACIDS

Fatty acids are oxidized in the mitochondria. A fatty acid is degraded step by step by the sequential removal of two-carbon units. Coenzyme A (CoA) is linked to the carboxyl carbon of the fatty acid as the first step in the oxidation process, forming the fatty acyl CoA derivative. Each two-carbon unit is liberated from the fatty acid as acetyl CoA. The mechanism is summarized in Fig. 9.7, in the inset of which is shown the succession of reactions

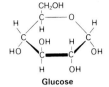

Glucose

CH$_3$CH$_2$CH$_2$CH$_2$CH$_2$CH$_2$CH$_2$CH$_2$CH$_2$CH$_2$CH$_2$CH$_2$CH$_2$CH$_2$CH$_2$COOH
Palmitic acid (a fatty acid)

Fig. 9.5 Glucose is in a more oxidized state than palmitic acid.

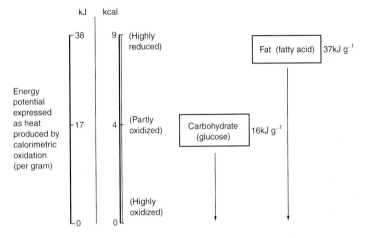

Fig. 9.6 More energy is released by oxidation of fatty acid than of glucose.

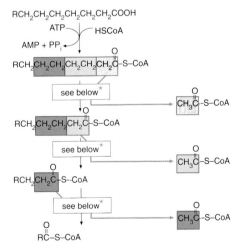

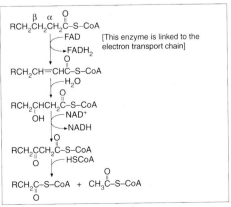

Fig. 9.7 The β-oxidation pathway of fatty acid catabolism.

that occurs for the removal of each two–carbon unit. First, a double bond is introduced at the β-carbon (hence the name of the pathway) by a flavoprotein that is a protein of the mitochondrial inner membrane. This is followed by addition of water across this double bond, oxidation of the secondary alcohol group to a carbonyl group and cleavage of the molecule by CoA to yield acetyl CoA and a fatty acyl CoA that is two carbons shorter than the starting material. The flavoprotein, fatty acyl CoA dehydrogenase, that initiates the oxidation process passes two electrons to the electron transport chain as indicated in Fig. 9.7 (inset), and the oxidation of the secondary alcohol yields a molecule of NADH. Both processes lead to ATP formation by oxidative phosphorylation (described below). The overall reaction requires the supply of half as many molecules of CoA as there are carbons in the fatty acid (Fig. 9.8), but the CoA is released at the first step of the citric acid cycle.

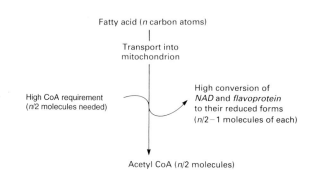

Fig. 9.8 $n/2$ molecules of acetyl CoA are formed from n carbons of fatty acid.

PEROXISOMAL FATTY ACID OXIDATION

In mammals, β-oxidation occurs in both mitochondria and peroxisomes. In mitochondria, it is confined to fatty acids up to 20 carbons long, its primary function being energy provision. In peroxisomes, it has special functions in retailoring very long-chain fatty acids and C_{27} bile acid intermediates, and degrading very long-chain fatty acids, branched chain acids, prostanoids and dicarboxylic acids. The sequence of reactions is similar in both organelles but the peroxisomal reactions are catalyzed by different acyl-CoA oxidases, which form H_2O_2 for the desaturation step, different multifunctional proteins (carrying out hydration plus dehydrogenation) and different thiolases. In human liver, there is an acyl-CoA oxidase for straight-chain fatty acids and one for β-methyl acids. There is also an α-oxidation enzyme deficiency of which leads to accumulation of phytanic acid, a plant acid that accumulates in Refsum disease. Failure to oxidize very long-chain fatty acids occurs in adrenoleukodystrophy. These disorders of peroxisomal metabolism may result from deficiency either of individual enzymes or of peroxisomal membrane proteins leading to deficient transport or impaired peroxisome formation.

THE GLYCOLYTIC PATHWAY

The oxidation of glucose to pyruvate is termed glycolysis. As shown in Fig. 9.9,

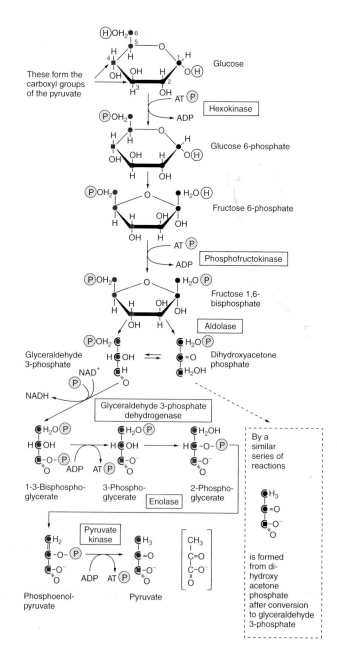

Fig. 9.9 The glycolytic pathway. Fluoride inhibits enolase, and is added to blood collection tubes to prevent glycolysis.

the first reaction of the pathway brings about the phosphorylation of C-6 of the glucose molecule by hexokinase. The resulting glucose 6-phosphate is converted to fructose 6-phosphate by glucose-6-phosphate isomerase, and fructose 1,6-bisphosphate is then formed by phosphofructokinase. The action of aldolase splits the fructose 1,6-bisphosphate to the two three-carbon compounds, glyceraldehyde 3-phosphate and dihydroxyacetone phosphate; these two molecules exist in an equilibrium catalysed by triose-phosphate isomerase. Glyceraldehyde 3-phosphate is then converted to 1,3-bisphosphoglycerate in a reaction that involves oxidation of C-1 to a carboxyl group with linkage to phosphate to form an anhydride; both reactions are achieved within a single enzymic mechanism, utilizing orthophosphate as the substrate for the phosphorylation. This remarkable step yields a molecule with a very high potential for further reaction, a potential that is utilized immediately in the formation of ATP and 3-phosphoglycerate. This formation of the phosphate anhydride by an enzyme of the cytosol is termed substrate-level phosphorylation to distinguish it from oxidative phosphorylation.

After conversion of 3-phosphoglycerate to 2-phosphoglycerate, another remarkable mechanism comes into play that leads again to substrate level phosphorylation. The enzyme enolase removes water across the C-2,3 bond, and thereby creates another reactive phosphate which is immediately utilized in phosphorylating ADP to ATP. Thus, as outlined in Fig. 9.10, the glycolytic pathway has a net yield of two ATP molecules. In addition, it yields one molecule of NADH, which, if the hydrogen is transported into the mitochondrion via the glycerophosphate shuttle (see p. 141), can give rise to a further three ATP molecules by oxidative phosphorylation.

REACTIONS OF PYRUVATE

To be further metabolized, the pyruvate produced by glycolysis must be converted to acetyl CoA (Fig. 9.11). This is achieved by the enzyme pyruvate dehydrogenase. This enzyme is a complex of three subunits, the reactions of which have already been described in the section on thiamine diphosphate (p. 102). In addition, pyruvate can be converted to oxaloacetate by pyruvate carboxylase, a reaction

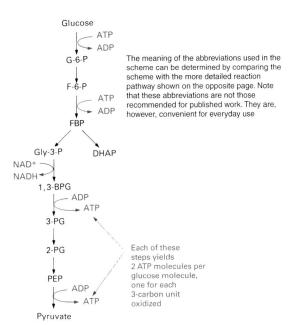

The meaning of the abbreviations used in the scheme can be determined by comparing the scheme with the more detailed reaction pathway shown on the opposite page. Note that these abbreviations are not those recommended for published work. They are, however, convenient for everyday use

Each of these steps yields 2 ATP molecules per glucose molecule, one for each 3-carbon unit oxidized

Fig. 9.10 There is a net yield of 2 moles of ATP from each mole of glucose oxidized by glycolysis.

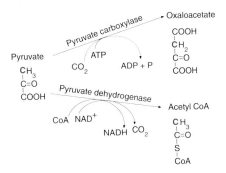

Fig. 9.11 Pyruvate is metabolized to acetyl CoA by pyruvate dehydrogenase and to oxaloacetate by pyruvate carboxylase.

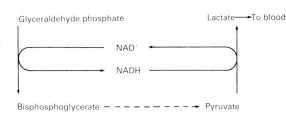

Fig. 9.12 Lactate dehydrogenase reduces NAD^+ to NADH to sustain glycolysis in anaerobic metabolism.

requiring biotin (described in more detail on p. 104). The regulation of all these activities will be discussed in a later section (Chapter 13).

METABOLISM OF LACTATE

Lactate is produced by red blood cells as an end-product of glycolysis, the pathway on which the erythrocyte depends for ATP formation. As these cells possess no mitochondria, the NADH formed by glyceraldehyde phosphate dehydrogenase cannot be oxidized by the respiratory chain, and reacts with pyruvate to form lactate, a reaction catalysed by lactate dehydrogenase, which thereby regenerates

NAD^+ for the continued operation of the glycolytic pathway, as shown in Fig. 9.12.

A similar situation results in white muscle when muscular activity is so great that the amount of NADH produced exceeds the capacity of the muscle mitochondria to oxidize it, a situation that leads to what is termed anaerobic oxidation. It should be appreciated that a sprinter is actually using about ten times more oxygen during a sprint than at rest. Despite this, the lactate produced is in excess of the amounts that can be oxidized.

The lactate produced by muscle is taken up from the blood by liver and used as a substrate for gluconeogenesis, as indicated on p. 148.

THE CITRIC ACID CYCLE

OUTLINE OF THE CITRIC ACID CYCLE

Oxaloacetate and acetyl CoA condense to form citrate, and a succession of enzymes then act on the citrate to convert it to oxaloacetate, a process that removes two carbons as CO_2, as shown in Fig. 9.13. In addition, eight hydrogen-atom equivalents are removed. The oxaloacetate that is thereby regenerated reacts with a further molecule of acetyl CoA and the process is repeated. Thus, theoretically, one molecule of oxaloacetate can function in the oxidation of an infinite number of molecules of acetyl CoA. It is as if the oxaloacetate is functioning as a catalyst, being continually regenerated after each turn of the reaction sequence. As will be explained below, the hydrogen atoms that are removed can be oxidized through the electron transport chain, yielding ATP. This sequence of reactions occurs in virtually every type of cell, with rare exceptions such as the erythrocyte. The cycle is shown in more detail in Fig. 9.14.

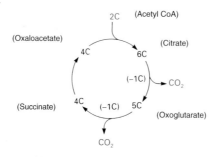

Fig. 9.13 Two carbons are removed as CO_2 in each turn of the citric acid cycle.

Note how the reactions for oxidation of succinate to oxaloacetate, shown in the inset, are similar to those involved in fatty acid oxidation.

An important general point of enzymology was made as a result of the study of citrate synthase, the enzyme that forms citrate from oxaloacetate and acetyl CoA. Citrate is a non-chiral molecule (p. 9), having a plane of symmetry, and at first sight it would appear that it could bind to the enzyme in either of two ways,

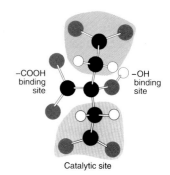

Fig. 9.15 Citric acid is metabolized stereospecifically.

as the outer carboxyl groups seem essentially equivalent. However, it became evident that, if the molecule is presented to a surface that can recognize both the hydroxyl group and the carboxyl group on the central carbon so that these can only bind at unique sites, then the two outer carboxyl groups become distinguishable, the same carboxyl always binding at the catalytic site, as shown in Fig. 9.15.

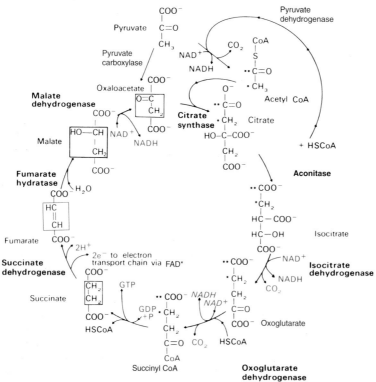

*FAD of succinate dehydrogenase

Note the reaction sequence

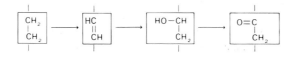

Fig. 9.14 The citric acid cycle reactions.

INTERACTIONS OF GLYCOLYSIS AND THE CITRIC ACID CYCLE WITH OTHER PATHWAYS

These major oxidative pathways also function as routes linking other pathways. In a number of cases the enzymes of the glycolytic pathway connect the pathway with others involved in fatty acid and triacylglycerol biosynthesis, and the metabolism of amino acids. These links are indicated in Fig. 9.16. The citric acid cycle also acts as a junction linking pathways of carbohydrate, lipid and amino acid metabolism, as shown in Fig. 9.17. In particular, oxaloacetate is a key substance to and from which glycolysis and gluconeogenesis lead, and oxaloacetate and oxoglutarate link to amino acid metabolism. Citrate is exported from the mitochondrion for lipogenesis.

THE ELECTRON TRANSPORT CHAIN

STRUCTURAL ASPECTS OF MITOCHONDRIA AND THE ELECTRON TRANSPORT CHAIN

The mitochondrion has an inner compartment, known as the matrix, which is surrounded by a membrane known as the inner membrane, as shown in Fig. 9.18 (also p. 3 and p. 47). Most of the enzymes of the electron transport chain are integral proteins of the inner membrane. There is an outer membrane surrounding the entire mitochondrion, and the space between the inner and outer membranes is termed the intermembrane space. The inner membrane invaginates into the matrix to give areas of intermembrane space permeating the central areas of the mitochondrion. These invaginations are known as cristae (see p. 138).

The inner membrane is not freely permeable but contains transport enzymes that translocate ATP, ADP and other anions (see p. 141). NADH and other nicotinamide nucleotides cannot cross the inner membrane. The outer membrane is freely permeable to ATP, ADP and other small molecules.

In simple outline, electron transport involves the removal of hydrogen atoms from oxidizable substrates, notably NADH, succinate and fatty acid; these hydrogen atoms enter the electron transport chain, a system of membrane-bound complexes (Fig. 9.19) and each is soon split to yield a proton and an electron. The electrons then pass through a series of enzymes known as cytochromes, finally reacting with

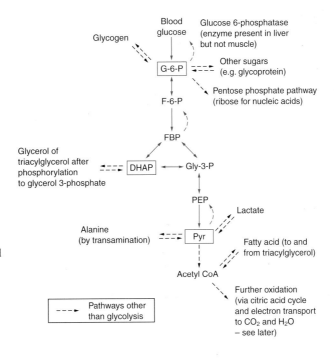

Fig. 9.16 The glycolytic pathway interconnects lipid and protein metabolism.

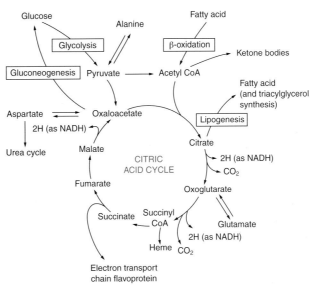

Fig. 9.17 The citric acid cycle acts as a hub between protein, carbohydrate and lipid metabolism.

dioxygen (molecular oxygen, O_2) and the protons that were released earlier, to form water. Figure 9.19 gives a schematic of this process for NADH and succinate.

OXIDATION OF NADH AND SUCCINATE

NADH produced by the citric acid cycle diffuses to the electron transport chain, where the flavoprotein enzyme, NADH dehydrogenase, oxidizes it to NAD^+. This involves transfer of a hydride ion to the enzyme flavin, in this case FMN, which then also accepts a proton to form $FMNH_2$. A hydride ion consists of a hydrogen nucleus with two associated

electrons, and can be denoted as H^-. Hydride ions do not have an independent existence, but sometimes represent the moiety transferred in biological reduction processes, as is the case here.

Succinate dehydrogenase, the citric acid cycle enzyme that converts succinate to fumarate, is an integral protein of the mitochondrial inner membrane associated with the enzymes of the respiratory chain. It is a flavoprotein, having FAD as coenzyme, and is the only membrane-bound enzyme of the citric acid cycle, linking the cycle directly to the respiratory chain.

$FMNH_2$ and $FADH_2$ are oxidized by enzymes that transfer the hydrogen atoms

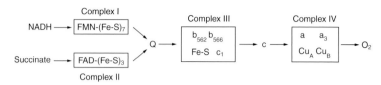

Fig. 9.19 Outline of the electron transport chain. Cytochromes are represented by b_{562}, b_{566}, c_1, c, a and a_3. Fe–S, iron–sulfur complexes; Cu, copper ions.

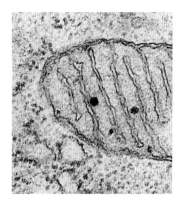

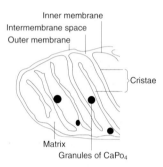

Fig. 9.18 The ultrastructure of the mitochondrion.

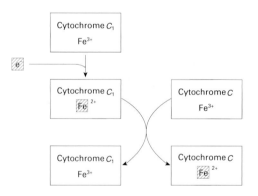

Ubiquinone, oxidized form
(Coenzyme Q, CoQ)

Ubisemiquinone

Dihydroubiquinone, ubiquinol (QH₂)

Fig. 9.20 The structure of ubiquinone.

Cytochrome C_1
Fe^{3+}

Cytochrome C_1
Fe^{2+}

Cytochrome C
Fe^{3+}

Cytochrome C_1
Fe^{3+}

Cytochrome C
Fe^{2+}

Fig. 9.21 Electrons pass from one cytochrome heme group to another.

to a molecule of ubiquinone, also known as coenzyme Q (abbreviated to Q), thereby forming reduced ubiquinone (QH₂, also called ubiquinol); the structures of these compounds are shown in Fig. 9.20. Ubiquinone also accepts hydrogens transferred from other molecules that have been oxidized by the electron transport chain, as in β-oxidation or the oxidation of glycerol 3-phosphate. Ubiquinone is a lipid-soluble molecule capable of diffusing through the hydrophobic core of the inner membrane, but it is also bound as a component of complexes II and III (see below), functioning within the complex. Up to this point, the molecules being oxidized transfer two electrons, but electron transfer through the cytochromes is a one-electron process. Ubiquinone has the property that it can form a semiquinone, ubisemiquinone in Fig. 9.20, when it transfers a single electron. This facilitates the transition from two–electron transfer to one-electron transfer, which is necessary as the electrons pass to the subsequent enzymes of the chain, the cytochromes.

THE CYTOCHROMES AND THEIR REDOX POTENTIALS

The enzymes known as the cytochromes were discovered during the 1930s. At that time, a hand-held spectroscope was often

used to detect absorption of frequencies in the range of visible light, a dark band appearing in the spectrum at the wavelength of any absorbed light. Cytochromes were so named as being cellular chromophores that caused such a band to appear. Each cytochrome consists of a complex assembly of protein subunits harbouring one or more heme molecules, often together with iron–sulfur complexes or, in the case of cytochrome *c* oxidase, copper ions. The heme is structurally related to that of hemoglobin, but in the cytochromes the iron atom undergoes oxidation and reduction between the ferric and ferrous forms as electrons pass from one cytochrome to another, as shown in Fig. 9.21. The heme of heme *b* is the same as that of hemoglobin, as also is that of heme *c*, but in the latter case the vinyl

groups are engaged in linkage to cysteines of the protein. In heme *a*, there are differences in the heme side-chains.

As with any enzyme reaction, the reaction of one cytochrome with another involves free energy change. This free energy change yields the potential for phosphorylation of ADP to ATP that is associated with electron transport in the functioning cell. The reactions taking place between components of the electron transport chain can be demonstrated in vitro. Figure 9.22 illustrates an apparatus in which the potential difference between the solutions in two half-cells can be measured by means of electrodes connecting solutions of the reactants through a salt bridge. If such reactions are carried out at standard temperature (298 K) and pressure (1 atm), using 1-M solutions of reactants,

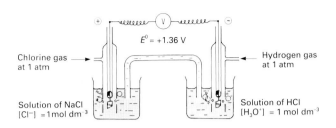

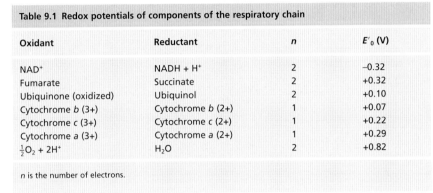

Fig. 9.22 The measurement of redox potentials.

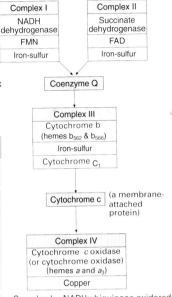

Table 9.1 Redox potentials of components of the respiratory chain

Oxidant	Reductant	n	E'_0 (V)
NAD^+	$NADH + H^+$	2	-0.32
Fumarate	Succinate	2	+0.32
Ubiquinone (oxidized)	Ubiquinol	2	+0.10
Cytochrome b (3+)	Cytochrome b (2+)	1	+0.07
Cytochrome c (3+)	Cytochrome c (2+)	1	+0.22
Cytochrome a (3+)	Cytochrome a (2+)	1	+0.29
$\frac{1}{2}O_2 + 2H^+$	H_2O	2	+0.82

n is the number of electrons.

Complex I   NADH:ubiquinone oxidoreductase
Complex II   Succinate:ubiquinone oxidoreductase
Complex III   Ubiquinol:cytochrome c oxidoreductase
Complex IV   Ferrocytochrome c: oxygen oxidoreductase

Fig. 9.23 The respiratory chain complexes.

the electronmotive force, as represented by the voltage recorded on the voltmeter, is an index of the standard oxidation–reduction potential of the reaction, or standard redox potential (E'_0). By convention, the standard redox potential of the $H^+ : H_2$ couple (1 M H^+ in equilibrium with H_2 gas at 1 atm) is defined as 0 V, and all other redox potentials can be related to this. Using such techniques, standard oxidation–reduction potentials can be determined; some are listed in Table 9.1. The standard free energy change ΔG^0, is related to ΔE, the change in the standard oxidation potential, by the equation:

$$\Delta G^{0\prime} = nF \Delta E'_0$$

where n is the number of electrons involved and F is the Faraday constant (96 500 coulombs). The units of $F\Delta E$ are coulomb–volts, or joules (4.18 J = 1 cal). The overall span of the respiratory chain is 1.14 V. Thus the standard free energy change associated with the oxidation of 1 mole of NADH can be calculated:

$$\Delta G^{0\prime} = (-2 \times 96\,500 \times 1.14)/4.18$$
$$= -52.6 \text{ kcal mol}^{-1}$$
$$= -220 \text{ kJ mol}^{-1}$$

ORGANIZATION OF THE COMPONENTS OF THE ELECTRON TRANSPORT CHAIN

Attempts to isolate the components of the electron transport chain revealed the nature of the complexes within which they are contained. Using mild solubilizing techniques, four complexes can be separated, as shown in Fig. 9.23. The available evidence indicates that the components isolated react in the sequence shown in this figure. NADH and succinate are oxidized by complexes I and II, respectively, reducing ubiquinone. Electrons then pass through complex III, cytochrome c and complex IV, complex IV then being oxidized by O_2.

PROTON PUMP ACTIVITY OF CHAIN COMPONENTS

As explained above, a feature of the oxidation process is the separation of the hydrogen atoms into protons and electrons; this process is important for the formation of ATP by the process of oxidative phosphorylation, as explained below. As part of this process, the protons released are pumped out of the inner membrane into the intermembrane space, as shown in Fig. 9.24. Complexes I, III and IV can function as pumps that bring this about, thereby creating a chemical and electrical gradient across the membrane. The face of the membrane to which protons are pumped is sometimes referred to as the P–side (P signifying positive), the face on the matrix side of the membrane being referred to as the N–side (N for negative). Much of our knowledge of the functioning of the chain has been obtained using inhibitors, and the sites of action of several of these are shown in Fig. 9.24.

OXIDATIVE PHOSPHORYLATION

THE NEED FOR OXIDATIVE PHOSPHORYLATION

Many kinds of chemical and physical work require the provision of ATP. Oxidative catabolism is an exothermic process, and the large negative free energy change with which the overall process is associated can be coupled to systems that phosphorylate ADP to ATP. One such system is the electron transport chain, and the overall negative free energy change of this process is sufficient for the formation of about three ATP molecules, if NADH is the oxidized substrate, or two if succinate is oxidized. The mitochondrial ATPase complex can be visualized at high magnification under the electron microscope using negative staining with phosphotungstate (see Fig. 9.25).

ATP SYNTHESIS

ATP is synthesized from ADP and P by the H^+-transporting ATP synthase, the general structure of which is shown in Fig. 9.26. It consists of two major complexes, known as F_0 and F_1. Each complex is composed of a number of subunits, F_0 having seven in eukaryotes, and F_1 having five different types of subunit, three each of α and β, and one each of γ, δ and ϵ, making nine in all. The core of the F_1 complex consists of the γ subunit surrounded by the six α and β subunits arranged alternately. ATP

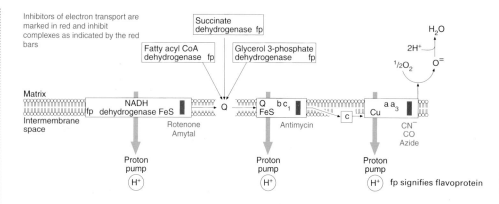

Inhibitors of electron transport are marked in red and inhibit complexes as indicated by the red bars

Fig. 9.24 Three respiratory chain complexes act as proton pumps.

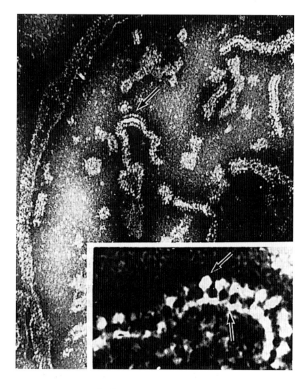

Fig. 9.25 The mitochondrial ATPase complex can be visualized as projections from the mitochondrial inner membrane (indicated by arrows).

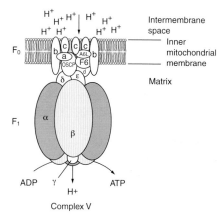

Fig. 9.26 The structure of the F_0/F_1 complex.

synthesis is thought to involve rotation of the $\alpha\beta$ subunits around the γ subunit. Joining the F_1 and F_0 complexes there is a region known as the stalk, consisting of the OSCP (oligomycin sensitivity conferral protein), F6, d, δ and ε subunits. F_0 consists of 12 c subunits, with 2 b, and one each of a and ABL. The precise structure of F_0 awaits full elucidation. Essential for the synthesis of ATP is the transport by the F_0/F_1 complex of protons from the intermembrane space into the matrix. Under certain conditions F_1 can function as an ATPase, hydrolysing ATP to ADP and P, and was often formerly referred to as the mitochondrial ATPase.

THE CHEMIOSMOTIC PROCESS

A scheme summarizing the process of proton pumping and ATP synthesis is

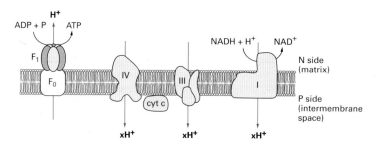

Fig. 9.27 The chemiosmotic potential drives oxidative phosphorylation.

shown in Fig. 9.27. The pumping of protons by complexes I, III and IV to the outside (P-side) of the inner membrane creates a protonmotive force as a result of the proton gradient and the associated electrical potential that is built up across the membrane by the increase in positive

charge. This electrochemical potential is maintained by the continual pumping of protons across the membrane, and tends to be dissipated by the action of the ATP synthase, because this enzyme uses the electrochemical energy to drive ATP synthesis, with concomitant flow of protons back to the matrix. Each of the pumping sites (complexes I, III and IV) pumps sufficient protons to support the synthesis of approximately one molecule of ATP for each pair of electrons passing along the chain. This mechanism is known as the chemiosmotic process. Each pair of electrons reduces one atom of oxygen ($\frac{1}{2}O_2$). The stoichiometry can therefore be expressed as a P/O ratio (number of molecules of inorganic P per $\frac{1}{2}O_2$).

When NADH is oxidized, with all three pumping sites operational, the P/O ratio is accordingly approximately 3. It is possible to block the chain with antimycin and show that, provided an external electron-accepting molecule is added, complex I can support oxidative phosphorylation by itself with a P/O ratio of approximately 1. Succinate oxidation, during which electrons flow through only two pumping sites (complexes III and IV), yields a P/O ratio of approximately 2. These values are approximate because the stoichiometry of proton pumping in relation to ATP synthesis is observed with an accuracy of about 10% either side of these figures. Fig. 9.27 can be linked with Fig. 9.24 to appreciate the combined effect of electron flow and oxidative phosphorylation.

COUPLING OF ELECTRON TRANSPORT TO OXIDATIVE PHOSPHORYLATION

Yields of ATP representing high P/O ratios can only be obtained in vitro from mitochondrial preparations that are relatively undamaged by the isolation procedures. In such preparations, oxidative phosphorylation is said to be tightly coupled to electron transport. A high ATP/ADP ratio causes electron transport and oxidative phosphorylation to occur more slowly, indicating that in tight coupling the rate of electron transport is regulated by the rate of phosphorylation of ADP. This is termed respiratory control, and can be demonstrated by recording the utilization of oxygen with an oxygen electrode. The result of such an experiment, in which the effect of various additions to an incubation of tightly coupled liver mitochondria was recorded, is shown in Fig. 9.28. Initially, oxygen utilization was very slow, but on addition of the substrate succinate it increased, and became much more rapid on addition of ADP. This continued until the ADP concentration had decreased due to its conversion to ATP. Addition of further ADP restored oxygen utilization. In other

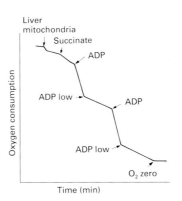

Fig. 9.28 Respiratory control revealed by the oxygen electrode.

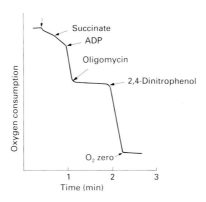

Fig. 9.29 Effects of uncoupling agent on respiration.

words, flow of electrons was controlled by the rate at which ATP could be synthesized.

UNCOUPLING AGENTS

Certain compounds can uncouple oxidative phosphorylation from electron transport. In the presence of such compounds, electron transport occurs at the maximum rate possible, but there is no phosphorylation of ADP. Uncoupling agents are thought to act by causing leakage of protons through the inner membrane, thus preventing the formation of an electrochemical gradient. One such compound is 2,4-dinitrophenol. Figure 9.29 shows an experiment of oxygen utilization by liver mitochondria initially in the tightly coupled state. Addition of succinate and ADP causes a similar response to that shown in Fig. 9.28. If oligomycin is then added, oxygen utilization ceases, because oligomycin inhibits the ATP synthase, without uncoupling it from electron transport, showing that, in tightly coupled mitochondria, blocking ATP synthesis stops electron flow. Addition of

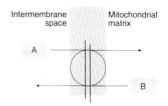

Fig. 9.30 Transport through the mitochondrial inner membrane by antiport.

Table 9.2 Mitochondrial antiporters	
A	**B**
Pyruvate	OH⁻
Phosphate	Malate
Citrate	Malate
Phosphate	OH⁻
ADP	ATP
Aspartate	Glutamate
Malate	2-Oxoglutarate

A and B refer to Fig. 9.30.

2,4-dinitrophenol then results in rapid electron transport and oxygen utilization, without ATP synthesis.

OTHER MITOCHONDRIAL TOPICS

TRANSLOCATION ACROSS THE INNER MITOCHONDRIAL MEMBRANE

It was mentioned earlier that the inner mitochondrial membrane is impermeable to nicotinamide nucleotides but that it contains systems that transport various anions while simultaneously carrying another molecule in the opposite direction, as shown in Fig. 9.30 (this is known as antiport; see p. 212). Some of these pairs of molecules are listed in Table 9.2.

THE GLYCEROL 3-PHOSPHATE SHUTTLE

Transport of hydrogen from the cytosol into the mitochondrion can be mediated by glycerol 3-phosphate interacting with a flavoprotein dehydrogenase in the inner mitochondrial membrane. NADH in the cytosol reduces dihydroxyacetone phosphate, forming glycerol 3-phosphate, a reaction catalysed by the soluble cytosolic glycerol-3-phosphate dehydrogenase. The mitochondrial membrane-bound enzyme interacts directly with the electron transport chain, and when it oxidizes the glycerol 3-phosphate back to dihydroxyacetone phosphate, the resulting $FADH_2$ passes hydrogen atoms directly to complex III, yielding a P/O ratio of 2. The overall reaction is thus the oxidation of cytosolic NADH by the electron transport chain, as shown in Fig. 9.31.

OXYGEN TOXICITY

Although oxygen is essential for most forms of life, it can give rise to highly toxic molecular species, especially when present as hyperbaric oxygen, i.e. oxygen at higher concentrations than in air at normal atmospheric pressure. One of the most reactive species is the superoxide ion, a free radical. A free radical is a molecule having an unpaired (and thus highly reactive) electron. Free radicals are discussed further in connection with vitamin E on p. 190. Another species of oxygen with high reactivity is known as singlet oxygen. Two forms of singlet oxygen occur: in one, both of the $\pi^\star$ 2p orbitals are occupied, each containing an electron but of opposite spin to each other; in the other form, only one of the $\pi^\star$ 2p orbitals is occupied, containing two electrons of opposite spins. The electron configurations of ground state oxygen and superoxide ion are shown in Fig. 9.32, the arrows indicating electrons and their direction of spin. Superoxide dismutase catalyses the reaction of two molecules of superoxide ion with two protons to form one molecule of O_2 and one of H_2O_2.

GLUTATHIONE AND OXYGEN TOXICITY

The tripeptide glutathione, the structure of which is shown in Fig. 9.33, is found in all mammalian cells except the neuron, and in many non-mammalian cell types. It is characterized by its γ-peptide bond, which is not attacked by peptidases, but is a substrate for γ-glutamyltransferase (see p. 89). The sulfhydryl is the functional group primarily responsible for the properties of glutathione, which is thus abbreviated, in the reduced form, as GSH. The oxidized form of two such molecules is denoted GSSG. One of the most important reactions in which glutathione participates, catalysed by glutathione peroxidase, inactivates hydrogen peroxide and other peroxides:

$2GSH + H_2O_2$ (or RO_2H) $\rightarrow$ GSSG + $2H_2O$ (or $ROH + H_2O$)

GSSG is then reduced back to GSH in a reaction with NADPH by the enzyme

glutathione reductase. In red blood cells, this NADPH is supplied by the pentose phosphate pathway. Glutathione is especially important in mitochondria because it reacts with and detoxifies reactive oxygen species formed in mitochondria. Experimental glutathione deficiency, caused by administering inhibitors of glutathione biosynthesis, brings about the death of newborn rats in 4–6 days. In adult animals, cataracts and mitochondrial swelling occur. The levels of ascorbate also fall dramatically, while administration of ascorbate in the diet alleviates the symptoms of glutathione deficiency. Ascorbate also reacts with

hydrogen peroxide and oxygen free radicals, and the dehydroascorbate that results is reduced back to ascorbate in a reaction with glutathione. These relationships are summarized in Fig. 9.34. In this figure, (O) represents peroxides and oxygen free radicals. Both ascorbate and dehydroascorbate can form the ascorbyl radical, semidehydroascorbate, which can be converted back to ascorbate by an NADH-dependent reductase system. Glutathione is synthesized by a specific enzyme pathway in the cytosol of nucleated cells, and transported into mitochondria through a transporter in the inner membrane (Fig. 9.35).

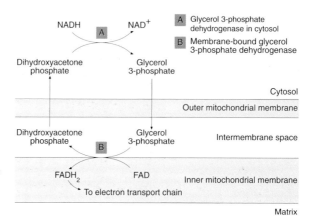

Fig. 9.31 The glycerol 3-phosphate shuttle.

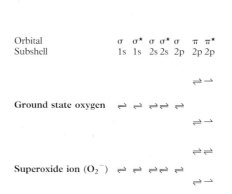

Fig. 9.32 The electron configuration of oxygen species.

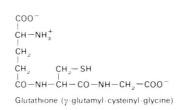

Glutathione (γ-glutamyl-cysteinyl-glycine)

Fig. 9.33 The structure of glutathione.

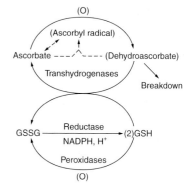

Fig. 9.34 Interaction between glutathione and ascorbate.

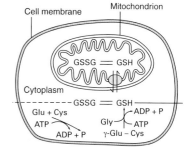

Fig. 9.35 Glutathione biosynthesis is by specific cytoplasmic enzymes.

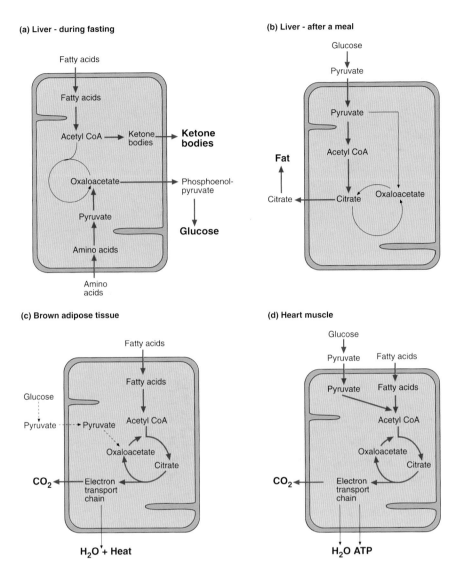

Fig. 9.36 Metabolism of mitochondria of different tissues.

TISSUE DIFFERENCES IN MITOCHONDRIAL FUNCTION

Figure 9.36 illustrates the way in which the flow of metabolites varies in the mitochondria of different tissues in various situations:

- Situation (a): liver during fasting. During a fast, large amounts of fatty acid and oxaloacetate are entering the liver, the fatty acid being converted to ketone bodies and the oxaloacetate acting as a precursor in gluconeogenesis (see Chapter 10).
- Situation (b): liver after a meal. In this situation, one of the main functions of liver is to carry out lipogenesis from ingested glucose. The glucose is degraded to acetyl CoA, which is exported from the mitochondria as citrate (p. 158).
- Situation (c): brown adipose tissue. This tissue has a special role in thermoregulation. Rapid oxidation that does not lead to work or other forms of useful energy leads to the production of heat. If there is some means of removing respiratory control, such as by constant hydrolysis of ATP, the effect will be similar to uncoupling oxidative phosphorylation. There will be unrestricted flow of electrons and oxidation of NADH, and a high rate of oxidative metabolism generating heat. In brown fat this results from the presence of an uncoupling protein.
- Situation (d): heart muscle. In cardiac muscle, constant contraction utilizes ATP, converting it to ADP. There are very large numbers of mitochondria in heart muscle, ensuring that oxidation by the heart is essentially always aerobic (in contrast to the anaerobic metabolism of skeletal muscle in some conditions, p. 135).

10

Carbohydrate and lipid metabolism in the fasting state

Although many tissues can use various sources of energy, the nervous system and red blood cells are dependent almost entirely on glucose, and maintenance of blood glucose levels is thus vital when an animal is starved. The liver plays a major role, releasing glucose rapidly from its store of glycogen (glycogenolysis). However, liver glycogen stores are comparatively small and the liver quickly starts converting amino acids, lactate and glycerol released from other tissues into glucose (gluconeogenesis). Although muscle stores of glycogen are relatively large, they can be used only within the muscle and do not contribute directly to blood glucose. Glucose sparing is achieved by many tissues switching to the use of alternative energy sources, e.g. muscles can use ketone bodies released from fat oxidation. The control of these processes and the role of insulin in health and disease are discussed.

METABOLISM IN THE FASTING STATE

METABOLIC REQUIREMENTS OF THE FASTING ANIMAL

When an animal is deprived of food, it has one overriding need – to maintain a supply of glucose to the blood, because a fall in blood glucose to below a critical level (about 2.5 mM in the human) leads to dysfunction of the central nervous system. In humans, this manifests as symptoms of hypoglycemia, such as muscular weakness and incoordination, mental confusion and sweating. If the blood glucose falls further, hypoglycemic coma and possibly death results.

The immediate source of blood glucose is the store of glycogen in the liver. This can be broken down to release glucose into the bloodstream within seconds, a process known as glycogenolysis. Muscle glycogen constitutes a much larger store of glucose but, as explained later (p. 148), does not directly contribute to blood glucose. Although glycogen is the immediate source of liver output of glucose, the liver can rapidly switch to producing glucose by de novo synthesis from amino acids that are released from muscle and metabolized in liver – a process known as gluconeogenesis. At the same time, ketogenesis begins; this is a process in the liver that converts fatty acids, released from adipose tissue, to ketone bodies, which can be utilized in some tissues to prevent excessive use of glucose. The release of fatty acids from the storage lipid, triacylglycerol, is known as lipolysis. These events are summarized in Fig. 10.1, and the pathways functioning within the tissues are indicated in Fig. 10.2. Initiation of these processes is dependent on the secretion of certain hormones, as discussed later (Chapter 13). Adrenaline and glucagon activate the enzymes that release glucose from liver glycogen. Glucagon also activates the process of gluconeogenesis. Glucocorticoids activate the release of amino acids from muscle, and adrenaline, adrenocorticotropin (ACTH) and growth hormone activate lipolysis.

GLYCOGEN AND ITS DEGRADATION

THE STRUCTURE OF GLYCOGEN

The main chains of glycogen consist of glucose units in α1-4 linkage, with branches formed by α1-6 links at approximately every six or seven glucose

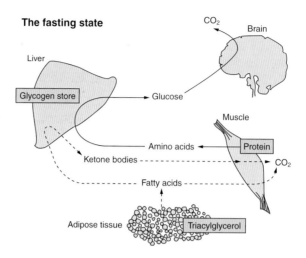

The fasting state

Fig. 10.1 Overview of tissue interactions in the fasting state.

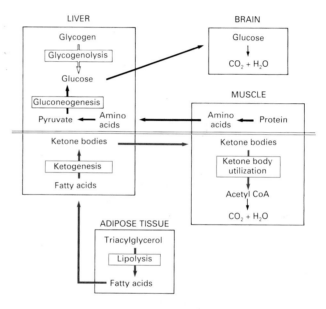

Fig. 10.2 Outline of fasting-state pathways.

units to give a branched structure as shown in Fig. 10.3. Figure 10.4 shows the detail of the α1-4 and α1-6 links in the glycogen molecule.

GLYCOGENOLYSIS

Both α1-4 and α1-6 links must be hydrolysed for extensive degradation of glycogen, but the α1-4 links are attacked first. The enzyme responsible for this, phosphorylase, removes terminal glucose units one by one by phosphorolysis, a reaction analogous to hydrolysis, except that phosphate is the attacking group rather than water, as shown in Fig. 10.5. The product is glucose 1-phosphate. Degradation of glycogen to glucose involves four enzyme reactions:

1. Phosphorylase, which hydrolyses α1-4 bonds.

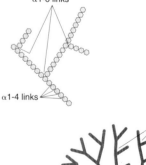

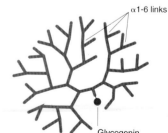

Fig. 10.3 The branched structure of glycogen.

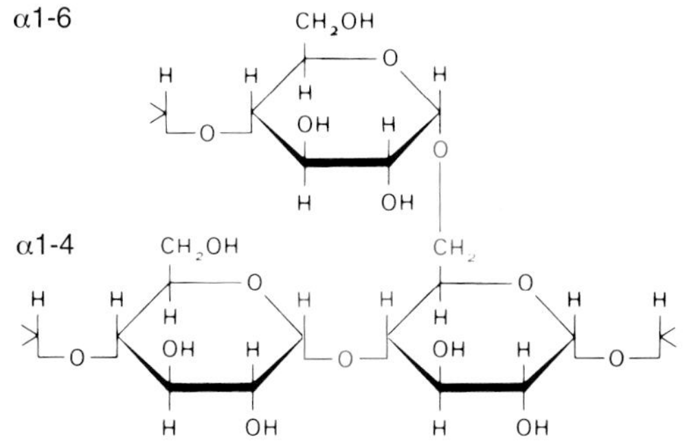

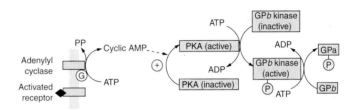

α1-6

α1-4

Fig. 10.4 α1-4 and α1-6 links of glycogen.

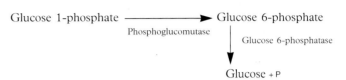

Fig. 10.6 'Debranching enzyme' activity is carried out by glucanotransferase (B) and 1-6-glucosidase (C).

Glucose 1-phosphate ⟶ Glucose 6-phosphate

Phosphoglucomutase

Glucose 6-phosphatase

Glucose + P

Fig. 10.7 Glucose 1-phosphate is converted to glucose via glucose 6-phosphate.

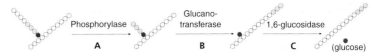

2. A debranching step, which removes α1-6 bonds.
3. Phosphoglucomutase, which converts glucose 1-phosphate to glucose 6-phosphate.
4. Glucose-6-phosphatase, which converts glucose 6-phosphate to glucose.

Phosphorylase action proceeds along the chain until it approaches a branch point. About three residues from the branch point its action ceases and glycogen-debranching enzyme hydrolyses the α1-6 bond. This enzyme has two activities associated with a single polypeptide chain: a transferase activity that transfers all except one of the remaining residues of the branch from the chain being degraded to the end of a longer chain, and 1,6-glucosidase activity that hydrolyses the α1-6 link, a reaction that releases free glucose, as shown in Fig. 10.6. Glycogen degradation to glucose then requires conversion of the glucose 1-phosphate released by phosphorylase to glucose 6-phosphate, and conversion of this to glucose by glucose 6-phosphatase. The effect of the combined action of all these enzymes is illustrated in Fig. 10.7. Glucose 6-phosphatase is not present in muscle, so

Fig. 10.8 The mechanism of activation of phosphorylase by cyclic AMP.

muscle glycogen cannot directly act as a source of blood glucose. Instead, it provides a source of energy for muscle contraction, the glucose 6-phosphate being acted on by enzymes of the glycolytic pathway (but see the Cori cycle below).

Glyogen is also degraded in lysosomes (p. 152).

THE REGULATION OF PHOSPHORYLASE

Cyclic AMP was first discovered during investigations of the mechanisms that activate phosphorylase. It was found that a heat-stable molecule in cell extracts was responsible for the increased activity of the enzyme found in adrenaline-stimulated

tissue; this molecule was identified as cyclic AMP. This activates cyclic AMP-dependent protein kinase (PKA), which then activates glycogen phosphorylase kinase, which in turn phosphorylates and activates phosphorylase (Fig. 10.8), converting it from glycogen phosphorylase *b* (Gp*b*) to glycogen phosphorylase *a* (Gp*a*), which is a more active form.

Glycogen phosphorylase is a homodimer of 97.4-kDa subunits, with pyridoxal phosphate bound to Lys-680. It conforms generally to the Monod–Changeux–Wyman model for allosteric enzymes (p. 94). Both the phosphorylated and unphosphorylated forms of the T state convert to active R forms but, whereas in the phosphorylated form this occurs

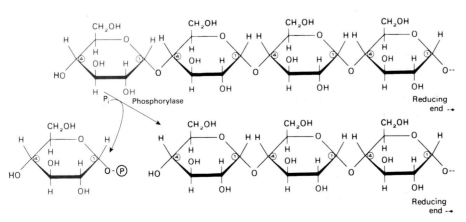

Fig. 10.5 The action of phosphorylase.

spontaneously, in the unphosphorylated form it requires the presence of allosteric modifiers such as glucose 6-phosphate. AMP opposes this action. Phosphatase 1 removes the phosphate from phosphorylase.

Phosphorylase kinase activates phosphorylase by phosphorylating it on Ser-14, in the N-terminal region, as shown in Fig. 6.34. The mechanisms by which the different forms of phosphorylase are regulated are shown in Fig. 10.9.

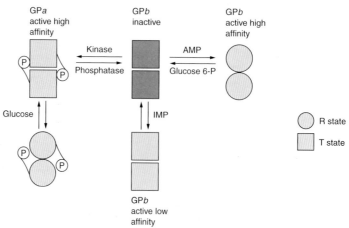

Fig. 10.9 The regulation of phosphorylase.

THE CORI CYCLE

The lack of glucose 6-phosphatase in muscle prevents the formation of free glucose in that tissue. However, muscle metabolism can contribute to blood glucose indirectly, in that lactate formed in muscle can be converted to glucose in the liver, as illustrated in Fig. 10.10. This sequence of reactions has been termed the Cori cycle, from the name of the husband and wife team who first realized its significance.

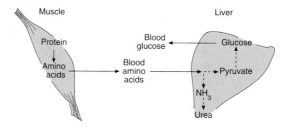

Fig. 10.10 The Cori cycle.

GLUCONEOGENESIS

THE GLUCONEOGENIC PATHWAY

During fasting, the supply of glucose to the blood is dependent on de novo synthesis in liver, utilizing the carbon skeletons of amino acids derived from muscle (Fig. 10.11); this process is known as gluconeogenesis. Protein breakdown in muscle to release the amino acids is activated by glucocorticoid hormones. The muscle to some extent assists the liver by converting many of the amino acids into alanine. When this arrives in the liver, the amino group is removed by transamination and converted to urea, and the resulting pyruvate enters the gluconeogenic pathway. Kidney and small intestine also possess the capacity for gluconeogenesis, but participate to a lesser extent than liver.

Compounds other than amino acids can act as substrates for gluconeogenesis, especially lactate, and to a lesser extent glycerol, after its conversion to glycerol 3-phosphate, which is then oxidized to dihydroxyacetone phosphate.

Many of the enzymes of gluconeogenesis also catalyse reactions in the glycolytic pathway that are readily reversible, but four enzymes act only in the gluconeogenic pathway (Fig. 10.12). They are:

1. Pyruvate carboxylase, which converts pyruvate to oxaloacetate. It is a

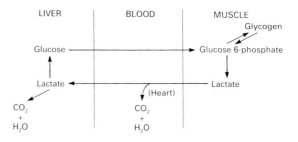

Fig. 10.11 Muscle amino acids provide carbon for gluconeogenesis.

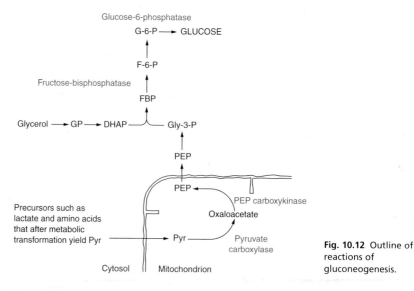

Fig. 10.12 Outline of reactions of gluconeogenesis.

mitochondrial enzyme that functions to provide oxaloacetate for gluconeogenesis, and also in other situations, such as for the citric acid cycle.

2. Phosphoenolpyruvate carboxykinase (PEPCK), which converts oxaloacetate to phosphoenolpyruvate (PEP). The requirement for GTP as one of the substrates, with GDP as a product,

ensures that at the concentrations that pertain in the cell, there is a negative free energy difference between the reactants and products, so that formation of the product phosphoenolpyruvate is favoured. There are both mitochondrial and cytosolic forms of this enzyme; in humans it is thought that the reaction occurs in the cytosol. In this case, oxaloacetate is transported out of the mitochondrion either as malate, after reduction by malate dehydrogenase, or as aspartate, after transamination, these being converted back to oxaloacetate by appropriate forms of similar enzymes in the cytosol (see Fig. 10.13). If PEPCK is mitochondrial, phosphoenolpyruvate is transported into the cytosol by a specific transporter.

3. Fructose-bisphosphatase, which is a cytosolic hydrolytic enzyme; thermodynamic considerations favour fructose 6-phosphate formation.

4. Glucose-6-phosphatase, which is a hydrolytic enzyme of the endoplasmic reticulum. Thermodynamically, glucose formation is favoured.

These enzymes, and their glycolytic counterparts, participate in three substrate cycles that are thought to be instrumental in regulating the glycolytic and gluconeogenic pathways. The effects of hormones, allosteric effectors and other control mechanisms on these enzymes, and those of glycogen synthesis and degradation, are considered in a later section (see Chapter 13).

KETONE BODY FORMATION AND UTILIZATION

KETOGENESIS

Gluconeogenesis is usually accompanied by ketogenesis. Almost all of the fatty acids of body tissues have an even number of carbon atoms, and yield acetyl CoA on degradation. They thus cannot contribute to the net synthesis of glucose. In general, they are not used as a fuel by the brain. The ketone bodies synthesized from them during fasting can be used by many tissues as a fuel, thus sparing the utilization of glucose. During a prolonged fast, even the brain adapts to the use of ketone bodies. An outline of the interactions between tissues is shown in Fig. 10.14. Ketone bodies are synthesized in the liver, which does not itself utilize them. The structures of the three compounds known as ketone

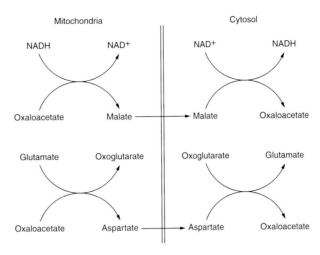

Fig. 10.13 Mechanisms for transporting oxaloacetate from mitochondrion to cytosol.

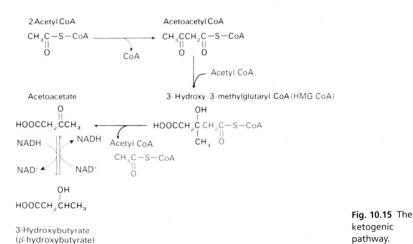

Fig. 10.14 Adipose tissue fatty acids provide carbon for ketone body formation.

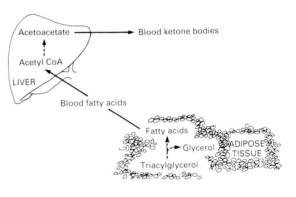

Fig. 10.15 The ketogenic pathway.

bodies – acetoacetate, 3-hydroxybutyrate and acetone – together with details of the pathway by which they are formed are given in Fig. 10.15. All of the enzymes of ketogenesis are mitochondrial. The scheme shows that three molecules of acetyl CoA are needed for the formation of hydroxymethylglutaryl CoA (HMG CoA),

one of these being released again on its conversion to acetoacetate.

3-Hydroxybutyrate dehydrogenase is a mitochondrial enzyme that maintains an equilibrium between 3-hydroxybutyrate and acetoacetate, and the relative concentrations of these compounds found in the blood are a direct reflection of the redox state of liver mitochondria. Some acetoacetate spontaneously decomposes to acetone.

HMG CoA is also an intermediate in cholesterol synthesis (p. 167), but in this case it is synthesized by a different, cytosolic, enzyme.

CLINICAL IMPLICATIONS OF KETONE BODIES

Ketone bodies are elevated in certain diabetic patients (see below). Clinical laboratory methods normally measure only acetoacetate; thus the variation in the relative amounts of acetoacetate and 3-hydroxybutyrate that occur with variations in the liver mitochondrial redox state affects the accuracy of the measurement as an indication of the total amount of ketone bodies.

KETONE BODY UTILIZATION

Ketone bodies produced in the liver circulate in the blood and are taken up and utilized by peripheral tissues such as muscle. During a prolonged fast, the brain adapts to the use of ketone bodies. Figure 10.16 shows the reactions involved. Most of these reactions relate to pathways that have already been discussed. The reaction that has not previously been described is that between acetoacetate and succinyl CoA, a citric acid cycle intermediate. This reaction forms acetoacetyl CoA and succinate. The succinate can be further metabolized by the citric acid cycle, and the acetoacetyl CoA is acted upon by thiolase to yield two molecules of acetyl CoA, which, with catalytic amounts of oxaloacetate, will then be metabolized by the citric acid cycle.

CONTROL OF THE BLOOD GLUCOSE IN HEALTH AND DISEASE

CONTROL OF THE BLOOD GLUCOSE

During a fast, the liver regulates with great precision and speed the amount of glucose secreted into the blood, to match the amount being removed. This ensures a constant blood glucose level during fasting. This is illustrated in the hypothetical situation shown in Fig. 10.17. A fasting person can leap suddenly out of a chair and run rapidly, with only minor effects on the blood glucose level, because of the speed with which the liver can increase

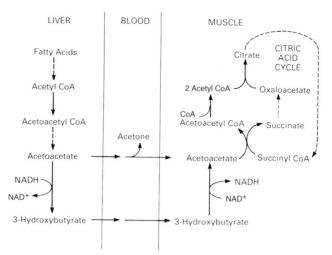

Fig. 10.16 Pathway for utilization of ketone bodies.

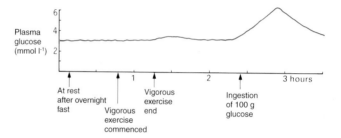

Fig. 10.17 Response of blood glucose to fasting exercise and ingestion of glucose.

glucose output. This is in contrast to the situation when glucose enters from the gut. When this happens, there is a rise in blood glucose concentration, the reduction of which is dependent on the secretion of insulin.

CLINICAL IMPLICATIONS – DIABETES MELLITUS, GLYCOGEN STORAGE DISEASE AND INSULINOMA

Disordered blood glucose concentration

Because of the constancy of blood glucose levels in a fasting healthy individual, any concentration that lies outside the normal range indicates a pathological situation, an elevated level being known as hyperglycemia and a depressed level as hypoglycemia. As explained at the beginning of this chapter, excessive hypoglycemia has immediate severe consequences. The effects of hyperglycemia are more long term. The condition that most commonly underlies hyperglycemia is diabetes mellitus, but other explanations are possible. A test that is often carried out to investigate the possibility of disordered blood glucose levels is the glucose

tolerance test. This test is carried out after an overnight fast. Glucose (75 g) is given orally and blood samples are then taken at intervals thereafter. The concentration of glucose, and sometimes other substances, is measured in these samples. In the example shown in Fig. 10.18, the levels of insulin and free fatty acids are also shown. In a young, healthy individual the concentration of glucose will have fallen to the normal level by 1.5 h. A significantly elevated level at 2 h normally indicates a diabetic condition.

Types of diabetes mellitus

Two forms of diabetes mellitus are recognized:

- type 1: the so-called juvenile type, because it often manifests itself in children and young adults
- type 2: or the maturity-onset type, because it often first manifests itself in mature adults, especially if they are obese.

The distinction between types 1 and 2 is somewhat blurred at some stages of the disease. In addition to these, a type of maturity-onset diabetes of the young

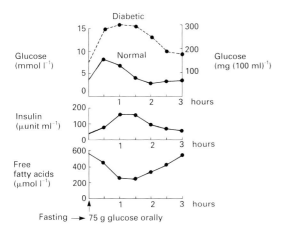

Fig. 10.18 The glucose tolerance test.

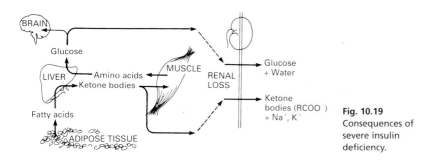

Fig. 10.19 Consequences of severe insulin deficiency.

excretion of the acidic ketone bodies results in the accompanying excretion of salts – potassium loss being a particularly severe consequence. Some of the ketone bodies are converted to acetone, which is expired and can be smelt on the breath.

Diabetic coma

Diabetic coma has its origin either in the effects of prolonged insulin deficiency, as described in the preceding paragraphs, or from poor management of recognized insulin-dependent diabetes.

In the former case, there is a state of long-standing hyperglycemia and the treatment involves administration of insulin, with correction of the associated electrolyte disorders, such as whole-body potassium depletion.

In the latter case, it results from severe hypoglycemia of sudden onset, due to failure to ingest adequate food after insulin administration. The treatment in this case is to give glucose-yielding nutrients. Clearly, administration of insulin in such a case would be disastrous and the correct diagnosis of the origin of the coma is thus of paramount importance.

(MODY) is known; this is a variant characterized by an autosomal-dominant mode of inheritance.

In type 1 diabetes there is a marked lack of secretion of insulin due to immune destruction of the β cells of the islets of Langerhans in the pancreas, as type 1 diabetes is considered to arise in many patients as a result of an autoimmune attack on the β cells by antibodies against this tissue formed by the patient's own immune system. The only effective treatment is the administration of insulin; thus this type is often referred to as insulin-dependent diabetes mellitus (IDDM).

Type 2 diabetes is discussed at the end of Chapter 12, as this calls for an understanding of lipid metabolism, which we deal with in the next two chapters.

Consequences of severe insulin deficiency

The classic acute diabetic crisis with blood insulin levels that have reached critically low values is characterized by:

- a high blood glucose
- very high concentrations of blood ketone bodies and free fatty acids
- loss of salts

- excessive urea excretion, excessive production of urine (polyuria)
- severe tissue wasting.

Eventually, the condition can result in diabetic coma and death.

As illustrated in Fig. 10.19, this condition can be seen as an example of the fasting situation of metabolism carried to the extreme, and its origins can be understood from a knowledge of that situation. In the absence of insulin, there is no regulator to keep the action of hormones such as the glucocorticoids, glucagon, ACTH and growth hormone within limits. There will then be a very high blood glucose concentration, which results from both the failure of tissues to take up glucose and the futile release of amino acids from muscle protein to support an unnecessary and pointless gluconeogenic response. This eventually leads to severe muscle loss with excessive excretion of urea. There will be continual release of free fatty acids from adipose tissue, leading eventually to almost complete loss of body fat and the secretion of large amounts of ketone bodies from the liver. Glucose is secreted from the kidney in large quantities and the high osmotic pressure caused by this results in excessive excretion of water by the kidney. The

Glycogen storage disease

A number of gene defects lead to conditions in which glycogen accumulates, with severe consequences for the health of the tissues, especially the liver; these are known generally as glycogen storage diseases. One of the most common is due to a deficiency of glucose 6-phosphatase, and is known as type 1 glycogen storage disease, or von Gierke disease. Because the metabolic lesion is precisely known, the symptoms present a model in which pathway interrelationships with carbohydrate metabolism can be studied. The symptoms include, after only a short fast, severe hypoglycemia. There is also at times mild ketosis, and mild lactic acidosis. The schemes shown in Fig. 10.20 illustrate some of the effects of the deficiency at the molecular level.

Fig. 10.20A shows that, in the fasting state, the mobilization of amino acids to act as precursors for gluconeogenesis leads to the formation of pyruvate in the liver, which in turn leads to formation of glucose 6-phosphate, and, as this cannot be exported as glucose, much of it will be channelled into glycogen, which accumulates. The resulting hypoglycemia exacerbates this situation because more amino acids will be released as the body

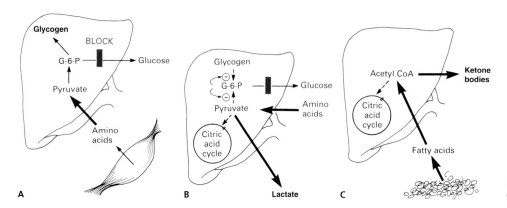

Fig. 10.20 Metabolic events in glucose 6-phosphate deficiency.

Table 10.1 Types of glycogen storage disease

Type	Name	Enzyme affected	In which tissue	Remarks
I	Von Gierke disease	Glucose-6-phosphatase	Liver, kidney	Low fasting blood glucose, enlarged liver with elevated glycogen levels
II	Pompe disease	Acid maltase	Several, including heart, skeletal muscle and liver	Glycogen accumulates in lysosomes; cardiomyopathy, muscular hypotonia
III	Limit dextrinosis	Debranching system*	Liver or muscle	Phosphorylase acts on α1-4 bonds until an α1-6 bond is reached. The resulting molecule is called a limit dextrin
V	McArdle disease	Phosphorylase	Muscle	Muscular pain, weakness and stiffness after only mild exercise
VI		Phosphorylase	Liver	Has some features similar to type I but, as gluconeogenesis is not blocked, hypoglycemia may not be so severe

*The deficiency can be in either the glucanotransferase or 1,6-glucosidase activities and can be in liver or muscle or both.

tries to correct the hypoglycemia, resulting in yet more glycogen synthesis.

Fig. 10.20B indicates that feedback processes resulting from accumulation of glucose 6-phosphate will tend to promote accumulation of pyruvate, and this will lead to the formation of lactate which will enter the blood.

Fig. 10.20C indicates that failure to form glucose, and the resulting severe hypoglycemia if glucose is not quickly ingested, will result in exaggerated release of fatty acids from adipose tissue, and a ketosis will follow.

A number of other glycogen storage diseases are known, some of which are summarized in Table 10.1. Pompe disease, in which there is a deficiency of lysosomal acid maltase (α-1,4-glucosidase), reveals that lysosomal degradation of some glycogen occurs and that serious consequences result from its failure. In this disease glycogen degradation in the cytosol is normal and glycogen accumulates only in the lysosomes.

HYPERINSULINEMIA

Excessive secretion of insulin occurs in cases of insulinoma, a tumour of the pancreatic islet cells. Severe hypoglycemia may result on fasting, due to the partial blocking of the action of fasting-state hormones by insulin, as illustrated in Fig. 10.21.

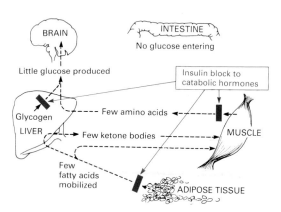

Fig. 10.21 Consequences of oversecretion of insulin.

Carbohydrate and lipid metabolism in the absorptive state

Ingested food that is surplus to an animal's immediate needs is converted into fat and glycogen for storage as energy reserves for use in periods of food deprivation. The processes operative in this metabolic state are glycogenesis, i.e. the biosynthesis of glycogen from glucose, and those elements of the lipogenic pathways involved in the biosynthesis of triacylglycerols from fatty acids. In addition, carbohydrates and lipids with structural roles must be synthesized. A variety of fatty acids are needed in cell membranes, including polyunsaturated fatty acids of the n-3 and n-6 families. The precursor fatty acids for these must be provided in the diet and are known as essential fatty acids.

THE PROCESS OF ABSORPTION

OVERVIEW OF THE ABSORPTIVE STATE

Ingested food supplies the immediate needs of an animal for precursors to be used in essential synthesis of structural compounds and as oxidative substrates. It is not uncommon, however, in modern industrial societies, for food in excess of these needs to be eaten. Similarly, for an animal in the wild, a meal eaten after a fast might well be larger than is needed for the animal's immediate needs. In both of these cases, food that is surplus to immediate needs will be converted into compounds that can be stored as an energy reserve for use during a subsequent period of food deprivation. Two important energy reserves are fat – in the form of triacylglycerol – and glycogen.

Figure 11.1 summarizes the events occurring during the absorptive state. Carbohydrates that have been ingested are broken down in the digestive tract to yield monosaccharides, which are then absorbed into the blood. A major component is glucose, which is taken up by liver and muscle and, if not oxidized to carbon dioxide and water, is converted to glycogen and also triacylglycerol. Ingested lipids are hydrolysed in the gut mainly to fatty acids and monoacylglycerol (in the case of triacylglycerols), and these are resynthesized to triacylglycerol or phospholipid and incorporated into plasma lipoproteins. The triacylglycerols in these lipoproteins are processed and then laid down in fat stores in adipose tissue, as described in subsequent sections. In this metabolic state, one hormone, insulin, is secreted and exerts major effects on the pathways involved in these steps.

THE DIGESTION OF FOOD

Before food can be absorbed from the digestive tract it must be processed to convert it into a form appropriate for absorption. The enzymes responsible for this are summarized in Fig. 11.2. Carbohydrates are hydrolysed by amylases. This process starts in the mouth, as saliva contains appreciable amounts of amylase, and is continued in the small intestine. Proteins are hydrolysed by proteolytic enzymes, termed endopeptidases, secreted into the stomach (pepsin) and intestine (trypsin, chymotrypsin). Lipids are hydrolysed by lipases and phospholipases. Apart from salivary amylase, which is secreted by the salivary glands in the

The Fed State

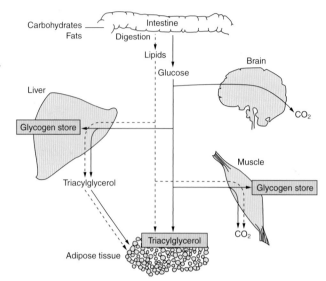

Fig. 11.1 Tissue interaction in the absorptive state.

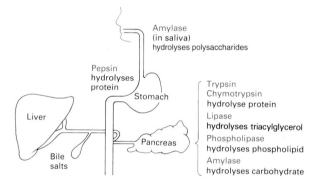

Fig. 11.2 The enzymes of digestion.

mouth, and pepsin, which is secreted by cells of the stomach wall, all of these enzymes are secreted by the exocrine cells of the pancreas into the intestine, in response to hormones that are secreted when food is ingested. The hydrolysis of lipids is facilitated by the presence of bile salts, which are secreted by the liver in bile.

PROTEIN DIGESTION

The enzymes pepsin, trypsin and chymotrypsin are secreted as the zymogens pepsinogen, trypsinogen and chymotrypsinogen, respectively. These are converted to the active enzymes by stomach hydrochloric acid, in the case of pepsin, and by enterokinase, in the case of trypsin. Trypsin converts chymotrypsinogen to the active enzyme. Each of these enzymes shows specificity with regard to the peptide bonds it attacks, as summarized in Fig. 11.3. Pepsin attacks bonds on the carboxyl side of hydrophobic residues such as phenylalanine, tyrosine and leucine. Trypsin attacks the carboxyl side of bonds of basic residues, and chymotrypsin attacks

on the carboxyl side of aromatic residues. Two other enzymes remove single residues from either the N-terminus, in the case of leucine aminopeptidase, or the C-terminus, as with carboxypeptidase A. The result is that the proteins are degraded to a mixture of small peptides and amino acids, which are then absorbed.

CARBOHYDRATE DIGESTION

Amylases are of two types: the α-amylases and the β-amylases. Both types break α1-4 bonds, but β-amylases cause inversion of the bond in the maltose units that are released, so that their product is β-maltose. β-Amylases are found mainly in plants and bacteria and remove maltose units from the non-reducing end of the substrate; they are thus termed exoamylases. The α-amylases in saliva and pancreatic juice break internal α1-4 bonds, and thus are endoamylases; they hydrolyse amylose and amylopectin – major polysaccharides of plants – and glycogen. The product is mainly maltose (Fig. 11.4) but the trisaccharide maltotriose, containing three α1-4-linked

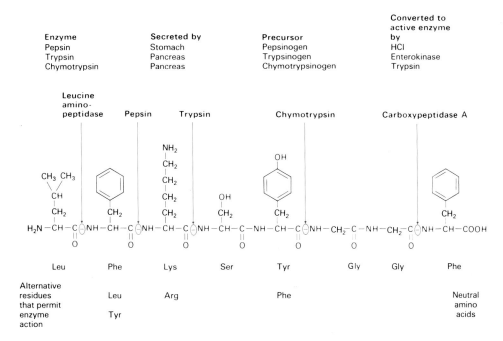

Enzyme	Secreted by	Precursor	Converted to active enzyme by
Pepsin	Stomach	Pepsinogen	HCl
Trypsin	Pancreas	Trypsinogen	Enterokinase
Chymotrypsin	Pancreas	Chymotrypsinogen	Trypsin

Fig. 11.3 Specificity of proteolytic enzymes.

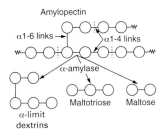

Fig. 11.4 The action of α-amylase.

glucose units, is also formed. Because α-amylases do not break α1-6 bonds, products from amylopectin include oligosaccharides known as limit dextrins. The enterocyte can only absorb free glucose, so these oligosaccharides are hydrolysed further to glucose monomers by oligosaccharidases of the intestinal surface brush border membrane. These include sucrase, which hydrolyses sucrose to glucose and fructose, and lactase, which hydrolyses lactose to galactose and glucose.

CLINICAL IMPLICATIONS – LACTOSE INTOLERANCE

A deficiency of intestinal disaccharidases is not uncommon in humans. Of these, lactase is located in the villus enterocytes of the small intestine, and is responsible for digestion of lactose in milk. Lactase activity is high during infancy, but in most humans lactase activity declines after the weaning phase. In many healthy humans, sufficient lactase activity persists throughout adult life to permit digestion of lactose in adults.

This dominantly inherited genetic trait is known as lactase persistence. The distribution of different lactase phenotypes in human populations is highly variable and is controlled by a polymorphic element cis-acting to the lactase gene. A putative single nucleotide change has been identified. Lactase persistence is most frequent in Northern Europeans and certain African and Arabian nomadic tribes, who have a history of drinking fresh milk, less frequent in others, especially Chinese. Failure of lactase persistence gives rise to lactose intolerance, a condition causing flatulence and diarrhea, due to the fact that lactose is not absorbed, and passes to the colon where it is fermented by gut bacteria with production of gas, and the presence of osmotically active compounds causes water to be drawn into the intestine, causing diarrhea. More rarely, lactose intolerance might be due to a congenital lactase deficiency. It could also be due to other causes of poor lactose absorption, such as celiac disease. The use of lactose-free milk alleviates the problem. Poor lactose absorption can be associated with poor calcium absorption, and might be a risk factor for developing osteoporosis.

LIPID DIGESTION

Ingested fat consists of a variety of lipids, the bulk of which comprise phospholipids and triacylglycerols. About 15% of the triacylglycerol is hydrolysed in the stomach by a lipase secreted by the gastric chief cells. The remainder of the triacylglycerols and phospholipids are hydrolysed in the small intestine by enzymes secreted by the pancreatic acinar cells. These include a phospholipase (see p. 187) and a triacylglycerol lipase. This pancreatic lipase acts on micelles of triacylglycerol and bile salts (see p. 169). The bile salts act on large fat droplets to form small micelles. Together with colipase, a 10-kDa protein cofactor that is essential for activity, the lipase, a 46-kDa protein, inserts itself into the interface at the surface of the micelles; this is illustrated in Fig. 11.5 (which in fact shows the precursor, procolipase (in red), because it was used in the study shown). In A, in the absence of lipid, the lid region of the lipase covers the active site, but in the presence of lipid, shown in B, the lid is retracted towards procolipase.

The lipase removes the outer two fatty acids, leaving monoacylglycerol, as shown in Fig. 11.6. The fatty acids and the monoacylglycerol are transported into the cells lining the intestinal wall. After absorption, the fatty acids are converted to fatty acyl CoA. The fatty acyl CoA can then react with monoacylglycerol to reform triacylglycerol, which is then incorporated into chylomicrons (see Chapter 12). Triacylglycerol is also formed in the intestinal cells from glycerol 3-phosphate and fatty acyl CoA as described on p. 161.

GLUCOSE AS A PRECURSOR IN GLYCOGENESIS AND LIPOGENESIS

The biosynthesis of glycogen, known as glycogenesis, occurs in liver and muscle, and in the absorptive state the main

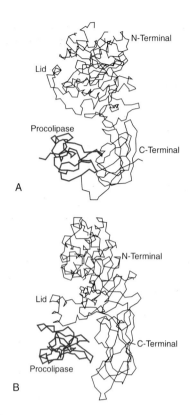

A

B

Fig. 11.5 The action of colipase.

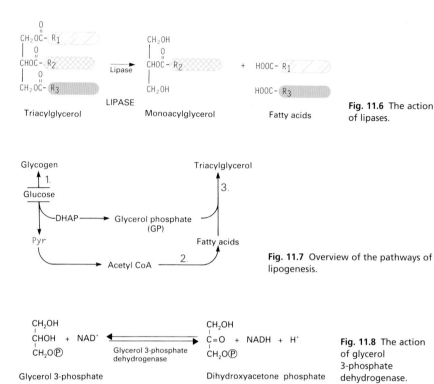

Fig. 11.6 The action of lipases.

Fig. 11.7 Overview of the pathways of lipogenesis.

Fig. 11.8 The action of glycerol 3-phosphate dehydrogenase.

Table 11.1 Classification of glucose transporters

Transporter	Distribution
GLUT 1	Widespread, but most abundant in red blood cells and brain microvessels
GLUT 2	Liver, enterocyte basolateral membranes and pancreatic β cells
GLUT 3	Almost exclusively in brain neurons and fetal muscle
GLUT 4	Insulin-sensitive tissues (e.g. skeletal and cardiac muscle, brown and white fat)
GLUT 5	Enterocyte luminal membranes, sperm, skeletal muscle and adipocytes. It is a fructose transporter, either in addition to, or in preference to, a glucose transporter

precursor is glucose derived from the blood. Lipogenesis occurs in liver and adipose tissue. Blood glucose is an important precursor in the absorptive state but triacylglycerol biosynthesis also results from the reassembly of ingested fatty acids into triacylglycerols of a different composition that is more appropriate for storage. The storage triacylglycerols contain mainly saturated and monounsaturated fatty acids for use as oxidation substrates, polyunsaturated fatty acids being stored as components of membrane phospholipids. The main pathways involved in the conversion of glucose to glycogen and triacylglycerol are summarized in Fig. 11.7. This shows (red numbers): (1) the formation of glycogen from glucose; (2) the synthesis of fatty acid from acetyl CoA; (3) the synthesis of triacylglycerol from fatty acids (after conversion to fatty acyl CoA) and glycerol 3-phosphate.

Triacylglycerol biosynthesis requires the provision of glycerol 3-phosphate, for the glycerol backbone of the lipid molecule. This is formed by glycerol-3-phosphate dehydrogenase, which reduces the glycolytic pathway intermediate dihydroxyacetone phosphate using NADH (Fig. 11.8).

GLYCOGENESIS

GLUCOSE TRANSPORTERS

One of the most important steps in glucose metabolism is its transport across the plasma membrane. In non-epithelial tissues, this occurs by facilitated diffusion (see p. 212), mediated by a family of glucose transporters. Five families of glucose transporters have been identified; these are designated GLUT 1 to GLUT 5. Their distribution in tissues is detailed in Table 11.1. In addition, GLUT 6 is a putative gene but has no protein product, and GLUT 7 is an intracellular transporter in liver endoplasmic reticulum membrane.

The total capacity of the plasma membrane to transport glucose into the cell depends on the amount of the transporter in the membrane. This depends not only on the rate of synthesis but also on the distribution of the transporter between the membrane and certain specific intracellular storage sites. One of the actions of insulin in increasing uptake of glucose into muscle and adipose tissue is to recruit GLUT 4 from an intracellular site to the cell surface. There is a constant traffic of GLUT 4 molecules between the plasma membrane and the intracellular site. The mechanism by which insulin brings about the translocation of the transporter to the plasma membrane is discussed more fully in relation to the insulin receptor in Chapter 15.

INITIATION OF GLYCOGEN BIOSYNTHESIS

The precursor of glycogen is UDP-glucose. In the pathway from glucose to glycogen, glucose is first converted to

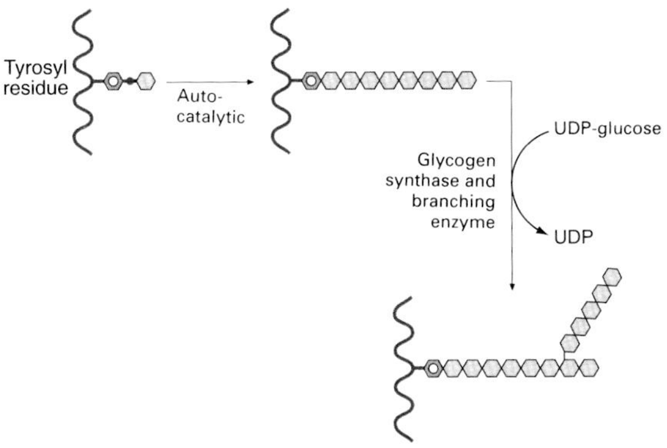

Fig. 11.9 The action of glycogenin.

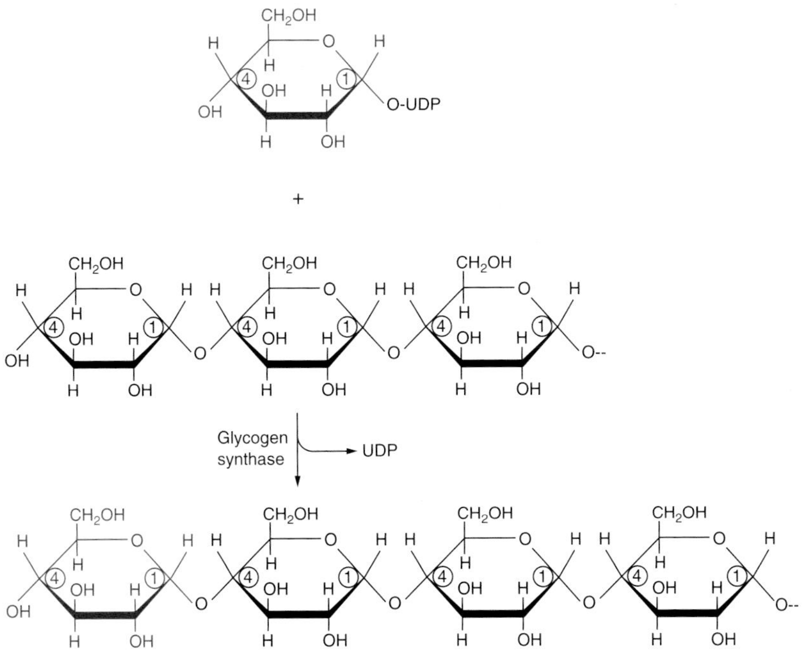

Fig. 11.10 Glycogen synthase adds glucose residues in α1-4 linkage.

glucose 6-phosphate, from which glucose 1-phosphate is formed; this reacts with UTP to form UDP-glucose. UDP-glucose then reacts with a glycogen precursor, glycogenin. This protein can catalyse the addition of a molecule of glucose to one of its own tyrosine residues, by a bond between the C-1 of the glucose and the tyrosine phenolic group. It can then catalyse the further addition to that glucose of about seven other glucose units in α1-4 linkage. The primer thus formed acts as a substrate for glycogen synthase (Fig. 11.9). Each glycogenin molecule carries one molecule of glycogen.

GLYCOGEN SYNTHASE

The main glycogen chains are synthesized by the addition of glucose units to C-4 of the terminal glucose at the non-reducing end of a pre-existing α1-4 chain primer. Note that the C-1 reducing group of each glucose unit added is involved in linkage to the existing chain. The action of glycogen synthase is outlined in Fig. 11.10. The enzyme is subject to a refined regulatory system as discussed in Chapter 13.

THE BRANCHING ENZYME

The branches in the glycogen molecule are introduced by an enzyme known as the branching enzyme. This enzyme breaks off a chain of six glucose units from the end of a growing α1-4 chain and transfers this hexasaccharide to another chain by forming an α1-6 bond between the free C-1 of the hexasaccharide and the C-6 of a glucose in the chain to which it is transferred, as illustrated in Fig. 11.11. The point of attachment is about six residues from a previous α1-6 link. The combined actions of glycogenin, glycogen synthase and the branching enzyme bring about the formation of a glycogen molecule. It should be appreciated that glycogen in a cell is polydisperse, i.e. it consists of molecules with a range of sizes, all at different stages of synthesis or degradation.

The sequence of reactions in glycogen biosynthesis is thus:

1. Linkage of about eight glucose residues to glycogenin.
2. Extension of α1-4 chains by glycogen synthase.
3. Formation of α1-6 bonds by branching enzyme.
4. Further extension of α1-4 chains by glycogen synthase.
5. Repetition of steps 3 and 4.

LIPOGENESIS

THE PENTOSE PHOSPHATE PATHWAY

Another pathway of carbohydrate metabolism that is of importance in the absorptive state (although it also has other functions) is the pentose phosphate pathway, or pentose shunt. It was given the name pentose shunt at the time it was being elucidated because it was seen as an alternative to glycolysis as a pathway of glucose degradation, but it is now seen as a pathway having special functions of its own. One of these functions is to provide pentoses for nucleotide and nucleic acid synthesis. Another function is to catalyse reduction of $NADP^+$ to NADPH to support biosynthetic processes, such as fatty acid biosynthesis, that require NADPH.

The pentose phosphate pathway occurs in the cytosol, and the reactions

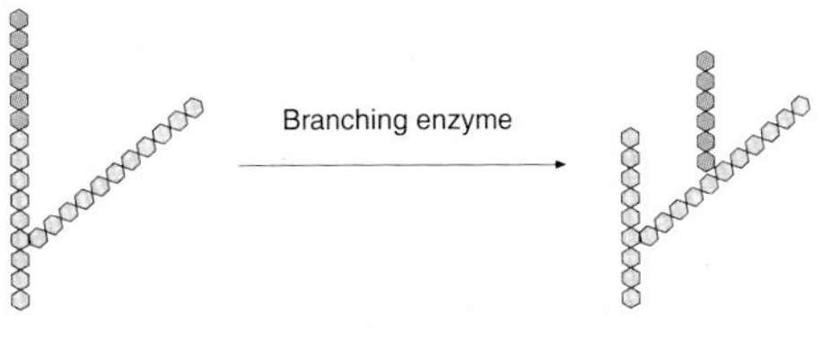

Fig. 11.11 Branching enzyme transfers a six-residue α1-4 chain to an α1-6 bond.

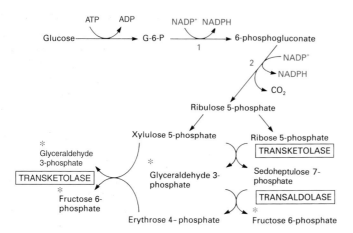

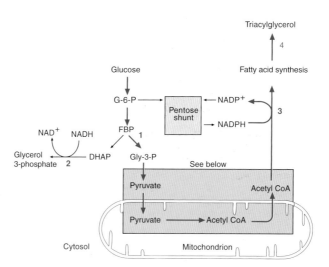

Fig. 11.12 The pentose phosphate pathway.

are outlined in Fig. 11.12. NADPH is a product of two dehydrogenases, glucose 6-phosphate dehydrogenase and 6-phosphogluconate dehydrogenase, which convert glucose 6-phosphate to the pentose, ribulose 5-phosphate. Ribulose 5-phosphate undergoes isomerization to both xylulose 5-phosphate and ribose 5-phosphate, and these two compounds serve as substrates for transketolase to yield sedoheptulose 7-phosphate and glyceraldehyde 3-phosphate. Transaldolase then converts these to fructose 6-phosphate and erythrose 4-phosphate. Transketolase also catalyses a reaction between xylulose 5-phosphate and erythrose 4-phosphate to form glyceraldehyde 3-phosphate and fructose 6-phosphate. Thus three pentose molecules (two of xylulose 5-phosphate and one of ribose 5-phosphate) yield two molecules of fructose 6-phosphate and one of glyceraldehyde 3-phosphate.

OVERVIEW OF THE CONVERSION OF GLUCOSE TO TRIACYLGLYCEROL

Lipogenesis from glucose involves the following steps:

1. Conversion of most of the glucose to acetyl CoA, via the glycolytic pathway and pyruvate dehydrogenase.
2. Formation of glycerol 3-phosphate from some of the dihydroxyacetone phosphate formed during glycolysis.
3. Biosynthesis of fatty acid and thence fatty acyl CoA from acetyl CoA.
4. Biosynthesis of triacylglycerol from fatty acyl CoA and glycerol 3-phosphate.

These steps are summarized in Fig. 11.13. An expanded view of the reactions

involved in the conversion of pyruvate to cytosolic acetyl CoA is also shown. These involve conversion of some of the pyruvate to oxaloacetate within mitochondria. The oxaloacetate and acetyl CoA condense to form citrate, which is then transported into the cytosol. This citrate is then cleaved

back to acetyl CoA and oxaloacetate, the acetyl CoA being used as substrate for fatty acid biosynthesis. The oxaloacetate is reduced to malate by cytosolic malate dehydrogenase and the malate then acts as substrate for the malic enzyme, which catalyses an oxidative decarboxylation to form pyruvate again. However, the latter two steps also effect the transfer of hydrogen from NADH to $NADP^+$ to form NADPH, which is then available for fatty acid biosynthesis, supplementing that provided by the pentose phosphate pathway, as described in the previous section.

FATTY ACID BIOSYNTHESIS

Fatty acid biosynthesis proceeds by the addition of two-carbon units derived from acetyl CoA. The first of the two-carbon units is derived directly from acetyl CoA, subsequent units being added through the intermediate, malonyl CoA. The reactions involved are summarized in Fig. 11.14. The acetyl group is first transferred from the

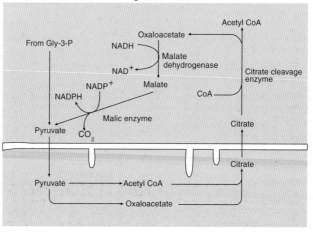

Fig. 11.13 Pathway interactions in lipogenesis.

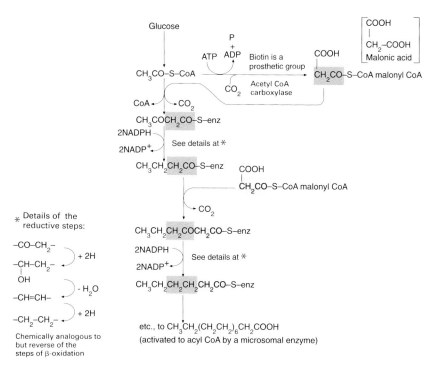

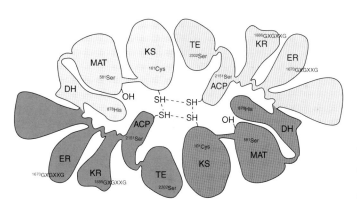

Fig. 11.14 The fatty acid synthase reaction.

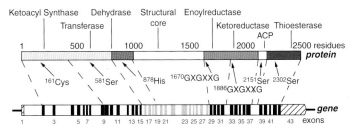

β-ketoacyl group attached to ACP. This four-carbon moiety is then transferred to the now-vacant adjacent cysteine and a further malonyl group is added to ACP. A similar sequence of reactions then ensues, resulting in elongation of the chain by two carbons, the sequence being continued until the synthesis of the fatty acid has been completed. In animals, synthesis continues until palmitic acid has been formed, and this is released and converted to palmitoyl CoA by an endoplasmic reticulum enzyme.

The structure of fatty acid synthase, depicted in Fig. 11.15, reveals the complexity that can be attained in multifunctional enzymes. All six of the enzymic activities are present on a single polypeptide chain of 2500 amino acid residues: ketoacylsynthase (KS), malonyl/acetyltransferase (MAT), dehydrase (DH), enoylreductase (ER), ketoreductase (KR) and thioesterase (TE). A map of the rat gene is given in Fig. 11.16. For the size of the protein, the gene is very compact (18 kilobases) having relatively short introns. This could possibly have arisen by the fusion of genes organized within a prokaryotic operon, and the hypothesis is supported by the fact that in a number of present-day prokaryotes similar genes are arranged in clusters within operons.

FATTY ACID STRUCTURES

Palmitic acid synthesized by fatty acid synthase is only one of a number of different fatty acids that are required by the animal body. The structures of some of the fatty acids commonly found in biomembranes and plant or animal oils are shown in Fig. 11.17. As indicated next to each name, fatty acids can be designated by a convention in which the total number of carbons in the chain precedes a colon, after which is given the number of double bonds. Thus palmitic acid is 16 : 0. In naming fatty acids, the position of the double bonds can be designated in either of the following ways:

Fig. 11.15 Fatty acid synthase has six activities within a single polypeptide chain.

sulfur atom of CoA to the sulfur atom of a cysteine residue in the enzyme fatty acid synthase, forming acetyl–enzyme. Malonyl CoA is formed by the addition of CO_2 to the methyl carbon of another acetyl CoA. In bacteria and plants, the fatty acid synthesizing system involves a separate polypeptide known as acyl carrier protein (ACP). In animals, ACP forms an integral part of the fatty acid synthase polypeptide chain. In all systems, ACP bears a pantetheine moiety, similar to that found in CoA. This is linked through a phosphate group to one of the ACP serines. In the synthesis of fatty acids, the malonyl group of malonyl CoA is transferred to this pantetheine sulfur, the acetyl group derived from acetyl CoA being on a neighbouring cysteine. Reaction between these groups

then occurs, in a way that results in the acetyl group being added to the methylene group of the malonyl residue. The carboxyl group that was added in the formation of malonyl CoA is lost in the reaction. The result is the formation of a four-carbon

Fig. 11.16 The fatty acid synthase gene has 43 exons.

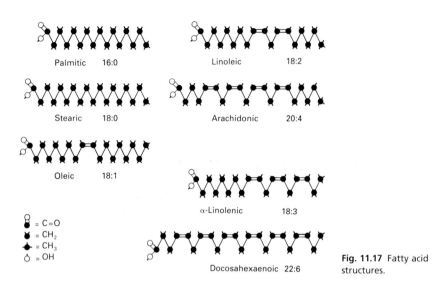

Fig. 11.17 Fatty acid structures.

$$\text{HOOCCH}_2\text{CH}_2\text{CH}_2\text{CH}_2\text{CH}_2\text{CH}_2\text{CH}_2\text{CH}_2\text{CH}_2\text{CH}_2\text{CH}_2\text{CH}_2\text{CH}_2\text{CH}_3$$

bonds cannot be inserted in this region

Fig. 11.18 Double bonds cannot be inserted within the nine carbons from the C-terminal of a fatty acid chain.

ω-6 family

Linoleic acid $\xrightarrow[\text{desaturation}]{\text{Elongation +}}$ γ-Linolenic acid → Arachidonic acid
(18:2 ω-6,9)   (18:3 ω-6,9,12)   (20:4 ω-6,9,12,15)

ω-3 family

α-Linolenic acid $\xrightarrow[\text{desaturation}]{\text{Elongation +}}$ Docosahexaenoic acid
(18:3 ω-3,6,9)   (22:6 ω-3,6,9,12,15,18)

ω-9 family

As double bonds can be inserted at ω-9–10, and points nearer to the carboxyl group than this, these acids can be synthesized from the saturated fatty acid palmitate, which in turn can be synthesized from acetyl CoA:

Palmitic acid → Stearic acid → Oleic acid → Eicosatrienoic acid
                                               (20:3 ω-9,12,15)

Fig. 11.19 Polyunsaturated fatty acid families.

1. From the carboxyl carbon, when the symbol Δ is used. In this system, linoleic acid is designated a $\Delta^{9,12}$ fatty acid.
2. From the terminal methyl carbon of the main chain, when the symbol n- (or ω-) is used. In this system, linoleic acid is designated n-6,9 or ω-6,9.

A number of desaturase enzymes are involved in the conversion of fatty acids to more highly unsaturated molecules. These are normally designated using the first of the conventions described above, the first double-bond carbon being used in the designation. Thus, Δ^4-desaturases insert double bonds between the C-4 and C-5 carbons. In addition, there are Δ^5-desaturases and Δ^9-desaturases. There are no mammalian desaturases that insert double bonds in the region shown in Fig. 11.18, i.e. between the C-9 and the methyl group. Thus, as mammals need fatty acids with double bonds in this part of the chain, precursors containing such double bonds must be taken in from the diet; these are therefore known as essential fatty acids. Linoleic acid and α-linolenic acids are examples of essential fatty acids, and are precursors of families of fatty acids that can be synthesized from them, as explained in the next section.

BIOSYNTHESIS OF LONG-CHAIN POLYUNSATURATED FATTY ACIDS

There are three major families of fatty acids; these are derived from palmitic acid, or from precursors with n-3 or n-6 double bonds. They are sometimes referred to as the palmitic acid (or oleic acid) family, the linoleic acid family and the α-linolenic acid family, respectively, according to the main precursor. These are called the n-9, n-6 or n-3 families or the ω-9, ω-6 or ω-3 families. These families of fatty acids are synthesized by a combination of the desaturase enzymes mentioned above, and elongation enzymes that can add two-carbon units to the carboxyl end of fatty acyl CoA molecules, using acetyl CoA as the two-carbon donor. An outline of the families that can result is shown in the scheme in Fig. 11.19.

ESSENTIAL FATTY ACID DEFICIENCY

If essential fatty acids are not provided in the diet, animals that require them develop a condition known as essential fatty acid (EFA) deficiency, with certain characteristic symptoms, such as a scaly skin. More importantly, the reproductive system is seriously affected. Under these conditions, increased amounts of polyunsaturated fatty acids of the n-9 family are synthesized, which replace those of the n-6 and n-3 families. In this condition, appreciable amounts of an eicosatrienoic acid, 20 : 3 $\Delta^{5,8,11}$, appear in the serum lipids, and the presence of this acid, which is present only in very small quantities in animals on EFA-adequate diets, can be used as an index of essential fatty acid status. The n-9 polyunsaturated fatty acids synthesized during EFA deficiency can substitute for those of the n-6 and n-3 families in many functions. Many tissue culture cell lines can survive happily without any fatty acids having the n-6 or n-3 structure. These latter are needed for specialized functions in higher animals, particularly the biosynthesis of prostaglandins and related eicosanoids.

TRIACYLGLYCEROL BIOSYNTHESIS

Triacylglycerols are synthesized in the final stage of lipogenesis. The initial steps involve addition of two fatty acyl CoA molecules to glycerol 3-phosphate to form phosphatidic acid. This is hydrolysed to diacylglycerol, which in turn is acylated to form a triacylglycerol, as shown in Fig. 11.20.

THE SECRETION OF TRIACYLGLYCEROL FROM THE LIVER

Considerable amounts of triacylglycerols are synthesized in the liver during the absorptive state, and these are exported to

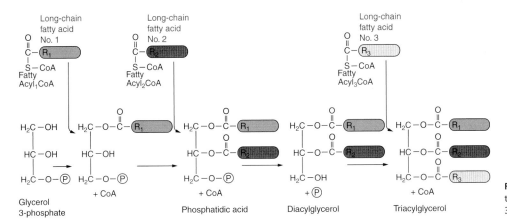

Fig. 11.20 The biosynthesis of triacylglycerol from glycerol 3-phosphate.

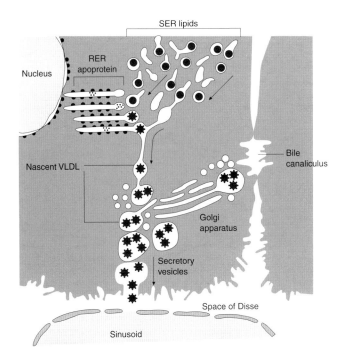

Fig. 11.21 VLDL is extruded into the space of Disse from secretory vesicles.

be taken up and stored in adipose tissue. The triacylglycerols are secreted from the liver in the form of lipoproteins; these are described in more detail in Chapter 12. The class of lipoprotein into which liver triacylglycerol is packaged is known as very low density lipoprotein (VLDL). The enzymes of triacylglycerol biosynthesis are in the smooth endoplasmic reticulum. The triacylglycerol moves into the Golgi apparatus where, together with cholesterol and phospholipids, it is formed into lipoprotein particles (see Fig. 11.21) with specific proteins, known as apolipoproteins (or, more simply, as apoproteins; see p. 164 for the meaning of apoprotein). In the case of VLDL, the proteins incorporated are apoprotein B-100 (apo B-100) and several forms of apo C (see Chapter 12), which have been synthesized in the rough endoplasmic reticulum. The lipoproteins found in plasma contain a number of other apoproteins, all of which are synthesized in the rough endoplasmic reticulum of liver, apo A and apo E being secreted from the liver in high density lipoprotein (HDL) particles. As depicted in Fig. 11.21, vesicles then bud off from the Golgi membranes and extrude the lipoprotein into the bile canaliculi.

CLINICAL IMPLICATIONS

The clinical implications of this chapter are dealt with extensively in Chapter 12.

Plasma lipoproteins, cholesterol metabolism and atherosclerosis

12

All lipid is transported in the blood in the form of plasma lipoproteins, the most important of which are very low density lipoprotein, low density lipoprotein and high density lipoprotein. Low density lipoprotein, formed in plasma from very low density lipoprotein, delivers cholesterol from the liver to peripheral tissues. It contains the highest amount of cholesterol and is associated with a familial form of ischemic heart disease. This has concentrated attention on the role of cholesterol in atherosclerosis, a precipitating factor in myocardial infarction. High density lipoprotein transports cholesterol away from peripheral tissues.

The only pathway for the metabolism of excess cholesterol is by conversion to bile acids. Some cholesterol is contained in bile. Therapeutic strategies for lowering plasma cholesterol involve sequestering bile acids to prevent their reabsorption from the gut and the use of drugs to inhibit liver cholesterol biosynthesis.

The clinical implications of combined obesity, elevated blood lipids, elevated blood sugar and the etiology of diabetes are described.

PLASMA LIPOPROTEINS AND CHOLESTEROL METABOLISM

THE COMPOSITION OF PLASMA LIPOPROTEINS

All the lipids that circulate in the blood do so as large assemblies of lipid and protein, termed lipoproteins. Two of these types of molecule are formed in liver: very low density lipoproteins (VLDL) and high density lipoproteins (HDL). Another class of lipoprotein consists of chylomicrons; these are synthesized in the intestine during fat absorption, and secreted into the lymphatic system and thence into the blood. The other major member of the plasma lipoproteins is low density lipoprotein (LDL), which is formed in the blood, mainly from VLDL. If plasma is subjected to electrophoresis and the electrophoresis strip stained for fat, a series of bands is observed relating to these lipoprotein classes, as shown in Fig. 12.1; this figure also gives some details of lipoprotein structure. An alternative system of nomenclature originates from this electrophoresis technique. HDL is the fastest moving component and thus was originally termed α-lipoprotein. The other band most prominent on the strip originated from LDL and was termed β-lipoprotein. A less prominent band, originating from VLDL and migrating ahead of LDL, was termed pre-β-lipoprotein. These analyses were often performed on fasting plasma, in which chylomicrons are absent. When present, chylomicrons remain near the origin.

Figure 12.2 shows the composition of lipoproteins in diagrammatic form. It also shows the different apolipoproteins associated with the different classes of lipoprotein. It includes an additional lipoprotein, IDL (intermediate density lipoprotein, see below), which is a product of metabolism in the plasma. The apolipoproteins can be further divided into sub-classes such as A-I, A-II etc., as shown in Fig.12.2, and as will be explained some of these have been shown to have specific roles.

The apo B of chylomicrons is a smaller molecule than that associated with VLDL, as explained on p. 36. Apo B synthesized by liver has an M_r of 514 000 and is designated B-100 to distinguish it from that synthesized by intestine, apo B-48, so-called because it is approximately 48% of the size of B-100.

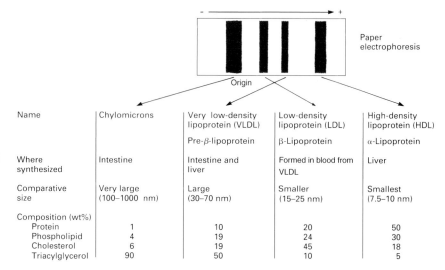

Fig. 12.1 Structure of the plasma lipoproteins.

Name	Chylomicrons	Very low-density lipoprotein (VLDL)	Low-density lipoprotein (LDL)	High-density lipoprotein (HDL)
		Pre-β-lipoprotein	β-Lipoprotein	α-Lipoprotein
Where synthesized	Intestine	Intestine and liver	Formed in blood from VLDL	Liver
Comparative size	Very large (100–1000 nm)	Large (30–70 nm)	Smaller (15–25 nm)	Smallest (7.5–10 nm)
Composition (wt%)				
Protein	1	10	20	50
Phospholipid	4	19	24	30
Cholesterol	6	19	45	18
Triacylglycerol	90	50	10	5

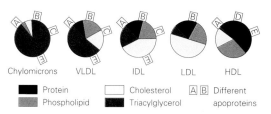

Chylomicrons   VLDL   IDL   LDL   HDL

■ Protein   □ Cholesterol   Ⓐ Ⓑ Different apoproteins
▨ Phospholipid   ■ Triacylglycerol

Fig. 12.2 Composition of the plasma lipoproteins. Subclasses: A–I, A–II, A–IV, B–100, B–48, C–I, C–II, C–III, C–IV and E.

Lipoprotein lipase: hydrolyses triacylglycerol in chylomicrons and VLDL to fatty acids and glycerol.

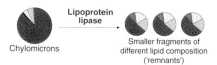

Chylomicrons → **Lipoprotein lipase** → Smaller fragments of different lipid composition ('remnants')

Fig. 12.3 Action of lipoprotein lipase on chylomicrons.

METABOLISM OF CHYLOMICRONS

The cells of the intestinal brush border synthesize triacylglycerols from the fatty acids and glucose absorbed from the gut after a meal. The triacylglycerols are packaged, with small amounts of cholesterol and phospholipid, into chylomicrons. Apolipoproteins are also required for the synthesis of the chylomicron particles, and include apo B-48, A-I, A-II and A-IV. Chylomicrons absorbed from the intestine enter the lymphatic system and, after a fatty meal, give a milky lymph, known as chyle (hence their name). They pick up apo C and apo E from HDL. In the circulation, if they are present in sufficient quantities, they confer on the plasma a milky appearance. The triacylglycerols they contain are degraded by an enzyme known as

lipoprotein lipase. Lipoprotein lipase is located on the outer surfaces of endothelial cells. The lipoprotein particles also pick up cholesteryl esters from HDL. The effect of lipoprotein lipase is to reduce the proportion of triacylglycerol in the particles (shown in Fig. 12.3), as well as to reduce their size, to give particles of lower triacylglycerol content and increased cholesteryl esters. These particles are referred to as remnants, and are further metabolized by being taken up intact into cells through specific receptors. The apo E that the chylomicrons acquire from HDL is important, as it is the ligand recognized by the receptor in the liver plasma membrane.

FORMATION OF LDL FROM VLDL

VLDL particles secreted into the plasma from liver or intestine are also acted on by

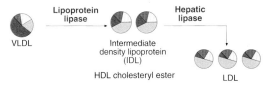

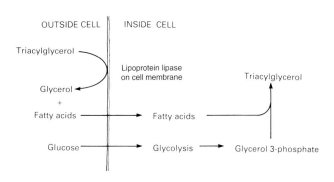

Fig. 12.4 Action of lipoprotein lipase on VLDL.

Lipoprotein lipase is activated by apoprotein C$_{II}$.

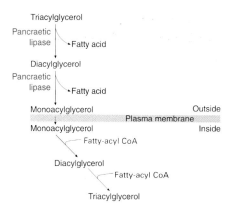

Fig. 12.6 Absorption of triacylglycerols involves breakdown and resynthesis.

Fig. 12.5 Uptake of fatty acids by peripheral tissues.

lipoprotein lipase, reducing the proportion of triacylglycerol they contain, thus also reducing their size. Apo C-II is important as an activator of lipoprotein lipase. These smaller particles accept cholesteryl esters from HDL, to form a lipoprotein class of smaller size, known as intermediate density lipoprotein (IDL). The cholesteryl esters are formed in HDL during its maturation, as explained below. The smaller VLDL and IDL particles are acted on by another lipase, which is located on the liver plasma membranes and known as hepatic lipase. This further degrades the triacylglycerols, reducing the amount of these in VLDL and IDL to low proportions. The result, as shown in Fig. 12.4, is the formation of LDL.

UPTAKE OF FATTY ACIDS BY CELLS

The fatty acids released by lipoprotein lipase are taken up by the cells of peripheral tissues, especially by adipose tissue (Fig. 12.5). The fatty acids are transported through the plasma membrane of cells and incorporated into intracellular triacylglycerols. These are synthesized as described on p. 161, and there is thus a requirement for the supply of glycerol 3-phosphate, derived by reduction of dihydroxyacetone phosphate produced by the glycolytic pathway. The glycerol released by lipoprotein lipase into the plasma is taken up by the liver and reacts with ATP to form glycerol 3-phosphate, as a result of the action of glycerol kinase. After oxidation to dihydroxyacetone phosphate it is metabolized by the glycolytic or gluconeogenic pathways.

In intestinal and liver cells, an alternative system also functions, in which fatty acyl CoA is added to monoacylglycerol (Fig. 12.6).

FORMATION OF HDL

An HDL precursor particle is formed in the liver by enzymic systems in the Golgi apparatus that are related to those previously discussed and which combine apoproteins synthesized in the rough endoplasmic reticulum with lipids synthesized in the smooth endoplasmic reticulum. These precursor particles contain two forms of apo A – apo A-I and apo A-II – as the main apoproteins together with apo E. They are discoidal in shape and rich in unesterified cholesterol and phosphatidylcholine (also

known as lecithin). After secretion into the plasma, these precursors are acted upon by the enzyme lecithin–cholesterol acyltransferase (LCAT, pronounced 'el cat') transferring a fatty acid from lecithin to cholesterol. As a result, the molecule becomes more enriched in cholesteryl esters, some of which are transferred to the maturing LDL particles. These processes yield the mature HDL, which is more spherical in shape. Figure 12.7 summarizes the formation of LDL and HDL in plasma.

FUNCTIONS OF APOLIPOPROTEINS

Some functions of apolipoproteins, additional to their structural role, are detailed in Table 12.1.

OVERVIEW OF LIPOPROTEIN METABOLISM

Figure 12.8 summarizes and brings together the various metabolic events concerned in lipoprotein traffic that have

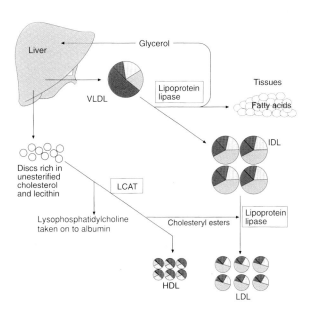

Fig. 12.7 Lipoprotein metabolism in plasma.

Table 12.1 Functions of apolipoproteins

Apoprotein	Function
A-I	Activates lecithin–cholesterol acyltransferase
B-100	Recognized by receptors on liver cells and other cells within the peripheral circulatory system, and plays an important role in the uptake by these cells of lipoproteins that carry this apoprotein
C-II	Activates lipoprotein lipase. A deficiency of this apoprotein has in some cases been associated with elevated plasma triacylglycerol levels
E	Liver cells carry receptors for apo E; this is important for efficient uptake by the liver of the lipoproteins in which it occurs

CHOLESTEROL BIOSYNTHESIS

The level of circulating cholesterol has received attention as a factor in the etiology of human disease, especially atherosclerosis. Cholesterol is synthesized from acetyl CoA in the liver. Figure 12.9 outlines the enzymic pathway that brings about the synthesis of squalene from cytosolic 3-hydroxy-3-methylglutaryl CoA (HMG CoA). These steps will not be discussed in detail but the first enzyme indicated in the figure, HMG-CoA reductase, plays a pivotal role in regulating the synthesis of cholesterol. The intermediates farnesyl diphosphate and geranyl diphosphate are important molecules in their own right (see, for example, p. 201).

Metabolism of isopentenyl phosphate (not shown in detail here) results in the formation of the 30-carbon compound, squalene, from six five-carbon

been discussed. LDL is a major vehicle for the distribution of cholesterol from the liver to other tissues of the body where, as unesterified cholesterol, it forms an essential constituent of the plasma membrane. The cholesterol content of LDL (as esterified cholesterol) is the highest of any lipoprotein. LDL interacts with the membranes of peripheral tissues to transfer cholesterol to them. HDL, on the other hand, has the capacity to remove cholesterol from these membranes, and these two lipoproteins appear to function in maintaining cholesterol levels in the body, together with other mechanisms discussed below.

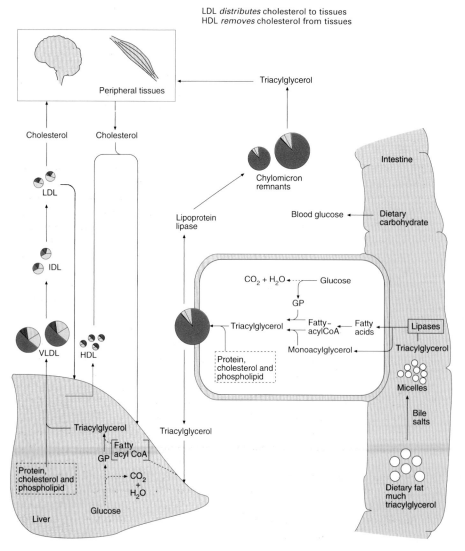

Fig. 12.8 Overview of lipoprotein metabolism. GP, Glycerol 3-phosphate

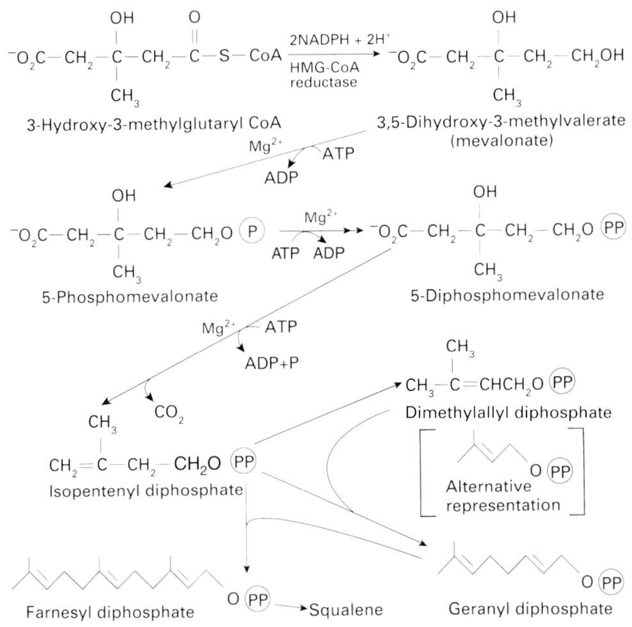

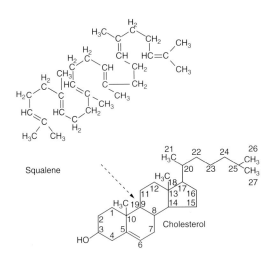

Fig. 12.9 The biosynthesis of prenyl compounds.

3-Hydroxy-3-methylglutaryl-CoA reductase (HMG-CoA reductase) is an important key enzyme that regulates cholesterol synthesis.

Fig. 12.10 The formation of cholesterol from squalene.

intermediates, and this molecule can then be transformed into cholesterol (Fig. 12.10). Although the major site of cholesterol synthesis is the liver, other tissues, such as the adrenal cortex, reproductive organs and skin fibroblasts (which are much used in culture to study cholesterol metabolism), can synthesize cholesterol. The regulation of this pathway is discussed in a later section (see Chapter 13).

LIPOPROTEIN RECEPTOR TRAFFIC

Lipoproteins have a limited life in the plasma. They are not only secreted into the circulation but are constantly being taken up by cells and removed from the circulation. They are then degraded, in the case of the proteins to constituent amino acids, in the case of the lipids to fatty acids and glycerol-based residues. Cholesterol cannot be oxidized to carbon dioxide and water; the regulation of its levels is dealt with in a subsequent section (p. 169). This continual synthesis and degradation is an important part of the mechanism for regulating the levels of circulating lipoproteins.

The process is illustrated in Fig. 12.11, in which the metabolism of LDL and its receptor is used as an example. Similar processes are involved in the metabolism of HDL and chylomicron remnants. The plasma membranes of liver cells, and of some cells of the mononuclear phagocyte system, contain receptors that recognize apoproteins B or E. In the case of LDL, apo B-100 is the important ligand. This is

recognized by a specific receptor that accumulates in coated pits, which are invaginations of the plasma membrane coated on the inner surface with clathrin, a protein that is described in more detail on p. 210. On binding LDL, the membrane pinches off into vesicles, which become organelles known as endosomes, and these deliver their contents to lysosomes. This vesicular uptake system is considered in more detail in Chapter 15. The lysosomes carry out the degradative processes mentioned above. Some of the cholesterol is re-esterified and stored as cholesteryl esters, and some is excreted as bile acids as explained below.

As shown in Fig. 12.11, new LDL receptors eventually progress from the rough endoplasmic reticulum, through the Golgi apparatus, to the plasma membrane, where as unoccupied receptors they accumulate in clathrin-coated pits ready to bind further apo B-100.

This system is regulated by elaborate control mechanisms described in Chapter 15. As indicated in Fig. 12.11, this includes inhibition of LDL receptor synthesis and of HMG-CoA reductase activity at times of oversupply of cholesterol. The inhibition of LDL receptor synthesis causes a reduction in the number of LDL receptors in the liver plasma membrane, thereby reducing further uptake of cholesterol.

BILE ACID BIOSYNTHESIS

The only way that excess cholesterol can be removed from the body is through excretion in bile, either directly or after its conversion to bile acids. The pathway for the synthesis of the bile acids is complex and will not be described in detail. It involves a number of modifications of the cholesterol molecule, which are summarized in Fig. 12.12. Two distinct series of bile acids are synthesized, yielding cholic acid and chenodeoxycholic acid, respectively. From these, deoxycholic acid and lithocholic acid can be synthesized by gut bacteria. The structures are shown in Fig. 12.12. 7α-Hydroxylase, the enzyme introducing the 7α-hydroxyl into the molecule, is a regulatory enzyme in bile acid synthesis.

In cholic acid, all three hydroxyl groups project from the same face of the molecule (see Fig. 12.13). The synthetic reactions are directed to achieving this. Thus the hydroxyl group already on the molecule, the 3β-hydroxyl group of cholesterol, must be inverted to a 3α-hydroxyl group in cholic acid.

167

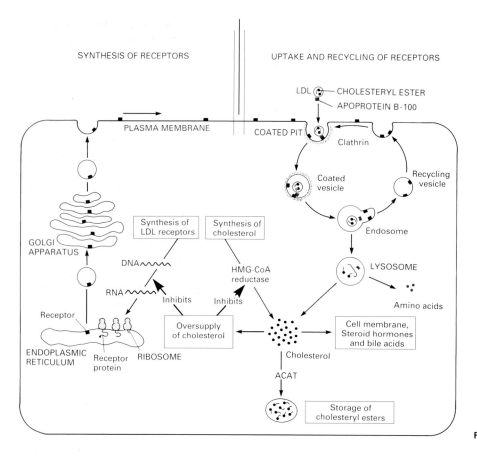

SYNTHESIS OF RECEPTORS

UPTAKE AND RECYCLING OF RECEPTORS

Fig. 12.11 Recycling of the LDL receptor.

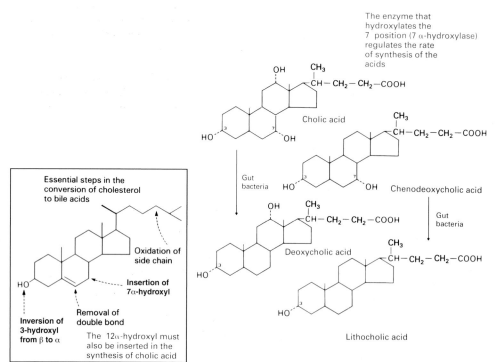

Fig. 12.12 The biosynthesis of bile acids.

The bile acids are excreted in conjugated form, as taurocholic acid or glycocholic acid. In taurocholic acid, taurine is linked to cholic acid by an amide linkage between the carboxyl group of cholic acid and the amino group of taurine. Taurine ($H_2NCH_2CH_2SO_3H$) is formed by the decarboxylation of cysteine and oxidation of the sulfhydryl group to a sulfonic acid group ($-SH \rightarrow -SO_3H$). Glycocholic acid has glycine linked to cholic acid in a similar manner.

BILE

Bile is a complex solution of salts and protein, containing micelles composed of cholesterol, phospholipids and bile salts. Bile is formed in the liver and secreted

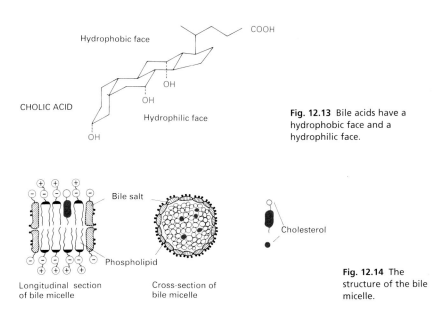

CHOLIC ACID

Hydrophobic face

COOH

OH

OH

Hydrophilic face

OH

Fig. 12.13 Bile acids have a hydrophobic face and a hydrophilic face.

Bile salt

Phospholipid

Cholesterol

Longitudinal section of bile micelle

Cross-section of bile micelle

Fig. 12.14 The structure of the bile micelle.

Table 12.2 Normal and abnormal bile differ comparatively little in composition

Component	Normal bile (%)	Abnormal bile (%) (taken from a patient with cholesterol gallstones)
Lecithin	74	71
Bile salts	20	13
Cholesterol	6	16

down the bile duct into the gall bladder, from where it passes into the intestine. Here the bile salts facilitate the degradation of ingested fats.

The structure of bile micelles is illustrated in Fig. 12.14. Bilayers of phospholipid (similar to those in cell membranes, see p. 200), in which cholesterol is embedded, form a disc with an ionic flat surface above and below. Around the edge of these discs, bile acids bind through their hydrophobic face to the hydrophobic side-chains of the phospholipids, the hydrophilic face of the bile salts being presented to the aqueous environment as a hydrophilic surface. This is possible because of the stereochemistry of the bile acids, illustrated in Fig. 12.13. They are a specialized form of detergent but whereas most detergents have a hydrophilic and a hydrophobic *end*, bile acids have a hydrophilic and a hydrophobic *face*. This results from the orientation of the hydroxyls towards the same face of the molecule.

CLINICAL IMPLICATIONS – GALLSTONES

The composition of bile micelles is critical and imbalance can lead to crystallization of

cholesterol in the gall bladder, leading to the formation of gallstones. This can result from relatively small differences in composition, as indicated in Table 12.2. Stones containing bile pigments, either alone or in mixed stones with cholesterol are also found.

WHOLE-BODY REGULATION OF CHOLESTEROL METABOLISM

Control of the level of total body cholesterol depends on the rate of its excretion in bile, as cholesterol or as bile salts, in relation to the rate of synthesis in the liver. The rate of synthesis is regulated by feedback inhibition on HMG-CoA reductase by excess cholesterol, as already described. Thus, if large amounts of cholesterol are entering the liver as a result of ingestion of cholesterol, the rate of synthesis will be inhibited. The excessive amounts of cholesterol can then be decreased by excretion in bile directly or as bile salts. The systems involved are summarized in Fig. 12.15. It is fortunate for individuals living on cholesterol-rich foods typical of those in the diets of prosperous nations that cholesterol absorption from the gut is not very efficient. However, the bile acids secreted into the intestine are reabsorbed very efficiently, and thus would not offer a means for the excretion of cholesterol unless mechanisms existed that reduced the effect of this. These mechanisms include conversion of bile acids by gut bacteria to forms that are not reabsorbed, and conjugation of reabsorbed bile acids in the kidney to forms that are excreted by that organ.

All of the cholesterol circulating in the blood is contained in lipoproteins, and the central role of cholesterol in lipoprotein metabolism is illustrated in Fig. 12.16.

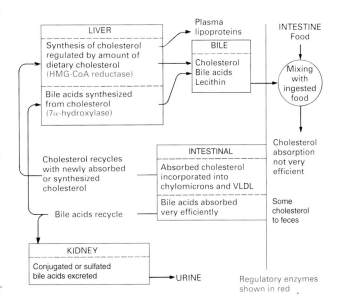

Fig. 12.15 Overview of whole-body metabolism of cholesterol.

LIVER

Synthesis of cholesterol regulated by amount of dietary cholesterol (HMG-CoA reductase)

Bile acids synthesized from cholesterol (7α-hydroxylase)

Cholesterol recycles with newly absorbed or synthesized cholesterol

Bile acids recycle

KIDNEY

Conjugated or sulfated bile acids excreted

Plasma lipoproteins

BILE

Cholesterol
Bile acids
Lecithin

INTESTINAL

Absorbed cholesterol incorporated into chylomicrons and VLDL

Bile acids absorbed very efficiently

INTESTINE
Food

Mixing with ingested food

Cholesterol absorption not very efficient

Some cholesterol to feces

URINE

Regulatory enzymes shown in red

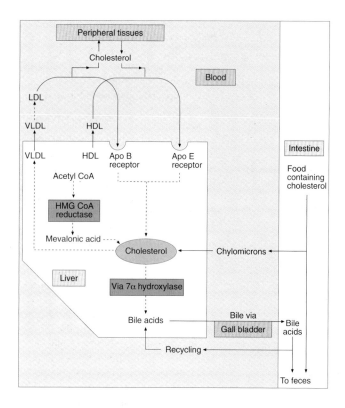

Fig. 12.16 The role of plasma lipoproteins in cholesterol metabolism.

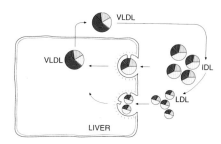

Fig. 12.17 The recycling of VLDL, IDL and LDL.

explained below, as a result of uptake of LDL by macrophages that results from excessively high levels of circulating LDL. The plaques are particularly hazardous if they occur in the coronary artery. In some cases they become so large that they occlude the artery to the point that if a blood clot occurs at that place (possibly induced by the plaque itself) severe ischemia results, causing a myocardial infarct. In heterozygotes, the higher incidence of myocardial infarcts is delayed to middle age.

Uptake of LDL by macrophages

A receptor in the macrophage plasma recognizes LDL that has undergone modification as a result of circulating in the plasma for a prolonged period, with resultant lipid peroxidation. In cases where elevated levels of LDL persist, these macrophages will take up LDL molecules continually, to the point that they become engorged with lipid. They can be seen in histological sections as 'foam cells' deposited in arterial walls. They store esterified cholesterol in lipid droplets, but with predominantly an oleoyl group rather than the linoleoyl group that is commonly found in plasma esterified cholesterol. The details are shown in Fig. 12.19. The modified LDL is internalized in vesicles (2) and degraded in lysosomal particles (3). The LDL is totally degraded, the protein being hydrolysed to amino acids. Phospholipids and triacylglycerols

CLINICAL IMPLICATIONS – ELEVATED BLOOD LIPIDS AND ATHEROSCLEROSIS

Hyperlipidemia

Hyperlipidemia – the presence of elevated levels of lipid in the blood – results from a number of conditions. It can be caused quite commonly as a secondary disorder in a number of conditions, such as alcoholism, hypothyroidism, diabetes or the use of drugs. The following sections consider the classification of the hyperlipidemias and the causes of specific hyperlipidemia.

Familial hypercholesterolemia

As previously stated, the plasma lipoprotein with the highest content of cholesterol is LDL. This continuously recycles back into the liver through the apo B-100 receptor. IDL is also taken up by liver through receptors recognizing apo B-100 and apo E (see Fig. 12.17), and much IDL is removed from the circulation before it is converted to LDL, an event that helps to regulate the plasma LDL level. Not only is the activity of HMG–CoA reductase regulated by the cholesterol entering the liver but, as indicated above (see Fig. 12.11), the rate of biosynthesis of the apo B-100 receptor, and thus the number of receptors, is down-regulated by the rate of uptake of LDL.

Some individuals inherit a defect in the biosynthesis of functional apo B receptors, leading to lack of these receptors in the plasma membrane and inability to remove LDL from the blood. This gives rise to familial hypercholesterolemia and is classified as type II hyperlipidemia. In the homozygote, there is a severe deficiency that leads to exceptionally high levels of LDL (and thus of cholesterol) in the blood (see Fig. 12.18). In the heterozygote, one allele is functional, so the condition is less severe. In the homozygote, the condition is sufficiently severe for atherosclerosis to develop to such an extent that it is apparent in children and young adults, leading in some cases to death at an early age. Atherosclerosis is the term given to a thickening of the walls of arteries by so-called plaques, consisting of lipid-laden macrophages with associated fibrosis and calcification. These are formed, as

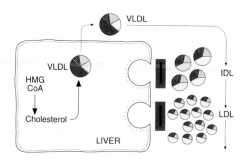

Fig. 12.18 The effect of defective lipoprotein receptors on plasma lipoproteins.

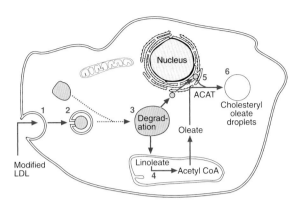

Fig. 12.19 The metabolism of lipoproteins by macrophages. See text for details. ACAT, acylcholesterol acyl transferase

are degraded to fatty acids and glycerol 3-phosphate or glycerol, and cholesteryl esters to cholesterol and fatty acids. The fatty acids, indicated by linoleate (4), are degraded in mitochondria to acetyl CoA from which oleate is formed. In the endoplasmic reticulum, oleate and cholesterol form cholesteryl oleate (5) which accumulates in lipid droplets (6).

THERAPEUTIC STRATEGIES FOR LOWERING PLASMA CHOLESTEROL

There is overwhelming evidence that lipid-lowering therapy limits the progression of atherosclerosis and reduces coronary artery disease and events associated with it. Statins such as compactin and lovastatin inhibit HMG-CoA reductase and thus restrict the production of LDL, the vehicle that delivers cholesterol to tissues, and which accumulates in foam cells when present in plasma at high levels for long periods (see above). They also lower triacylglycerol-rich lipoproteins and raise HDL. Attention has previously concentrated on reducing LDL cholesterol with statins, but recent evidence also stresses the importance of raising HDL levels and reducing triacylglycerol-rich lipoproteins. The fibrates, another important class of drug, have a major impact in lowering plasma triacylglycerol-rich lipoproteins and raising HDL levels. They enhance lipoprotein lipase, apo A-I and apo A-II transcription and reduce that of apo C-III. Their action is discussed more fully below (see Clinical implications – combined obesity, elevated blood lipids, elevated blood sugar, diabetes type 2, p. 173). Fibrates and statins have complementary lipid modifying and pleiotropic effects so that their combination should provide the highest cardiovascular benefit. This hypothesis is currently being tested in the Lipid in Diabetes Study, an outcome trial comparing monotherapy with fenofibrate and cerivastatin with combination therapy.

The effect of these drugs can be enhanced by simultaneously administering an agent that prevents the reabsorption of bile acids, thus increasing the conversion of cholesterol to bile acids. If an anion-exchange resin (one that is used therapeutically is known as cholestyramine) is administered by mouth, this will pass through the intestine, binding bile acids that are present and causing them to be excreted in the feces (Fig. 12.20).

CLASSIFICATION OF HYPERLIPIDEMIA

The simplest classification of hyperlipidemia consists in distinguishing elevated cholesterol levels and elevated

triacylglycerol levels. Elevated cholesterol levels are associated with more serious consequences, as explained above, but elevated triacylglycerol levels also correlate, less strongly, with disease. In many cases, this classification is sufficient. However, as the bulk of blood lipids are contained in the lipoproteins, hyperlipidemias have also been classified into types of hyperlipoproteinemia, first described by Fredrickson. This classification is shown in Table 12.3. Inspection of the compositions of the various lipoproteins (p. 164) makes it clear how these distinctions arose.

Diagnosis of the type of hyperlipoproteinemia can be achieved by electrophoresis of the plasma proteins, followed by detection of the lipoproteins by use of a stain for lipids. Some examples are shown in Fig. 12.21. A more extensive analysis can be obtained using an analytical ultracentrifuge. Patterns obtained from solutions containing different lipoprotein mixtures are shown in Fig. 12.22. At the salt densities used, the lipoproteins move towards the centre of the rotor, i.e. they float at rates determined by the density of the particles. The abscissa is marked in units that indicate the rate at which the different components of the solution float, termed Svedberg flotation units. The ordinate indicates the amount of any component at the different points in the

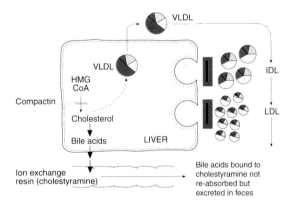

Fig. 12.20 Strategies for lowering plasma cholesterol.

Table 12.3 Classification of the hyperlipidemias

Fredrickson type	Lipoprotein elevated	Cholesterol level	Triacylglycerol level
I	Chylomicrons (also possibly VLDL)	+	+ + +
IIa	LDL	+ + +	±
IIb	LDL and VLDL	+ +	+ +
III	'Floating' LDL	+ + +	+ + +
IV	VLDL	±	+ +
V	VLDL and chylomicrons	+	+ + +

±, normal to slightly increased; + +, moderately increased; + + +, greatly increased.

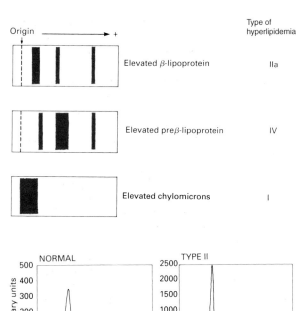

Origin ——————→ +

Elevated β-lipoprotein — IIa

Elevated preβ-lipoprotein — IV

Elevated chylomicrons — I

Type of hyperlipidemia

Fig. 12.21 Diagnosis of hyperlipidemia by electrophoresis.

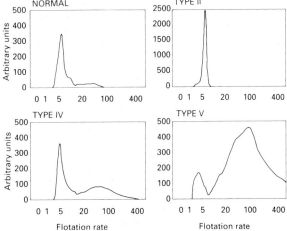

NORMAL

TYPE II

TYPE IV

TYPE V

Flotation rate

Flotation rate

Arbitrary units

Fig. 12.22 Lipoproteins in the ultracentrifuge.

rotor cell. As can be seen, there is a continuous spectrum of particles of different densities within any density range. Note the very high levels of LDL in familial hypercholesterolemia (classified as type II hyperlipidemia), such that the scale of the ordinate has to be altered.

'GOOD' AND 'BAD' CHOLESTEROL?

Increased awareness of the role of HDL in transporting cholesterol from tissues to liver for processing led to the realization that measurements of total serum cholesterol as an index of atherogenic risk could be misleading, and that there was a need for the separate measurement of LDL and HDL cholesterol. Elevated HDL cholesterol might in fact be a favourable indicator. Impetus has been given to this concept by the discovery of a mutation in apoA-I in a population in the village of Limone sul Garda in Italy, a polymorphism known as apo A-I(Milano), or apo A-I$_M$, after the clinic in which it was identified. Apo A-I$_M$ is the result of a point mutation, (R173C, arginine to cysteine substitution at position 173). This mutation appears to

confer high protection against cardiovascular disease to this small population. Laboratory and clinical evidence has been adduced that introduction of this mutant into animals and humans can reduce plaque formation, though the exact nature of the protective effect is still a matter of discussion

DIETARY POLYUNSATURATED FATTY ACIDS AND BLOOD LIPIDS

The types and quantities of different fatty acids (i.e. the fatty acid profile) of the diet are reflected in the fatty acid pattern of plasma lipoproteins. Increasing the amount of linoleate in the diet will increase the linoleate level in all the lipoprotein types, and therefore the ratio of polyunsaturated fatty acids to saturated fatty acids, which can be referred to as the P/S ratio. This leads to changes in the fatty acid patterns of the tissue lipids. Thus, in contrast to the situation with dietary protein or carbohydrate, the nature of an individual's dietary fat exerts a qualitative influence on bodily composition. The fatty acid patterns of different meats and oils are shown in Table 12.4. It can be seen that poultry and fish have comparatively high levels of polyunsaturated fatty acids. Not all oils used for cooking are equally rich in polyunsaturated fatty acids but oil generally contains more unsaturated fatty acids than the solid fats obtained from meat, which

Table 12.4 The fatty acid patterns of fats and oils

Fat or oil	16:0	16:1	18:0	18:1	18:2 (ω-6)	20:4 (ω-6)	20:5 (ω-3)	22:6 (ω-6)
Animal fat								
Beef	35	3	20	36				
Mutton	27		31	32				
Pork	30	3	11	42	11			
Rabbit	27	9	3	28	20			
Chicken	18	10	5	34	17			
Duck	21	6	6	49	16			
Turkey	23	7	8	32	25			
Fish								
Herring	15	12	2	21	3	1 (20:1 ω-9, 15%) (22:1 ω-11, 16%)	9	6
Sardine	16	9	3	11	1	2	17	13
Salmon	11	5	4	24	5	5	5	17
Oils								
Olive	10		2	78	7			
Corn	10		2	30	50			
Sunflower	6		6	18	69			

Compositions vary considerably from sample to sample. Only selected fatty acids are listed but values represent % of all fatty acids present.

have a low P/S ratio. The addition of oils such as corn oil or sunflower seed oil to the diet (e.g. by using them in cooking) is the only really effective way of significantly increasing the P/S ratio, accompanied by a reduction in the ingestion of highly saturated meats such as mutton, pork and beef.

Polyunsaturated fatty acids are frequently located at the *sn*-2 position of phospholipids, whereas saturated fatty acids predominate at the *sn*-1 position; however, despite this general rule, phospholipids with two unsaturated fatty acids or two saturated fatty acids are found. One of the latter, dipalmitoylphosphatidylcholine, is a lung surfactant, the concentration of which is a useful indicator of the maturity of the fetal lung.

CLINICAL IMPLICATIONS – COMBINED OBESITY, ELEVATED BLOOD LIPIDS, ELEVATED BLOOD SUGAR. DIABETES TYPE 2

Type 2 diabetes mellitus came to be recognized in individuals who had elevated blood sugar levels but also significant levels of circulating insulin. It is now considered to be a polygenic disease (see p. 51) closely associated with obesity, and together they constitute a major health problem worldwide. In the majority of cases, type 2 diabetes is now widely considered to be one component within a group of disorders sometimes called the metabolic syndrome. Factors characteristic of the metabolic syndrome, also known as dysmetabolic syndrome X, are abdominal obesity, atherogenic dyslipidemia (elevated triacylglycerol levels, small low density lipoprotein particles, low high density lipoprotein cholesterol levels), elevated blood pressure, and insulin resistance (with

or without glucose intolerance). Together, these contribute to a prothrombotic state, increasing the risk of cardiovascular disease.

People who develop type 2 diabetes usually pass through the phases of excessive adipogenesis (obesity), insulin resistance, hyperinsulinemia, pancreatic β cell stress and damage, leading to progressive decrease of insulin secretion and impaired glucose levels (both postprandial and fasting). Fasting glucose is presumed to remain normal as long as insulin hypersecretion can compensate for insulin resistance. The fall in insulin secretion leading to hyperglycemia occurs as a later phenomenon, and initially treatment with insulin is not required. Thus type 2 diabetes is often referred to as non-insulin-dependent diabetes mellitus (NIDDM).

The cause of insulin resistance is not known. Certainly, elevated free fatty acid levels, such as those found in obese persons, inhibit the utilization of glucose within muscle. Genetic defects leading to defective insulin receptor function might also contribute. Few defects of the insulin receptor are known (insulin is an important regulator of growth and development). Those that do occur are associated with severe insulin resistance leading to conditions such as leprachaunism, of which more than 100 cases are known. Mutations of downstream mediators such as IRS-2 (see p. 203) are thought more likely to contribute to insulin resistance.

Effects of transcription factors PPAR and LXR in diabetes type 2 and atherosclerosis

Attention has recently been focused on transcription factors that regulate a number of genes involved in lipid metabolism known as PPARs – peroxisome

proliferator-activated receptors. Activated PPAR-α stimulates the expression of genes involved in fatty acid and lipoprotein metabolism. Interest in PPARs is stimulated by the knowledge that PPAR-α activators, such as the fibrates (see also p. 171), decrease triacylglycerol concentrations by increasing the expression of lipoprotein lipase and decreasing apo C-III concentration. Furthermore, they increase HDL cholesterol by increasing the expression of apo A-I and apo A-II. PPAR-α activation by fibrates improves insulin sensitivity and decreases thrombosis and vascular inflammation.

Another group of transcription factors thought to be important in lipid metabolism are Liver X receptors (LXR). LXRs positively regulate genes involved in cholesterol metabolism. They also have effects on genes involved in fatty acid metabolism, and on SREBP (p. 183).

PPARs and LXRs are members of the family of nuclear receptors that act as transcription factors (p. 43). They possess characteristic conserved DNA-binding domains, including two zinc finger motifs (p. 43) and ligand-binding domains. Natural ligands for PPARs and LXRs appear to be fatty acids and cholesterol metabolites, respectively. Both receptors form heterodimers, PPAR/RXR and LXR/RXR, with the retinoid receptor RXR, and these function as transcriptional regulators in the presence of appropriate ligand complexes. It was the cloning of PPARα cDNA that led to realization that PPARα was a moelcular target of fibrates, such as clofibrate and gemfibrizol, which are PPARα activators that have long been used as lipid-lowering drugs.

This is an emerging area with important potential value in the investigation of the metabolic syndrome.

13

The action of hormones and other effectors in regulating glycogen and glucose metabolism, ketogenesis and lipogenesis

At the whole-body level, carbohydrate and lipid metabolism is regulated by hormones. In the fasting state, hormones having a major role are glucagon, adrenaline, glucocorticoids and adrenocorticotropin (ACTH). These variously stimulate the release of glucose from liver glycogen, amino acids from muscle protein and fatty acids from fat depots. In the absorptive state, insulin opposes the action of these hormones and is responsible for lowering the blood glucose level, for stimulating the uptake of glucose by muscle, and for activating pathways for the synthesis of glycogen and triacylglycerol. In the short term, these hormones act through second messenger systems, including cyclic AMP and the products of phosphoinositide-specific phospholipase C. These then stimulate protein kinases and protein phosphatases.

Enzyme systems are also controlled at the level of gene expression, and the structure of promoters and their interaction with specific transcription factors determines how and when the genes are activated or repressed.

WHOLE-BODY INTERACTIONS

OVERALL STRATEGY OF CONTROL

Integration of carbohydrate and lipid pathways is an important feature of metabolism in all species. This discussion concentrates on the situation in mammals. In these animals, hormones exert a dominant effect on these pathways.

When such an animal ingests a meal, carbohydrate and lipid intermediary metabolism is dominated by the influx of metabolites from the intestine. The most important metabolites from the point of view of the present discussion are glucose, derived from dietary carbohydrates, and triacylglycerols, derived from the fatty acids removed in the gut from the variety of lipids that have been ingested. In this situation, insulin is the main agent of control. As outlined in Fig. 13.1, its actions in this condition are to promote the synthesis of glycogen from glucose in muscle and liver, and the synthesis of triacylglycerols in liver and adipose tissue. It might at first sight seem surprising that triacylglycerols are being synthesized in the liver when they have already been synthesized in intestinal cells and absorbed as components of chylomicrons, as explained in the section on plasma lipoproteins. The chylomicrons, however, function simply as a transport vehicle for the absorbed fatty acids, which then have to be sorted and restructured in accordance with the needs of the host animal. The pattern of fatty acids in the diet is only partly reflected in the pattern in tissue lipids, as the liver and other tissues engage in a retailoring process, oxidizing some fatty acids and synthesizing others as necessary to maintain the proportions of the different fatty acids in appropriate lipids as required by the needs of the cell. The triacylglycerols of adipose tissue contain little polyunsaturated fatty acid. Although an appreciable amount of the absorbed fatty acid is taken up and incorporated into triacylglycerol directly by peripheral tissues, especially adipose tissue, the liver is the tissue primarily involved in the process of retailoring fatty acid patterns. The liver has the additional function of maintaining the appropriate concentrations of the different plasma lipoproteins, as explained in Chapter 12, and to this end will also be synthesizing phospholipid for VLDL and HDL from the ingested fatty acids. Excess carbohydrate is also converted by the liver to triacylglycerol by the lipogenic pathways, and this conversion of carbohydrate to a

storage fuel is a major function of liver in the absorptive state.

In contrast to the above situation, in the fasting state insulin action is moderated, and other hormones such as glucagon, glucocorticoids, adrenaline, ACTH (adrenocorticotropin) and growth hormone will be acting to direct metabolic pathways, as outlined in Fig. 13.2. The amount of glucose that can be derived from the breakdown of liver glycogen is limited, so it is also necessary for amino acid carbon to be mobilized from the muscles for conversion to glucose. The use by peripheral tissues of ketone bodies, synthesized from fatty acids mobilized from adipose tissue and converted to ketone bodies in the liver, reduces the amount of glucose used as fuel. The use of fuel from fat stores rather than from muscles is beneficial, because, in a long fast, muscles are essential for survival.

The hormones act mainly through the mechanisms discussed in Chapter 6 – namely, as second messengers and in protein phosphorylation. In addition, the pathways being considered are also subjected to non-hormonal regulation. For

instance, when muscle contracts, there is an immediate requirement for production of glucose 1-phosphate from muscle glycogen, together with an increase in glycolytic flux, if the supply of ATP is to be maintained, and control of this process is non-hormonal.

THE REGULATION OF GLYCOGEN METABOLISM

GLYCOGEN METABOLISM IN MUSCLE

The reactions involved in muscle glycogen metabolism are outlined in Fig. 13.3. The opposing actions of glycogen synthase and phosphorylase are dominant in this cycle, and the enzymology involved in their regulation is very complex. In addition, the contribution of glycogenin (see p. 157) might be important but has yet to be clarified. Glycogen synthase and phosphorylase are subject to regulation by protein kinases and phosphatases, as also are the kinases and phosphatases that act on them.

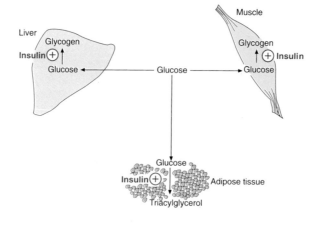

Fig. 13.1 The effect of hormones on tissue metabolism in the absorptive state.

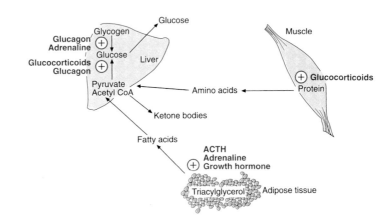

Fig. 13.2 The effect of hormones on tissue metabolism in the fasting state.

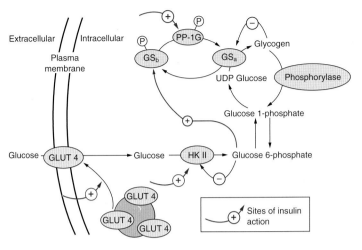

GSa Glycogen synthase a
GSb Glycogen synthase b
PP-1G Protein phosphatase 1G
HK II Hexokinase II
GLUT 4 Insulin-sensitive glucose transporter

Fig. 13.3 The action of insulin on muscle glycogen metabolism.

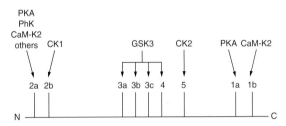

Fig. 13.4 Muscle glycogen synthase has nine phosphorylation sites.

Muscle glycogen synthase has nine phosphorylation sites, indicated in Fig. 13.4. These sites are phosphorylated by several kinases, including cyclic AMP-dependent protein kinase (PKA), casein kinase 2 and glycogen synthase kinase 3 (GSK–3). Liver glycogen synthase lacks phosphorylation sites 1a and 1b. A number of protein kinases have been classified as glycogen synthase kinases, because of their action in phosphorylating glycogen synthase at different sites; they include GSK-1, which is PKA, and GSK-2, which is phosphorylase kinase; GSK-5 is casein kinase 2. GSK-3 acts to phosphorylate three sites, probably after the other sites have been phosphorylated. Phosphorylation of the enzyme converts it from glucose 6-phosphate-independent GSa, formerly known as the I form, to a less active form, formerly known as the D form but now called GSb, which is glucose 6-phosphate dependent. The switch between the forms is not all-or-none, and probably intermediate forms are normally present in the cell, of differing states of phosphorylation, and with intermediate sensitivities to glucose 6-phosphate. Phosphorylase is phosphorylated by phosphorylase kinase on only one site, as

shown on p. 147; this converts it to a more active form that does not depend on AMP for activation. Thus the action of kinases tends to promote glycogenolysis.

Phosphorylase kinase is the largest of all the protein kinases. It is hexadecameric, consisting of a complex of four identical tetramers of α, β, γ, δ subunits, and is activated by PKA. The δ subunit of phosphorylase kinase is in fact the calmodulin molecule, which mediates the regulatory role of Ca^{2+} in this aspect of glycogen metabolism. Ca^{2+} also activates PKC, which is yet another kinase that phosphorylates glycogen synthase.

Protein phosphatase-1 (PP-1G) acts on glycogen synthase b and phosphorylase a. This protein phosphatase has a catalytic C subunit and a regulatory G subunit. The regulatory G subunit gives it its subclassification, and is responsible for binding it to glycogen.

Glycogen is found in large particles that include glycogen metabolizing enzymes such as glycogen synthase, phosphorylase, phosphorylase kinase and protein phosphatase-1, so the enzymes responsible for both the synthesis and breakdown of glycogen appear to be in contact with it,

and the direction of metabolism depends on the state of regulatory mechanisms.

THE EFFECT OF INSULIN ON GLYCOGEN METABOLISM IN MUSCLE

Insulin promotes glycogen synthesis in muscle by controlling the influx of glucose through the transporter GLUT 4 (see p. 156), molecules of which it recruits to the plasma membrane (see Fig. 13.3). The result is increased formation of glucose 6-phosphate. It also activates a protein kinase cascade, which has the following effects:

- Inhibition of GSK3, and thus activation of glycogen synthase (the phosphorylated form of glycogen synthase, GSb, is the less active form; thus, if the kinase is inhibited, phosphatase action will dominate and cause activation).
- Phosphorylation of PP-1G, activating it; this enhances conversion of GSb to GSa. It also stimulates action of the phosphatase on phosphorylase, which is thus inactivated (p. 147).
- Activation of glycogen synthase and inhibition of phosphorylase result in enhanced glycogen biosynthesis.

Further details of the mechanism by which insulin brings about these effects are on p. 203.

GLYCOGEN METABOLISM IN LIVER

Glucose influx into liver is not insulin dependent. GLUT 2 is the liver glucose transporter and delivers glucose to glucokinase, which regulates the rate of metabolism of glucose (Fig. 13.5). In liver, in contrast to muscle, PP-1G is inhibited by phosphorylase a, and this maintains phosphorylase in the more active form. It also prevents conversion of glycogen synthase to the more active form, thus favouring glycogen breakdown. The inhibition of PP-1G by phosphorylase a results from binding of phosphorylase a to the G subunit of PP-1G. The inhibition can be overcome by high glucose levels, as glucose binding to phosphorylase a makes phosphoserine-14 more accessible to phosphatase action, and the resulting less active phosphorylase b does not inhibit PP-1G. Thus glucose tends to activate glycogen synthesis. Adrenaline activates PKA to phosphorylate PP-1G, and this causes dissociation of subunits G and C. This inactivates the phosphatase and thus

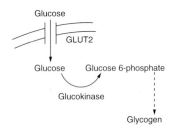

Fig. 13.5 Glucose uptake by liver is not insulin-dependent.

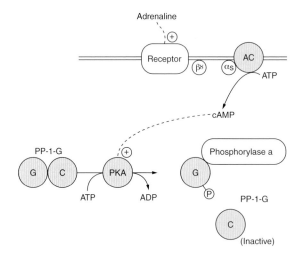

Fig. 13.6 The inactivation of PP-1G by cyclic AMP.

also glycogen synthase, while at the same time preventing conversion of phosphorylase to its less active form, consistent with the role of adrenaline in activating glycogen breakdown (Fig. 13.6).

REGULATION OF GLYCOLYSIS AND GLUCONEOGENESIS

OVERVIEW OF THE REGULATION OF GLYCOLYSIS AND GLUCONEOGENESIS

Figure 13.7 shows the enzymes involved in glycolysis and gluconeogenesis. The pathways of glycolysis and gluconeogenesis utilize common enzymes for certain stretches of the pathway and the enzymes that have been picked out for special attention for their regulatory role are those that are specific for one pathway or the other, that is to say the glucose/glucose 6-phosphate and fructose 6-phosphate/fructose 1,6-bisphosphate (Fru-6-P/Fru-1,6-P$_2$) substrate cycles and the conversion of phosphoenolpyruvate to pyruvate.

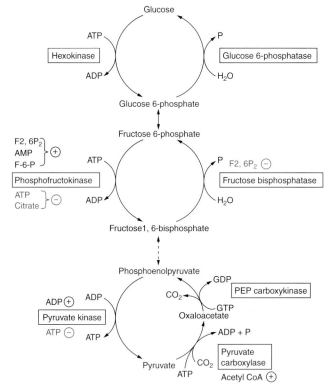

Fig. 13.7 Coordinated regulation of glycolysis and gluconeogenesis.

GLUCOSE PHOSPHORYLATION

Hexokinase phosphorylates glucose and other hexoses, and a number of isoforms are known. The liver contains four hexokinases (A–D or I–IV, according to the system of nomenclature as detailed on p. 96). As explained there, glucokinase is well adapted to respond to changes in blood glucose concentration around the physiological level. As it is the predominant hexokinase isoenzyme in liver, it exerts a major influence on liver glucose metabolism.

   Glucose-6-phosphatase is located within the lumen of the endoplasmic reticulum, and thus its substrate must be transported from the cytosol into the lumen to interact with it (Fig. 13.8).

FRUCTOSE 2,6-BISPHOSPHATE

The analogue fructose 2,6-bisphosphate plays an important role in the Fru-6-P/Fru-1,6-P$_2$ cycle. This is formed by the enzyme 6-phosphofructo-2-kinase, which, under appropriate conditions, can function also as a fructose 2,6-bisphosphatase, as shown in Fig. 13.9. This is a 49-kDa protein that when phosphorylated acts as a phosphatase, and when the phosphate is removed acts as a kinase. Fructose 2,6-bisphosphate activates phosphofructo-1-kinase and acts as a negative regulator of fructose 1,6-bisphosphatase. This is considered a major regulatory system of the Fru-6-P/Fru-1,6-P$_2$ cycle. In addition,

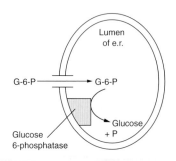

Fig. 13.8 Glucose 6-phosphatase is located in the lumen of the endoplasmic reticulum.

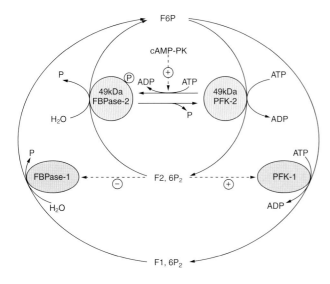

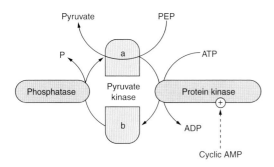

Fig. 13.9 Phosphofructokinase-2 regulates fructose 2, 6-bisphosphate concentrations.

Fig. 13.10 Pyruvate kinase is regulated by a cyclic AMP-dependent protein kinase.

has been extensively studied with regard to longer-term regulation of the pathway (see p. 180). Pyruvate carboxylase is activated by acetyl CoA.

INFLUENCE OF LIVER MORPHOLOGY ON REGULATION

Many examples have already been given in other chapters of the way in which compartmentation of enzymes within cell organelles contributes to the control of metabolism. The formation of macromolecular complexes is yet another way in which physical and structural organization exerts such an influence. The liver provides an example of the importance of morphology in regulating metabolism, in that different groups of apparently similar cells, the hepatocytes, express different levels of the enzymes typical of hepatocyte metabolism, as explained below. It is not yet clear how these differences are brought about at the transcriptional, post-transcriptional and post-translational levels.

Liver tissue consists of cells arranged in lobules. The lobules are ordered arrays of cells that surround a central vein, and are somewhat hexagonal in shape, as shown in Fig. 13.11. The outer edge of the lobules is known as the periportal zone and contains small vessels of the portal vein, which carries blood from the intestine to the liver. At the centre of each lobule there is a vessel of the central vein, draining blood and carrying it out of the liver. Histochemical staining for enzyme activity reveals that many enzymes are distributed in a graded concentration throughout the lobule, as for instance glutamine synthetase and the urea cycle enzymes. The latter are localized in a wide periportal zone that comprises more than 90% of all

however, a number of other allosteric effectors are known to act at this point, especially on PFK. These include, as activator, AMP and, as inhibitors, ATP and citrate. AMP inhibits fructose 1,6-bisphosphatase.

PYRUVATE AND PHOSPHOENOLPYRUVATE INTERCONVERSION

As described earlier, pyruvate kinase is the enzyme that converts phosphoenolpyruvate (PEP) to pyruvate in the glycolytic pathway, whereas for the reverse step during gluconeogenesis the two enzymes pyruvate carboxylase and PEP carboxykinase are required. Pyruvate kinase is present in liver at markedly higher activities than pyruvate carboxylase and PEP carboxykinase. It is an allosteric enzyme that exhibits homotropic cooperativity with regard to its substrate PEP, and is allosterically inhibited by ATP and alanine. In addition it is activated by fructose 1,6-bisphosphate. It is phosphorylated by both PKA and Ca^{2+}/calmodulin-dependent protein kinase (CAM kinase) (Fig. 13.10). Thus the

two major second messengers, cyclic AMP and Ca^{2+}, bring about its phosphorylation, which inhibits the enzyme. Both compounds phosphorylate an identical serine, in a sequence LRRASVAQLTQE, the underlined threonine also being phosphorylated by CAM kinase in vitro. PEP carboxykinase is not known to be regulated in a physiologically significant manner by allosteric effectors but its gene expression

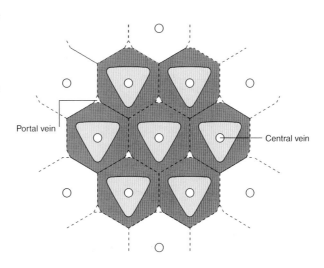

Fig. 13.11 Anatomical structure of liver lobules. Hepatic arteries lie near portal veins.

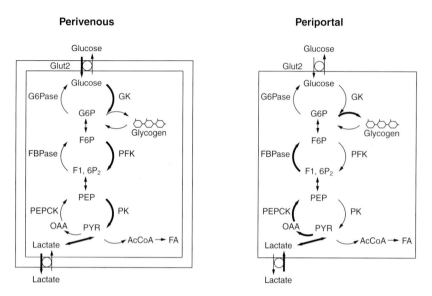

Perivenous

Periportal

Fig. 13.12 The distribution of the glycolytic and gluconeogenic enzymes within liver lobules.

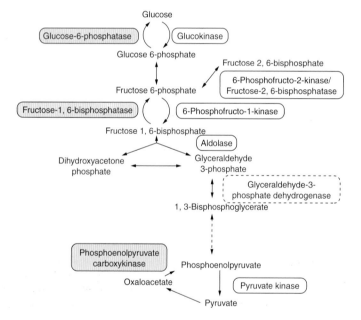

Fig. 13.13 Regulation of the glycolytic and gluconeogenic enzymes at the level of transcription.

TRANSCRIPTIONAL REGULATION OF GENES OF GLYCOLYTIC AND GLUCONEOGENIC ENZYMES

Long-term regulation of glycolysis and gluconeogenesis involves changes in gene expression and protein synthesis, and also the rate of degradation of enzyme protein. These changes have often been studied as a response to nutritional changes but hormones such as insulin have important roles in the growth and survival of cells, and many of the actions of hormones on genes of the glycolytic and gluconeogenic pathways are related to effects on growth and development. The enzymes of the glycolytic and gluconeogenic pathways known to be subject to transcriptional regulation are indicated in Fig. 13.13. Transcription of the enzymes indicated in pink is inhibited by insulin and stimulated by cyclic AMP. In the case of the enzymes without colour, transcription is stimulated by insulin and/or glucose and inhibited by cyclic AMP, except that for glyceraldehyde-3-phosphate dehydrogenase only stimulation by insulin has been observed.

All genes have sequences that bind general transcription factors. Some of these have been described on p. 42. Other regulatory sequences, known as response elements, bind specific transcription factors that function only in particular situations. These tissue-specific factors might, for example, include hormone receptors. A map of the promoter of PEP carboxykinase is given in Fig. 13.14 as a basis for illustrating the type of regulation exerted by metabolic events on gene transcription. The promoter has a negative insulin response element at about −410 bp that is not dependent on glucose, i.e. insulin itself is responsible for the inhibition of transcription exerted through this response element. It is well established that metabolic genes that are down-regulated by insulin are positively regulated by glucagon, and vice versa. Thus, the PEP carboxykinase gene is activated by cyclic AMP acting through the response element, CRE (see also p. 206), to which the CRE binding protein (CREB) binds after phosphorylation by PKA. The effect of CREB is dependent on binding of C/EBP to an additional element (P3) located at −240. The other factors in the region denoted as cyclic AMP-positive are positive regulators. The Fos/Jun dimer is important in growth regulation, as discussed in Chapter 16. Glucocorticoids exercise a permissive action on gene activation by glucagon, i.e. the presence of the glucocorticoid/glucocorticoid receptor

hepatocytes. The remaining 10% of hepatocytes, which comprise a zone one to two cells wide around the central vein, do not normally contain urea cycle enzymes, but they do contain a high concentration of glutamine synthetase, which is not present in the hepatocytes containing urea cycle enzymes. Such a clear-cut segregation is unusual; enzymes belonging to other complementary systems show considerable overlap. The suggestion has been made that the glutamine synthetase possibly scavenges any ammonia that has escaped the urea cycle enzymes, before the exit of metabolites from the liver lobules.

Another system that exhibits a gradient distribution in hepatocytes involves the pathways of glycolysis and gluconeogenesis. Figure 13.12 shows that enzymes of glycolysis are relatively enriched in perivenous hepatocytes. In periportal hepatocytes, gluconeogenic enzymes are relatively enriched, but not in so pronounced a manner. These experimental findings indicate that, although substrate recycling is a valid notion for the liver taken as a whole, it appears to be limited in extent at the single cell level as a result of this functional specialization of hepatocytes.

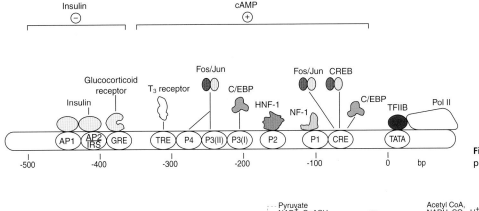

Fig. 13.14 The PEP carboxykinase promoter.

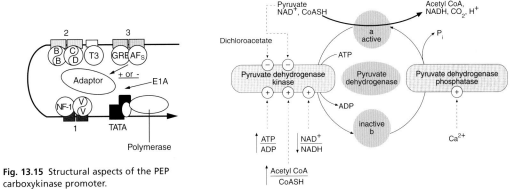

Fig. 13.15 Structural aspects of the PEP carboxykinase promoter.

Fig. 13.16 Regulation of the pyruvate dehydrogenase complex.

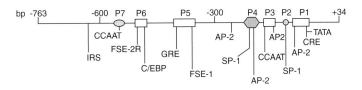

Fig. 13.17 The promoter of the pyruvate dehydrogenase complex E1α subunit.

complex bound to GRE is required for the action of glucagon on transcription via CREB.

CREB is part of a family of transcription factors containing the leucine zipper (p. 43). Through the leucine zipper, CREB will dimerize with itself, or with ATF-1, Fos or Jun. The type of interaction between transcription factors, the ability of these dimers to bind to the CRE elements and the degree of phosphorylation of the individual factors by PKA regulates transcription of specific genes.

The action of regulatory sequences remote from the initiation site might be achieved by the folding of the DNA so that the regulatory sequences come into proximity with the initiation site. This is illustrated for PEP carboxykinase in Fig. 13.15. In this figure, B represents C/EBP, C represents Jun, D represents Fos and V represents a site that can bind any of C/EBP, Fos, Jun or CREB. AF indicates accessory factors AP1 and AP2.

REGULATION OF LIPID METABOLISM

CONVERSION OF PYRUVATE TO ACETYL CoA

The conversion of pyruvate to acetyl CoA is a critical step in metabolism because, once it is taken, the carbon cannot be used for net carbohydrate biosynthesis but is committed either to lipid biosynthesis or oxidation to carbon dioxide and water. Thus, pyruvate dehydrogenase is a strongly regulated enzyme. The main regulatory mechanism involves a protein kinase/phosphatase couple, the phosphorylated enzyme being less active than the non-phosphorylated enzyme. This kinase is not cyclic AMP dependent but is specific to mitochondria and belongs to a unique family unrelated to the protein kinases of cytosol or plasma membrane. There are two forms, one of which is tightly bound to, and phosphorylates, the E1 subunit.

As shown in Fig. 13.16, the kinase is activated by a high ATP/ADP ratio and a high acetyl CoA/HSCoA ratio, and also when the NAD^+/NADH ratio decreases. It is inhibited by pyruvate, so that as pyruvate levels rise its conversion to acetyl CoA is stimulated. The protein phosphatase is activated by Ca^{2+}. Dichloroacetate is used as a drug to alleviate lactic acidosis. It inhibits the kinase, thereby increasing pyruvate oxidation.

The genes encoding the different subunits of the pyruvate dehydrogenase complex are regulated by a variety of transcription factors. Figure 13.17 shows the promoter-regulatory region of the human E1α subunit. This reveals several CAAT boxes, together with consensus sequences for various known transcription binding/recognition sites, including SP1 binding, AP-2 binding, fat-specific elements, glucocorticoid-responsive element and cyclic AMP-responsive element. A TATA box is also present.

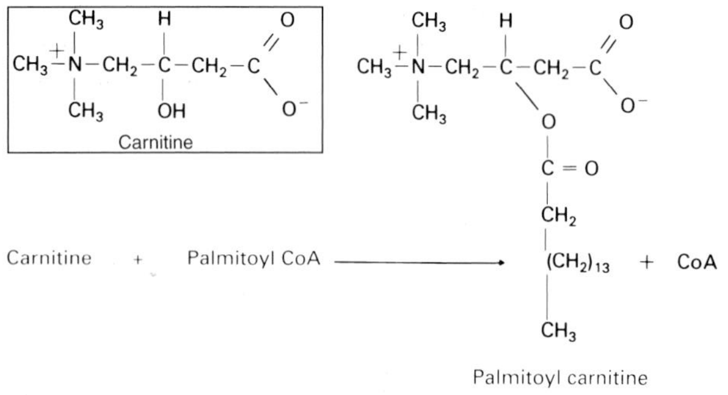

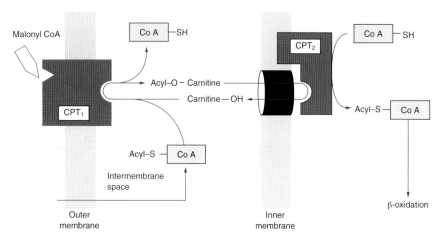

Carnitine + Palmitoyl CoA ⟶ Palmitoyl carnitine + CoA

Fig. 13.18 The structure of palmitoyl carnitine.

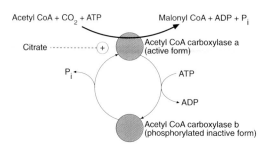

Fig. 13.19 The carnitine palmitoyltransferase isoenzymes transport fatty acyl CoA into mitochondria.

CARNITINE AND ITS FUNCTION

Fatty acids are transported across the inner mitochondrial membrane as esters of carnitine, a quaternary ammonium hydroxyacid. The carnitine acyl esters are formed in a reversible reaction catalysed by the enzyme carnitine palmitoyltransferase, as shown in Fig. 13.18. Two forms of this enzyme exist in mitochondria, one in the outer membrane, known as CPT_1, and one in the inner membrane, CPT_2. In liver mitochondria, CPT_1 largely has the function of converting acyl CoA esters into acylcarnitine esters, while CPT_2 is concerned with the formation of acyl CoA esters by reaction of CoA with acylcarnitines, after they have been transported through the inner membrane by the acylcarnitine:carnitine antiporter, as shown in Fig. 13.19. The acyl CoA esters formed within the mitochondrial matrix are then metabolized by the β-oxidation pathway. CPT_1 plays an important role in the regulation of fatty acid metabolism. It is strongly inhibited by malonyl CoA, so when levels of malonyl CoA are high, as in situations in which lipogenesis is activated, acyl CoA molecules will not enter mitochondria for oxidation, but will be retained in the cytosol for triacylglycerol synthesis.

CLINICAL IMPLICATIONS – CPT DEFICIENCY

Deficiency of either CPT I or CPT II can occur. Symptoms include hypoglycemia and hyperammonemia due to hepatic involvement and lethargy due to muscular involvement. Severe defects manifest in infancy, with early death, but late-onset forms occur with some mutation. Carnitine palmitoyltransferase II deficiency is the most common inherited disorder of mitochondrial long-chain fatty acid oxidation. In young adults, the 'classic' myopathic form occurs and is characterized by recurrent episodes of rhabdomyolysis triggered by prolonged exercise, fasting or febrile illness.

REGULATION OF LIPOGENESIS

The pathway of lipogenesis involves transport of acetyl CoA, formed by pyruvate dehydrogenase, out of the mitochondrion. In the cytosol, acetyl CoA is converted to malonyl CoA by acetyl-CoA carboxylase. This enzyme is sensitive to nutritional state, its concentration decreasing in starved rats and increasing on refeeding. It is regulated by phosphorylation state, as shown in Fig. 13.20. Malonyl CoA is an inhibitor of CPT_1, thus restricting entry of fatty acyl groups into the mitochondrion.

COORDINATED REGULATION OF LIPID METABOLISM IN LIVER

As explained in Chapter 3, operons are not found in eukaryotes. However, transcription of groups of genes of related function can be coordinately controlled by regulatory elements. A good example of this is the group of genes involved in lipid metabolism in liver, which regulate VLDL and cholesterol synthesis. Transcription of these genes is regulated in response to the need for the liver to synthesize sterols, and the promoter regions of these genes contain regulatory sequences known as sterol regulatory elements (SRE). SRE-binding proteins (SREBP) act as the associated transcription factors. A list of proteins known to be responsive to SREBP is given in Table 13.1, and can be seen to embrace proteins involved in a wide

Table 13.1 Proteins encoded by genes responsive to SREBP

- Acetyl-CoA carboxylase
- Apoprotein B-100
- Fatty acid synthase
- HMG-CoA reductase
- HMG-CoA synthase
- Isopentylfarnesyldiphosphate synthase
- LDL receptor
- Microsomal triglycerol transfer protein
- Squalene synthase

Fig. 13.20 The regulation of acetyl-CoA carboxylase.

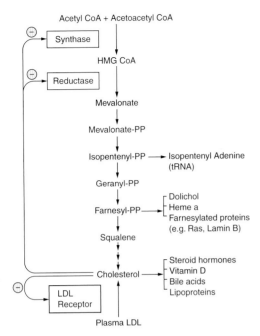

Fig. 13.21 Effects of the mevalonate pathway.

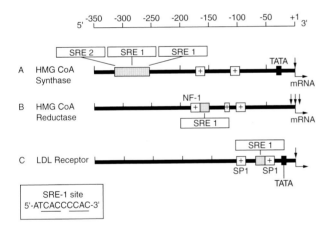

Fig. 13.22 Steroid response elements of the genes of HMG-CoA synthase, HMG-CoA reductase and the LDL receptor.

synthesis of the LDL receptor, HMG–CoA reductase and HMG–CoA synthase. This inhibitory action is exerted through SRE in the 5′ flanking regions of the genes; Fig. 13.22 shows details of the promoter structure of the three genes. SREBP bind to sequences that contain a direct repeat of 5′-PyCAPy-3′ (Py = any pyrimidine).

SREBP are synthesized as precursors having membrane-spanning domains that locate them in the endoplasmic reticulum. A cytosolic domain constitutes the SREBP, and contains a DNA-binding region in the form of a basic helix-loop-helix zipper. When mammalian cells are starved of cholesterol, the SREBP is released from the membrane of the endoplasmic reticulum by proteolysis and enters the nucleus, where it activates transcription of genes having SRE.

POST-TRANSCRIPTIONAL REGULATION OF LIPOPROTEIN METABOLISM

Of equal or greater importance to transcriptional regulation are other means of regulating the amounts of proteins involved in lipid metabolism. These include protein degradation, especially in the case of HMG-CoA reductase and apo B-100. HMG-CoA reductase is an integral protein (see Chapter 15) of the endoplasmic reticulum and its regulation is linked, in a way not yet understood, to flux through the mevalonate pathway. It is possible that farnesyl diphosphate acts as a degradation signal. When flux through the mevalonate pathway increases, degradation of HMG–CoA reductase increases, as a result of proteasome activity (see p. 48). In the case of apo B-100, it is known that, if any of the lipids required for the assembly of VLDL are lacking, the apoprotein is not effectively translocated through the endoplasmic reticulum membrane during synthesis and is degraded cotranslationally, i.e. it is broken down as it is synthesized.

spectrum of lipid metabolic functions. The mevalonate pathway is intimately involved in this regulatory system. Not only is it thought to produce compounds that act as transcriptional regulators, but also has far-reaching effects on cell function through its links with other systems, as illustrated in Fig. 13.21. These include, for example, the farnesylation of proteins, such as the *ras* oncogene product. This figure also indicates the inhibitory action that overactivity of this pathway has on the

Phospholipids, other lipid substances and complex carbohydrates

14

Complex lipids and carbohydrates have important roles both as structural entities and as active modulators of metabolic activity. Glycerophospholipids are composed of a glycerol moiety esterified with one or two fatty acids and a phosphate group that in turn is esterified to a nitrogenous base or inositol. Further derivatives of these exist. Sphingolipids are derivatives of the nitrogenous base sphingosine. The simplest sphingolipid is ceramide, which is sphingosine in amide linkage with a fatty acyl group. The phospholipids are degraded by hydrolysis catalysed by phospholipases.

The lipid-soluble vitamins include vitamins A, D, E and K. Prostaglandins and leukotrienes are formed from polyunsaturated fatty acids, of which the most important is arachidonic acid. The clinical implications of the use of anti-inflammatory drugs is described.

The steroid hormones are synthesized from cholesterol. The clinical effects of defects of steroid hormone metabolism are described. The complex carbohydrates consist of polymers of a variety of monosaccharides, including amino sugars and sialic acid. The hydroxyl groups are often sulfated. These polysaccharides form part of glycoproteins and glycolipids, the biosynthesis of which involves dolichyl phosphate, on which the carbohydrate chain is built before it is transferred to protein in the Golgi apparatus.

PHOSPHOLIPIDS

THE STRUCTURE OF PHOSPHOLIPIDS

The phospholipid structure is based on one of the isomers of glycerol phosphate. The designation of the carbon atoms depends on a system of stereospecific numbering, and to denote this the abbreviation *sn* is used. Under this system, the glycerol phosphate that is involved in lipid metabolism is named *sn*-glycerol 3-phosphate. Thus carbons C-1 and C-2 are often referred to as the *sn*-1 and *sn*-2 carbons, respectively (see Fig. 14.1).

In phospholipids a fatty acyl group is in ester linkage to each of the C-1 and C-2 hydroxyl groups, and a phosphoryl group is esterified to the C-3 hydroxyl group. Another group is often esterified to this phosphoryl group, and this can be either inositol or one of the three nitrogenous compounds, choline, serine or ethanolamine, as shown in the structures in Fig. 14.2. The phosphate together with the nitrogenous compound (or the inositol) is referred to as the headgroup. In phosphatidylglycerol, the nitrogenous compound is replaced by glycerol, esterified to the phosphate by one of its primary alcohol groups. An important phospholipid in mitochondria is cardiolipin, in which two molecules of phosphatidic acid are linked through a molecule of glycerol, each of the phosphate groups being esterified to one of the primary alcohol groups of the glycerol.

The simplest phospholipid has no nitrogenous or other group attached to the phosphoryl group. It is diacyl-*sn*-glycero-3-phosphate, i.e. *sn*-glycerol 3-phosphate esterified with fatty acyl groups at C-1 and C-2. Its common name is phosphatidic acid, and its derivatives are thus phosphatidyl esters, so that the choline ester of phosphatidic acid is known by the generic name, phosphatidylcholine.

Phospholipids can have any of a number of different fatty acids esterified at C-1 and C-2. Thus many different forms are possible for each phospholipid, each of these being referred to as a phospholipid species. 1-Palmitoyl-2-linoleoyl-*sn*-glycero-3-phosphocholine and 1-stearoyl-2-arachidonoyl-*sn*-glycero-3-phosphocholine are two phosphatidylcholine species. Polyunsaturated fatty acids tend to be found on C-2 and saturated fatty acids on C-1. Phosphatidylserines, phosphatidylethanolamines and phosphatidylinositols can be similarly specifically named if their fatty acyl constituents are known.

BIOSYNTHESIS OF PHOSPHOLIPIDS

The biosynthesis of phospholipids starts with reactions in which two molecules of fatty acyl CoA are used to acylate a molecule of glycerol 3-phosphate to form phosphatidic acid, as occurs in the biosynthesis of triacylglycerols. In further transformations, intermediates containing a nucleotide moiety as an activating group are involved. Figure 14.3 shows the structure of one such molecule, cytidine diphosphocholine, and indicates the pathway by which it is formed by reaction of phosphocholine with CTP. Other such molecules are cytidine diphosphoethanolamine and cytidine diphosphodiacylglycerol, in each case the structure being analogous to that of CDP-

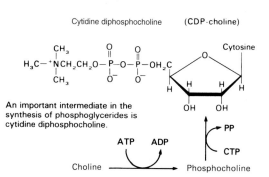

Cytidine diphosphocholine   (CDP-choline)

An important intermediate in the synthesis of phosphoglycerides is cytidine diphosphocholine.

Fig. 14.3 The biosynthesis of CDP-choline.

Fig. 14.1 *sn* numbering of glycerol 3-phosphate.

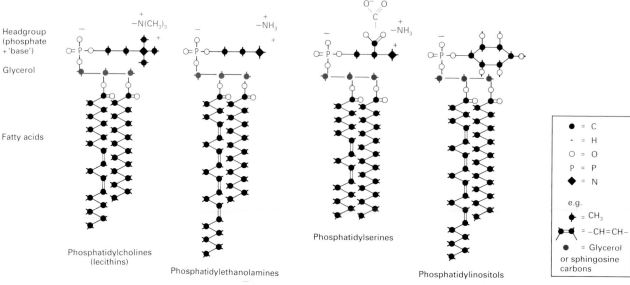

Phosphatidylcholines (lecithins)

Phosphatidylethanolamines

Phosphatidylserines

Phosphatidylinositols

● = C
- = H
○ = O
P = P
◆ = N

e.g.
◆ = CH₃
✳ = −CH=CH−
● = Glycerol or sphingosine carbons

Fig. 14.2 The structure of glycerophospholipids.

choline, having an ester bond between the terminal phosphate of CDP and the hydroxyl group of ethanolamine and diacylglycerol, respectively. The reactions by which several phospholipids are formed are outlined in Fig. 14.4.

PHOSPHOLIPASES

Phospholipids are degraded by phospholipases, enzymes that hydrolyse one or other of the bonds between different moieties of the phospholipid molecule. Thus, as shown in Fig. 14.5 for phosphatidylcholine, phospholipase A_1 enzymes hydrolyse the ester bond at C-1, and phospholipases A_2 hydrolyse the ester bond at C-2. If just one fatty acid is removed, the resulting compound is called a lyso compound (e.g. lysophosphatidylethanolamine). Phospholipases B remove the residual fatty acid from a lyso compound. Phospholipases C break the bond between the diacylglycerol moiety and the headgroup. Thus, diacylglycerol and phosphocholine are formed from phosphatidylcholine. Phospholipases D hydrolyse the phosphatidyl bond to yield phosphatidic acid and the nitrogenous group. Phospholipases A_2 have a special significance in cell membranes, as the fatty acid they release from C-2 can be a polyunsaturated fatty acid, often arachidonic acid. Indeed, some of these enzymes show specificity for phospholipids containing arachidonoyl groups at C-2, and thus release substrate for prostaglandin and leukotriene biosynthesis.

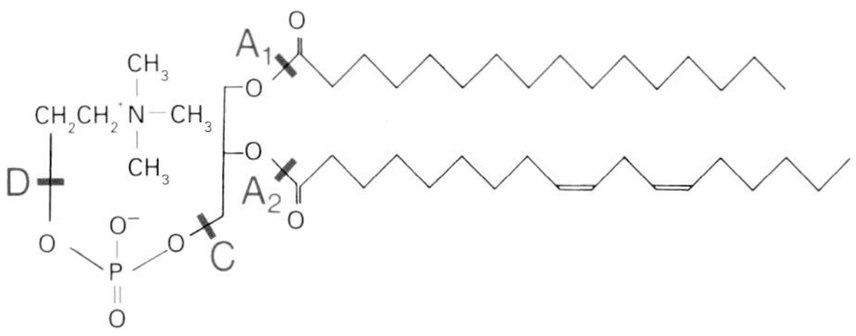

INOSITOL-CONTAINING PHOSPHOLIPIDS

Inositol-containing phospholipids, referred to generally as phosphoinositides, have received a great deal of attention recently for their role in cell signalling (see Chapter 15). As shown in Fig. 14.6, the simplest of these is phosphatidylinositol (PtdIns), which can be successively phosphorylated on positions 4 and 5 of the inositol ring to give phosphatidylinositol 4-phosphate (PtdIns$P$) and phosphatidylinositol 4,5-bisphosphate (PtdInsP_2). Phospholipases C specific for phosphoinositides are important, as explained in Chapter 15, in releasing diacylglycerol and phosphorylated inositol derivatives that function in cell signalling. In the case of PtdInsP_2, inositol 1,4,5-trisphosphate (InsP_3) is released. This type of enzyme is also termed a

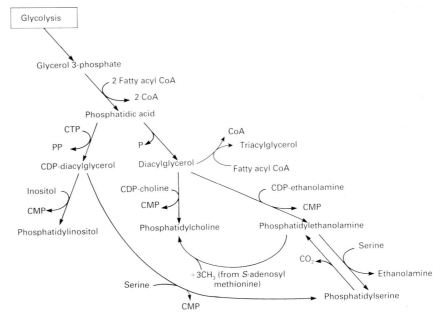

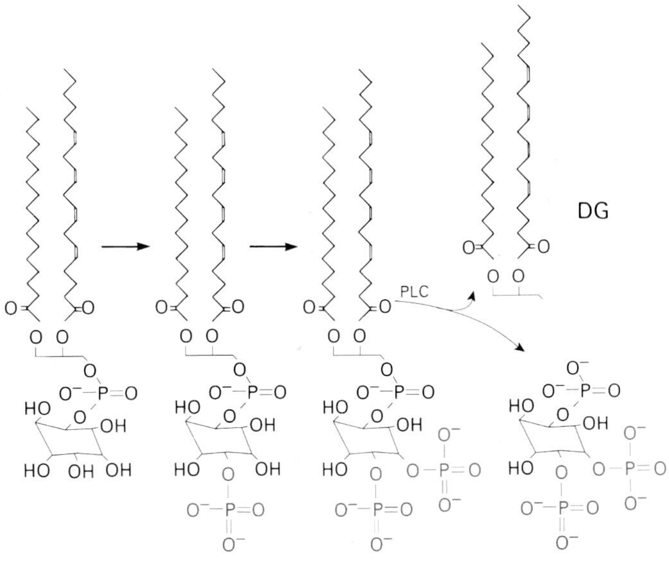

Fig. 14.4 The biosynthesis of phospholipids.

Fig. 14.5 The sites of action of phospholipases A, C and D.

Fig. 14.6 The phosphatidylinositols.

phosphodiesterase, because it attacks diesters of phosphoric acid, i.e. phosphoric acid with two of its acidic −OH groups involved in ester linkage.

SPHINGOLIPIDS

Sphingolipids are based on the amino alcohol sphingosine. A fatty acid is attached to the nitrogen in amide linkage and the terminal hydroxyl group is attached in glycosidic linkage to a sugar or chain of sugars, except in the case of sphingomyelin, when it is a phosphocholine group that is attached in ester linkage through its phosphate group. The structures of some of the sphingolipids are illustrated in Fig. 14.7. The gangliosides form an important group of sphingolipids. Sphingomyelin is also correctly termed a phospholipid, because it contains phosphorus. Cerebrosides and gangliosides contain no phosphorus but do contain carbohydrate structures, and thus are both sphingolipids and glycolipids. Some gangliosides contain sialic acid (see p. 195). Sphingomyelin is an important structural lipid in membrane bilayers, comprising 10–20% of the total phospholipid of the bilayer. As their name suggests, cerebrosides are found in appreciable quantities in the brain, especially in myelin, together with their sulfated derivatives, sulfatides. Gangliosides also are found in quantities in brain, from which they were first isolated. Cerebrosides and gangliosides are found in much smaller quantities in the plasma membranes of many cell types.

Sphinganine, the compound from which sphingolipid biosynthesis can be considered to start, is formed from palmitoyl CoA and serine, through the intermediate 2-ketosphinganine, as shown in Fig. 14.8. Sphingolipid biosynthesis then proceeds via ceramide (Fig. 14.9). This is formed by acylation of the amino group of sphinganine, followed by the introduction of a double bond at C-4. Ceramide can then react with either UDP-glucose or UDP-galactose, to form glucosylceramide or galactosylceramide, respectively. Alternatively, it can react with CDP-choline to form sphingomyelin. Glucosylceramide is also known as glucocerebroside, and galactosylceramide as galactocerebroside.

LIPID-SOLUBLE VITAMINS

VITAMIN A

The vitamer (form) of vitamin A present in food is retinal, which is converted to

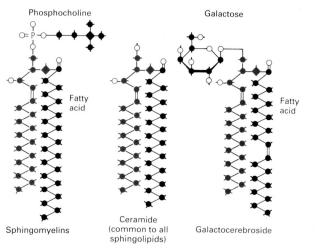

Fig. 14.7 The structures of sphingolipids.

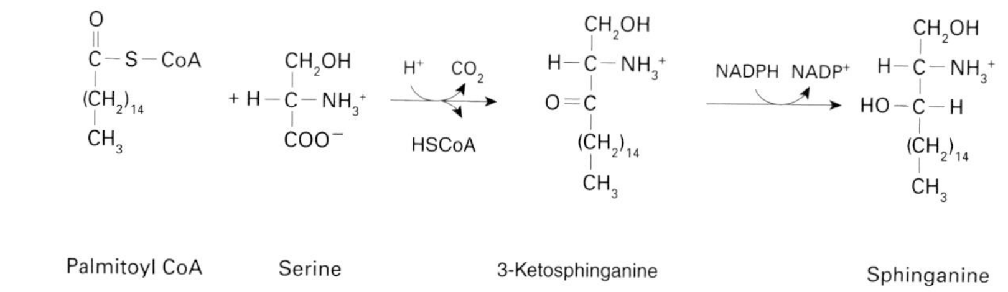

Fig. 14.8 The biosynthesis of sphinganine from palmitoyl CoA and serine.

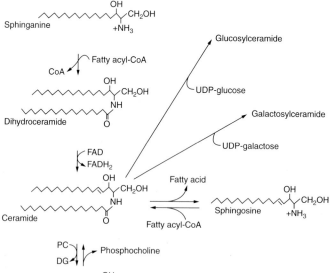

Fig. 14.9 The biosynthesis of ceramide, sphingomyelin and sphingosine. Pc, phosphatidycholine

11-*trans*-retinal by oxidation of the hydroxyl group to an aldehyde. The structures of 11-*trans*-retinal and 11-*cis*-retinal, the functional form of the vitamin in visual processes, are shown in Fig. 14.10. 11-*cis*-Retinal is formed from 11-*trans*-retinal by retinal isomerase. 11-*cis*-Retinal interacts with the protein opsin to form the visual pigment rhodopsin. If rhodopsin is exposed to light, the double bond at C-11 of *cis*-retinal isomerizes to *trans*, causing dissociation of rhodopsin to opsin and *trans*-retinal, which is then converted back to the *cis* form by retinal isomerase.

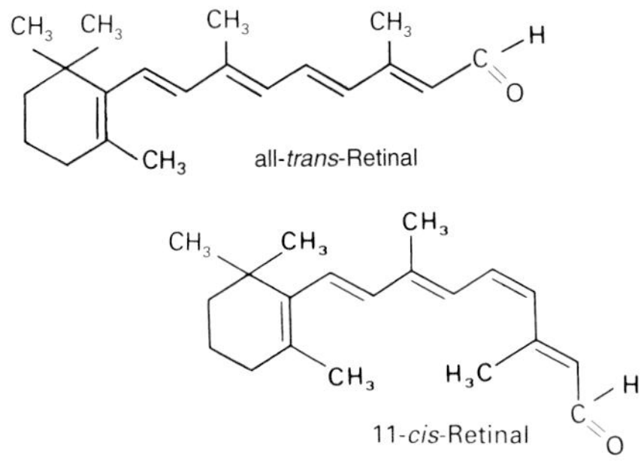

Fig. 14.10 The structures of all-*trans*-retinal and 11-*cis*-retinal.

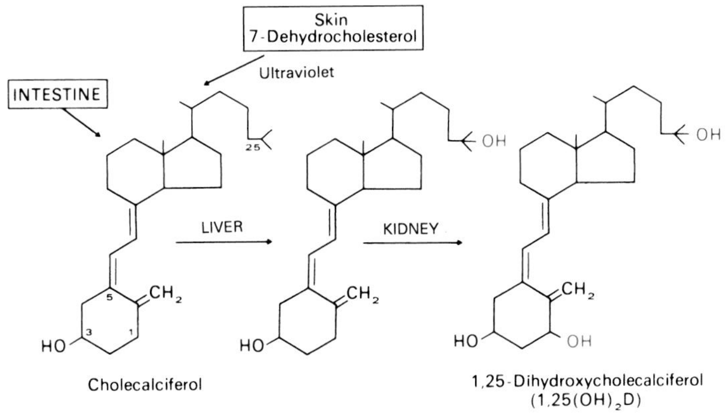

all-*trans*-Retinal

11-*cis*-Retinal

Fig. 14.11 The biosynthesis of 1,25-dihydroxycholecalciferol.

Skin
7-Dehydrocholesterol

INTESTINE

Cholecalciferol

1,25-Dihydroxycholecalciferol
(1,25(OH)₂D)

At least three different physiological functions are dependent on proper vitamin A nutrition:

1. Somatic function, including growth and differentiation of, for example, epithelial structures and bone.
2. Reproduction, including spermatogenesis, oogenesis, placental development and embryonic growth.
3. Visual processes, especially vision in the dark.

CLINICAL IMPLICATIONS – VITAMIN A TOXICITY

Excessive doses of vitamin A are highly toxic, and can prove fatal. Prolonged over-administration of vitamin A is thought to be teratogenic, i.e. to cause fetal abnormalities; this is a risk factor of importance in pregnant women because vitamin A and its derivatives are an effective treatment for acne.

VITAMIN D

Vitamin D is based on cholecalciferol, which is formed by the action of ultraviolet light on 7-dehydrocholesterol, a derivative of cholesterol stored in the skin. Cholecalciferol (Fig. 14.11) is converted in the liver to 25-hydroxycholecalciferol, which is then converted in kidney to the active form of the vitamin, 1,25-dihydroxycholecalciferol (1,25(OH)₂D). This is impaired in renal disease which may lead to osteoporosis. Vitamin D is involved with the hormones parathyroid hormone and calcitonin in regulating calcium metabolism, as summarized in Fig. 14.12.

Parathyroid hormone (PTH) is secreted by the parathyroids in response to a drop in the blood Ca²⁺ level. It increases production of 1,25(OH)₂D by kidney, increases Ca²⁺ resorption from bone and decreases Ca²⁺ excretion in urine. It thus tends to elevate blood Ca²⁺ levels. High serum Ca²⁺ levels block production of PTH.

1,25(OH)₂D increases Ca²⁺ absorption from gut. 1,25(OH)₂D also acts synergistically with PTH in response to low serum calcium levels to increase Ca²⁺ resorption from bone and thus to increase serum Ca²⁺ levels. When serum Ca²⁺ levels are high, the inhibition of PTH secretion reduces formation of 1,25(OH)₂D.

Calcitonin is produced by the C cells of the thyroid. It is secreted in response to an elevated serum Ca²⁺ level and inhibits bone resorption.

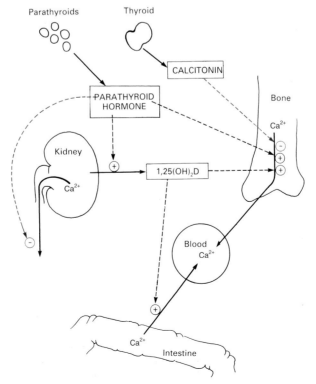

Fig. 14.12 The roles of parathyroid hormone, calcitonin and 1,25(OH)₂D in calcium metabolism.

CLINICAL IMPLICATIONS – RICKETTS

Dietary deficiency of vitamin D causes rickets, a disease in which there is defective bone formation, because of the defective intestinal absorption of Ca^{2+} that results from the deficiency.

In patients with Paget's disease, both bone resorption and bone formation are excessive, bone formation being coupled to bone resorption. Administration of calcitonin in this disease is very effective, as in addition to inhibiting bone resorption it has an inhibitory effect on osteoclast activity.

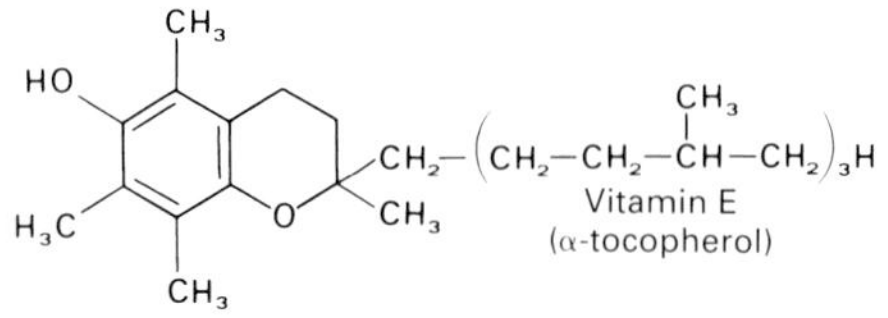

VITAMIN E AND FREE RADICALS

Vitamin E, α-tocopherol (Fig. 14.13), can act as an antioxidant by accepting an electron from a free radical to form a relatively stable intermediate. It can thus break the chain reaction that ensues when free radical formation occurs. Free radicals arise from a number of sources, such as ultraviolet radiation. Polyunsaturated fatty acids esterified in membrane phospholipids are susceptible to free radical attack, as shown in Fig. 14.14. The resulting hydroperoxide-containing phospholipids are recognized by phospholipases, which remove the modified fatty acids. These are converted to hydroxy fatty acids by glutathione peroxidase (see p. 142), which can then be oxidized by other enzyme systems.

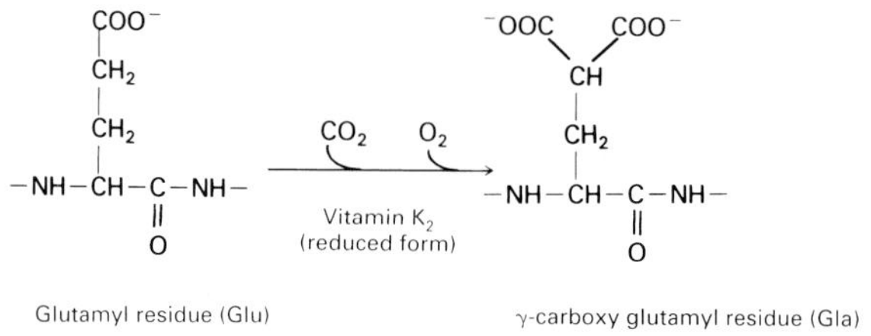

CLINICAL IMPLICATIONS – FREE RADICALS AND DISEASE

It has been postulated that damage by free radicals and reactive oxygen species such as H_2O_2 may be involved in a number of disease states. It seems beneficial to have regard to this possibility, and to include in the diet vegetables such as tomatoes that contain lycopenes, substances that can trap free radicals. If a diet rich in polyunsaturated fatty acids is administered, it should be accompanied by additional vitamin E because of the increased possibility of free radical formation. Selenium deficiency results in accelerated peroxidation of fatty acids, possibly because of a decrease in the levels of selenium-dependent glutathione peroxidase. Increased intake of vitamin E can mitigate the effects of selenium deficiency.

VITAMIN K

Vitamin K_2, menaquinone, is essential for normal blood clotting. It is a cofactor

Fig. 14.13 The structure of α-tocopherol (vitamin E).

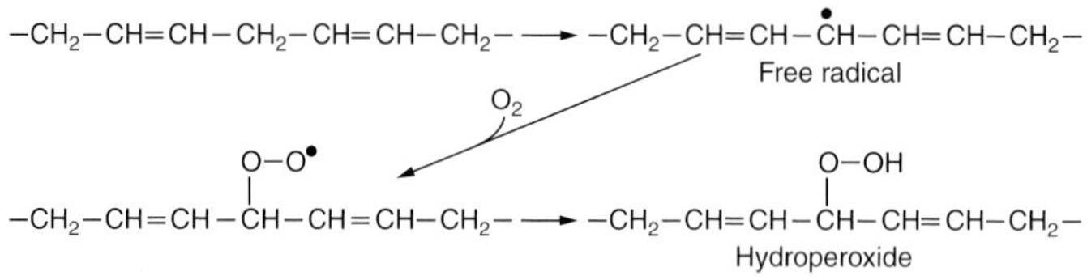

Fig. 14.14 The formation of free radicals and hydroperoxides.

Fig. 14.15 The formation of γ-carboxyglutamyl residues.

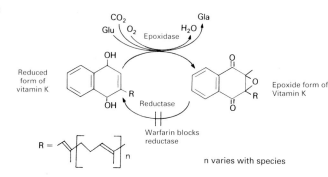

Fig. 14.16 The formation of vitamin K epoxide.

in post-translational formation of γ-carboxyglutamyl residues in certain proteins, including prothrombin, shown in Fig. 14.15. If as a result of vitamin K deficiency glutamyl residues of prothrombin cannot be γ-carboxylated, the blood-clotting mechanism functions imperfectly. When vitamin K reacts in the carboxylation of glutamyl residues to γ-carboxyglutamyl residues, it is oxidized to an epoxide form (see Fig. 14.16). This form is normally reduced back to vitamin K by a reductase.

Vitamin-K-dependent carboxylation of glutamyl residues occurs in a number of proteins in the blood coagulation cascade. The proteins that contain carboxyglutamyl residues are shown in red in Fig. 14.17. Carboxyglutamyl residues are also found in a number of tissue proteins. Carboxyglutamate-containing proteins bind Ca^{2+} strongly because of the

chelating properties of the γ-carboxyglutamyl group.

CLINICAL IMPLICATIONS – USE OF WARFARIN AS ANTICOAGULANT

Warfarin inhibits the reductase that reduces the epoxide form of vitamin K and thus mimics vitamin K deficiency. This is the basis of its clinical use as an anticoagulant. Care must be taken to monitor blood coagulation (prothrombin time) for the drug may cause serious internal bleeding, this explaining its use as a very effective rat poison. Warfarin is metabolized by a P450 enzyme. This is induced by phenobarbitone or chronic alcohol consumption, leading to enhanced metabolism of warfarin, with the patient requiring a larger dose to control anticoagulation. If, however, the patient then stops the phenobarbitone or alcohol

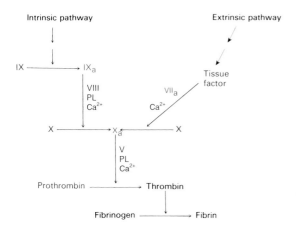

Intrinsic pathway   Extrinsic pathway

Fig. 14.17 The γ-carboxyglutamyl-containing proteins of the blood-clotting cascade.

intake, over-anticoagulation would result with serious consequences.

OTHER LIPID COMPOUNDS

PROSTAGLANDINS AND LEUKOTRIENES

The prostaglandins are synthesized in many tissues in minute amounts. They have a very short half-life, often around 1 or 2 min. The different prostaglandins have highly potent pharmacological actions that embrace contraction of smooth muscle, including that of the uterus. They also cause vasodilation and platelet aggregation. However, their actions are too numerous to summarize in any simple way, especially as the same prostaglandin can have different actions in different situations. It is, however, useful to indicate their structures and summarize their metabolism (see Fig. 14.18), because a number of widely used drugs depend for their action on their effects on these pathways.

Prostaglandins formed from arachidonic acid are synthesized from the two endoperoxides, PGG$_2$ and PGH$_2$, which are products of the enzyme prostaglandin-endoperoxide synthase, also known as cyclooxygenase. The different prostaglandin classes are distinguished by the substituents and nature of the ring structure, as shown in Fig. 14.19. As indicated in Fig. 14.20, prostaglandins of different series can be formed, depending on whether prostaglandin-endoperoxide synthase acts on arachidonic acid, dihomo-γ-linolenic acid (giving rise to the '1' series of prostaglandins) or α-linolenic acid (giving rise to the '3' series).

The most commonly found is the '2' series, formed from arachidonic acid.

Other enzymes, known as lipoxygenases, act on arachidonic acid to form hydroxylated derivatives of polyunsaturated fatty acids that have pharmacological activities. One such compound is 12-hydroxyeicosatrienoic acid (HETE), which is involved in the inflammatory response as a chemotactic agent and attracts cells to move up a chemical gradient. Of major significance are the leukotrienes, which are derived from the product of 5-lipoxygenase, which converts arachidonic acid to leukotriene A$_4$, a 20-carbon fatty acid in which an epoxide has been introduced at the 5,6-position. It has a characteristic triene structure with conjugated double bonds at positions 7,9,11 (as indicated in the name). The sulfhydryl group of glutathione can react at position 6 to give leukotriene C$_4$ (LTC$_4$), the structure of which is shown in Fig. 14.21. Leukotrienes that are formed from the action of 5-lipoxygenase on dihomo-γ-linoleic acid comprise another series based on LTC$_3$. The leukotrienes undergo metabolism that includes removal of glutamic acid from LTC$_4$ or LTC$_3$ to yield LTD$_4$ or LTD$_3$, respectively. The structure of LTC$_4$ was elucidated as a result of the isolation and identification of the so-called slow-reacting substance of anaphylaxis (SRS-A). The leukotrienes form part of an extensive system of related metabolites that have widespread and potent activity in the inflammatory response and cell signalling function.

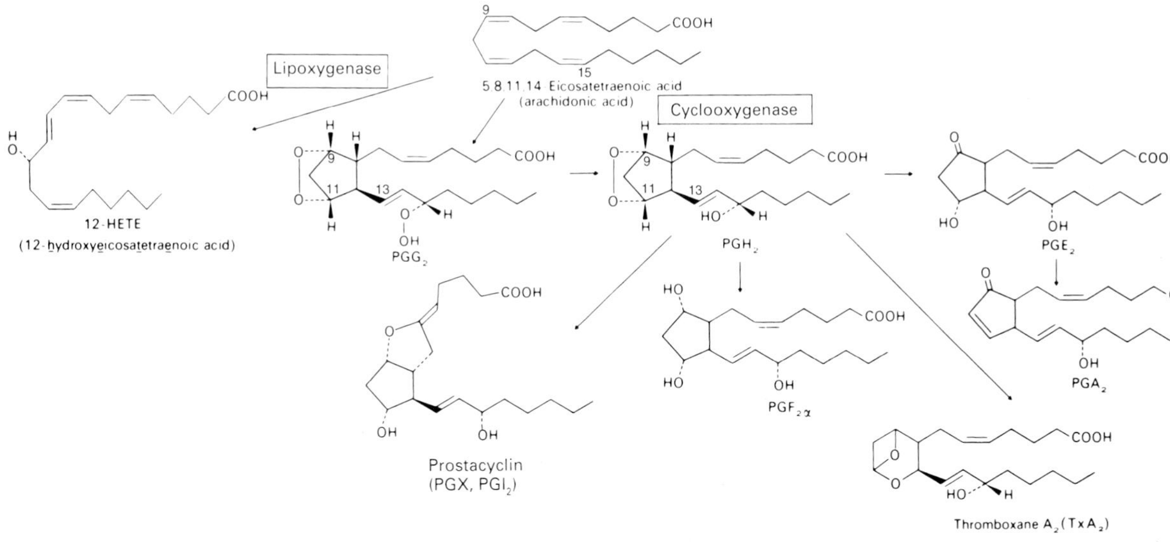

Fig. 14.18 The biosynthesis of the eicosanoids.

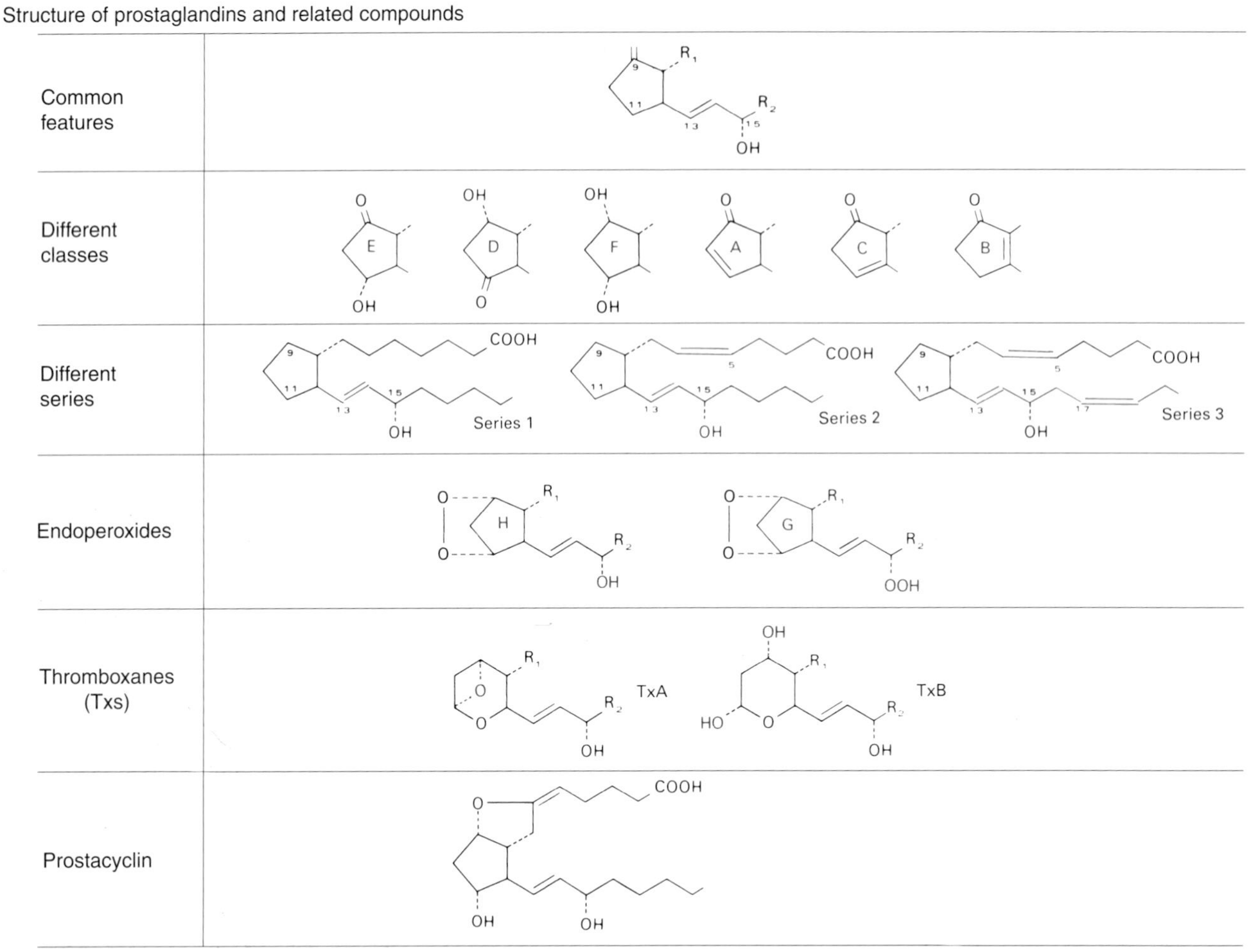

Structure of prostaglandins and related compounds

Fig. 14.19 Eicosanoid structures.

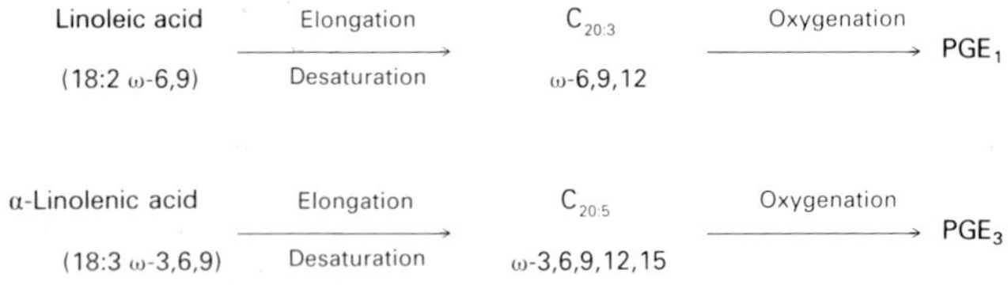

Fig. 14.20 Linoleic acid and α-linolenic acid act as precursors of different prostaglandin families.

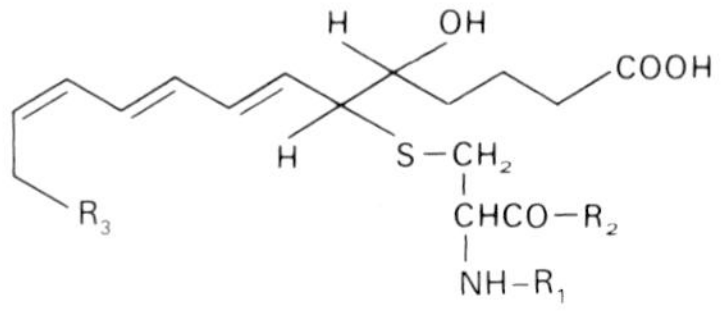

Fig. 14.21 The structures of leukotrienes.

CLINICAL IMPLICATIONS – NON-STEROIDAL ANTI-INFLAMMATORY DRUGS

Cyclooxygenase exists in at least two isoforms, COX-1 and COX-2. COX-1 is constitutively expressed in many cell types, while COX-2 is detectable only when induced by cytokines, growth factors and tumour promoters and is considered to be a major mediator of the inflammatory response. At low doses aspirin (N-acetylsalicylic acid) is analgesic and antipyretic. It irreversibly inhibits COX-1 by acetylating an active site serine. At much higher doses it is anti-inflammatory and inhibits COX-2. Aspirin and a group of drugs of similar action, of which indomethacin was the progenitor, are known as non-steroidal anti-inflammatory drugs (NSAIDs). At sufficiently high dose they inhibit all types of cyclooxygenase. An undesirable side effect of these drugs is the inhibition of gastric production of prostaglandins by COX-1, as this leads to the formation of ulcers. New NSAIDs have therefore been developed that are selective inhibitors of COX-2. These can be used to reduce chronic inflammation without having the effects on the stomach shown by COX-1 inhibitors.

There is evidence that regular use of low-dose aspirin can reduce the risk of heart attacks, as at this dosage it inhibits platelet COX-1, preventing formation of TXA_2, a potent thrombotic agent. The platelet COX-1 cannot be resynthesized in the platelets in which it has been inhibited, as platelets have no ability to synthesize protein, so the enzyme will only exist in newly formed platelets. Daily dosage thus effectively inhibits most platelets. The use of paracetamol as an analgesic has the advantage that it only weakly inhibits cyclooxygenase in peripheral tissues, is not anti-inflammatory and is less irritant on the stomach. It accumulates in the central nervous system in which it does inhibit cyclooxygenase.

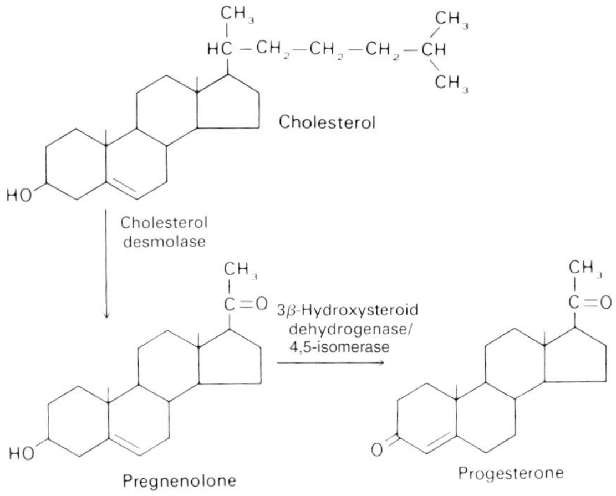

STEROID HORMONES

Steroid hormones are primarily synthesized in the adrenal cortex and the gonads, with some conversion occurring in other tissues. Cholesterol acts as a precursor to the steroid hormones, which comprise:

1. testosterone and dihydrotestosterone, male sex hormones or androgens
2. estradiol, a female sex hormone or estrogen
3. progesterone, a pregnancy-maintaining hormone or gestagen
4. cortisol, a glucocorticoid
5. aldosterone, a mineralocorticoid.

Synthetic analogues of all these are used clinically to replace deficiencies of the natural hormone or to achieve additional effects.

The initial step in the synthesis of all steroid hormones is the formation of pregnenolone from cholesterol, as indicated in Fig. 14.22. Formation of androgens occurs via two pathways. One is by conversion to 17α-hydroxypregnenolone and dehydroepiandrosterone (DHA). This route is favoured in the adrenal gland. The alternative route, via progesterone, is favoured in the gonads.

Testosterone is formed in the Leydig cells of the testes in males under stimulation by luteinizing hormone (LH) from the pituitary gland and this is in turn stimulated by gonadotrophin-releasing hormone (GnRH) from the hypothalamus. Testosterone inhibits release of these hormones in a feedback control system. Testosterone is made to a small extent in females in the ovary. Synthetic preparations include testosterone enanthate. The so-called androgenic-anabolic steroids are testosterone analogues misused as performance enhancers by athletes.

Estradiol is formed from androgens in the ovary under the influence of both LH and follicle-stimulating hormone (FSH). During the menstrual cycle, estrogen feedback is first negative and then becomes

Fig. 14.22 The conversion of cholesterol to progesterone.

positive, to initiate the LH surge that leads to ovulation. Estradiol is made to a small extent in males in the testis and other tissues. Synthetic analogues include estradiol valerate.

Progesterone is formed in the developing corpus luteum of the ovary and is made in large quantities in pregnancy. Synthetic forms include norethisterone and levonorgestrel. Synthetic estrogens and gestagens are used in the contraceptive pill. The natural hormones testosterone and estradiol are also given as adhesive skin patches, for example in hormone replacement therapy for post-menopausal women.

Formation of aldosterone and cortisol takes place in the adrenal cortex (Fig. 14.23). Three zones can be distinguished within the cortex. These are the zona glomerulosa, zona fasiculata and zona reticularis. The zona glomerulosa produces aldosterone, which acts on cells of the distal nephron in the kidney to increase the reabsorption of sodium, with resulting excretion of potassium and hydrogen ions. Its secretion is regulated by the renin–angiotensin system. Renin is secreted by the kidney in response to osmotic changes. It is an enzyme, cleaving a precursor peptide, angiotensinogen to angiotensin I. Angiotensin-converting enzyme (ACE) cleaves this to produce angiotensin II, which stimulates aldosterone secretion. Both aldosterone and angiotensin II actions result in a rise of blood pressure. The most used aldosterone analogue is fludrocortisol. An ACE inhibitor, captopril, is a useful drug used for the control of hypertension.

The zona fasiculata produces cortisol. This has wide effects, including increase of blood sugar concentration via stimulation of gluconeogenesis. Secretion is stimulated by the pituitary hormone, adrenocorticotrophic hormone (ACTH).

ACTH secretion is in turn stimulated by corticotrophin-releasing hormone (CRH) released by the hypothalamus. Cortisol acts at both pituitary and hypothalamic levels to limit these hormones in a feedback regulatory system. Synthetic analogues include betamethasone (Fig. 14.24) and prednisolone, and these are commonly used for their anti-inflammatory and immune suppressive actions. A potent analogue, dexamethasone, is used for testing the function of the pituitary–adrenal feedback regulatory system.

The zona reticularis produces dehydroepiandrosterone (DHA), a weak androgen. It is present in relatively high concentrations in blood. This has led to speculation about possible physiological roles, but this remains controversial.

CLINICAL IMPLICATIONS

Inherited defects of steroid hormone metabolism

Inherited disorders of enzymes in the cortisol biosynthetic pathway result in failure of feedback inhibition of adrenal steroidogenesis (Fig. 14.25). This begins in utero so that the newborn infant shows greatly increased steroid production from enlarged adrenal glands (congenital adrenal hyperplasia). Deficiencies of 11β-hydroxylase or 21-hydroxylase result in increase of 17-hydroxyprogesterone and increased androgen formation, which causes virilization of the female fetus, whereas deficiency of 3β-hydroxysteroid dehydrogenase results in virilization via excess production of DHA. Deficiency of 11β-hydroxylase also results in increase of deoxycorticosterone, a weak mineralocorticoid, causing hypertension, and this is also a consequence of 17-hydroxylase deficiency. In the latter disorder, no androgens or estrogens are

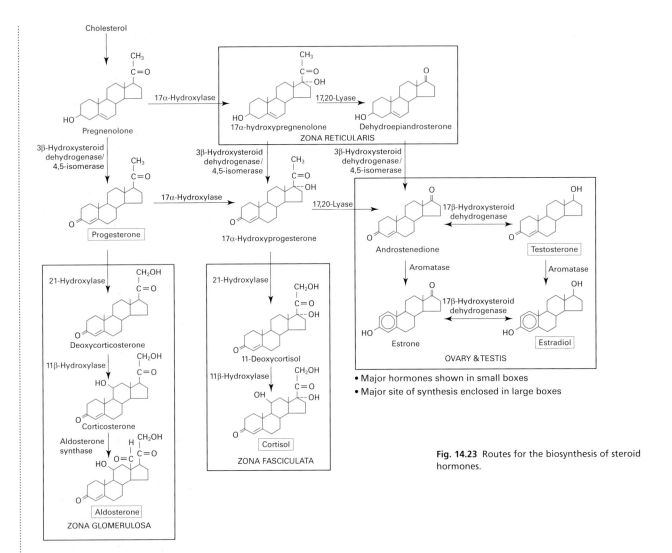

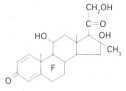

Fig. 14.23 Routes for the biosynthesis of steroid hormones.

- Major hormones shown in small boxes
- Major site of synthesis enclosed in large boxes

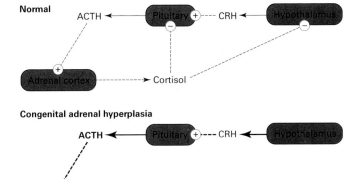

Fig. 14.24 The structure of betamethasone.

Fig. 14.25 The pathogenesis of congenital adrenal hyperplasia.

synthesized, resulting in failure of virilization in the male. Corticosterone, a weak glucocorticoid, is increased.

Aldosterone synthase deficiency results in renal salt loss and consequent stimulation of mineralocorticoid precursor synthesis via an increase of renin secretion.

Inherited defects of steroid hormone metabolism are summarized in Table 14.1.

COMPLEX CARBOHYDRATES

STRUCTURES OF COMPLEX CARBOHYDRATES

The term 'complex carbohydrate' is used to refer to oligosaccharides and polysaccharides containing a wide variety of sugars, often substituted with sulfate groups and including amino sugars. They form the carbohydrate moieties of glycoproteins and are also found as glycolipids based on ceramide, which provides another mechanism for binding some of the carbohydrates found on the outer surfaces of cells to the plasma membrane. Two sugars not previously

Table 14.1 Inherited defects of steroid hormone metabolism

Enzyme deficiency	Steroid hormone decreased	Steroid hormone increased	Clinical effects
11β-Hydroxylase	Cortisol	Deoxycorticosterone, testosterone	Virilization, hypertension
21-Hydroxylase	Cortisol ± aldosterone	Testosterone	Virilization ± salt loss
3β-Hydroxysteroid dehydrogenase	Cortisol, aldosterone, testosterone	DHA	Virilization of female, lack of virilization of male, salt loss, hypoglycemia
17-Hydroxylase	Cortisol, testosterone, estradiol	Corticosterone Deoxycorticosterone	Hypertension, lack of virilization of male
Aldosterone synthase	Aldosterone	Corticosterone	Salt loss

which these complex carbohydrates are ideally suited, and which many of them perform in physiological situations, is to act as recognition molecules.

Attachment of carbohydrate chains to proteins is either to a serine or threonine hydroxyl group, known as *O*-linked carbohydrate, illustrated in Fig. 14.29, or to the amide nitrogen of an asparagine residue, known as *N*-linked carbohydrate, illustrated in Fig. 14.30. The glycoprotein linkage illustrated in Fig. 14.29 is the structure of a mucin, the name originating in the fact that these were isolated originally from secretions of mucous cells (e.g. in saliva). This example is one of the blood group substances in which the antigenic activity resides in the carbohydrate moiety. It is found in both the glycoprotein and glycolipid forms. The gangliosides form an important group of sialic-acid-containing glycolipids that occur in brain, where they comprise about 6% of the lipid fraction. Small amounts are found on the surface of many other cells. The structure of ganglioside G_{M1} is shown in Fig. 14.31.

Fig. 14.26 The structures of α-L-fucose and sialic acid.

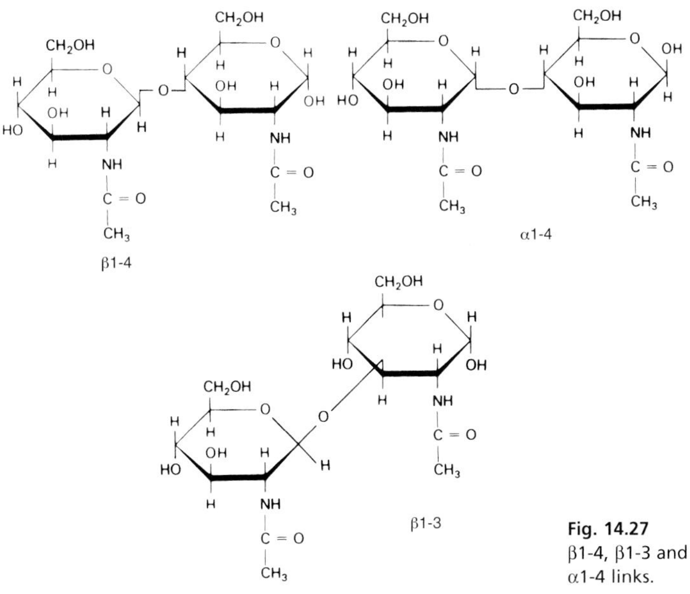

α-L-Fucose

N-Acetylneuraminic acid (sialic acid)

GLYCOPROTEIN AND GLYCOLIPID BIOSYNTHESIS

The biosynthesis of complex polysaccharides utilizes the lipid molecule, dolichyl phosphate (Fig. 14.32), formed by the action of dolichol kinase. To this is added sequentially different monosaccharide units derived from either nucleotide sugars or dolichyl diphosphosugars. In a typical synthesis, UDP-*N*-acetylglucosamine reacts with dolichyl phosphate to form dolichyl diphospho-*N*-acetylglucosamine and UMP, one of the phosphates of the UDP moiety having been transferred with the *N*-acetylglucosamine. A further *N*-acetylglucosamine from another molecule of UDP-*N*-acetylglucosamine is added to C-4 of the *N*-acetylglucosamine to form GlcNAc(β1–4)GlcNAc-diphosphodolichol. Five mannose residues are then added in reactions utilizing GDP-mannose as substrate, to give a branched structure shown within the box in Fig. 14.33. All these reactions take place in the endoplasmic reticulum with the growing oligosaccharide chain facing the cytoplasm. The dolichyl diphospho-oligosaccharide is then inverted through the membrane, so that the oligosaccharide protrudes into the lumen. Four further mannose units are then added, using dolichyl diphosphomannose, and then three glucose residues are added using dolichyl diphosphoglucose as substrate.

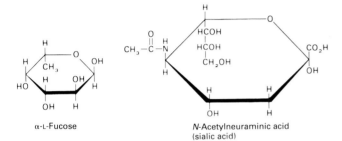

β1-4

α1-4

β1-3

Fig. 14.27 β1-4, β1-3 and α1-4 links.

described but found in these carbohydrate chains are fucose and sialic acid, shown in Fig. 14.26.

Apart from the α1-4 links common in the storage polysaccharides, the complex carbohydrates contain glycosidic linkages to any of the different hydroxyls of the constituent monosaccharide units, some of which are illustrated in Fig. 14.27. The three-dimensional structure will be profoundly affected by the type of linkage between molecules, so that the number of shapes that can be made by even a trisaccharide is very great. Figure 14.28 shows the substantial changes in three-dimensional shape that arise from relatively minor differences in structure. These examples are of blood group substances of the Lewis system. Because of the many shapes that can be formed, one role for

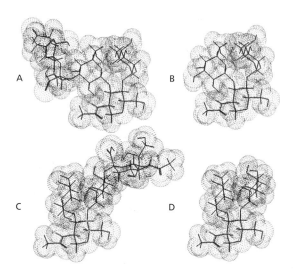

Fig. 14.28 Relatively small changes in complex carbohydrate structure influence molecular shape significantly. The structures represent the non-reducing ends of antigens of the Lewis blood group system, as follows:

(a) Sialyl Le^a Galβ1-3GlcNacβ1-
           | 2,3 | 1,4
          NeuAcα Fucα

(b) Le^a Galβ1-3GlcNacβ1-
              | 1,4
              Fucα

(c) Sialyl Le^x Galβ1-4GlcNacβ1-
           | 2,3 | 1,3
          NeuAcα Fucα

(d) Le^x Galβ1-4GlcNacβ1-
              | 1,3
              Fucα

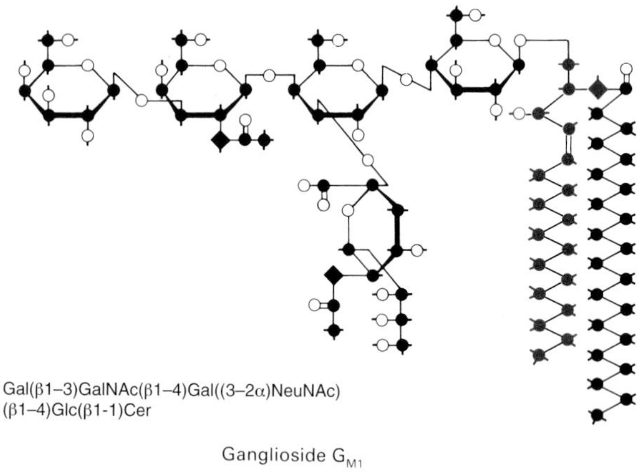

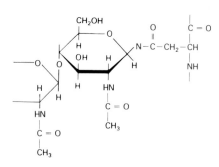

Submaxillary mucin (porcine A blood-group specificity)

GalNAc(α1—3)Gal(β1—3)GalNAc-O-Ser { or Thr }
              2   6
              α1   α2
             Fuc   NeuNAc

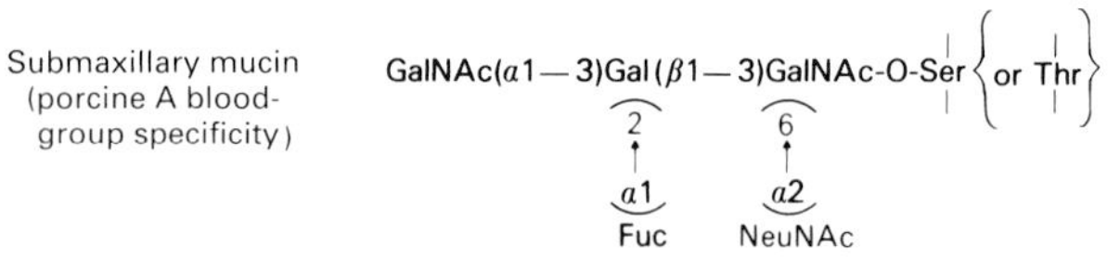

Gal NAc = N-acetylgalactosamine   Fuc = Fucose   Glc = Glucose
Gal = Galactose   NeuNAc = Sialic acid

Fig. 14.29 The structure of a submaxillary mucin with blood group A specificity.

Fig. 14.30 N-Linked oligosaccharides are attached to protein asparagine residues.

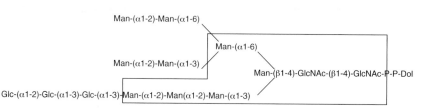

Gal(β1–3)GalNAc(β1–4)Gal((3–2α)NeuAc)
(β1–4)Glc(β1-1)Cer

Ganglioside G$_{M1}$

Fig. 14.31 The structure of ganglioside G$_{M1}$. For the meaning of symbols, see p. 186. Cer, ceramide.

$$H\text{-}[CH_2\text{-}\underset{CH_3}{C}=CH\text{-}CH_2\text{-}]_n\text{-}CH_2\text{-}\underset{CH_3}{CH}\text{-}CH_2\text{-}CH_2\text{-}O\text{-}\underset{O^-}{\overset{O^-}{P}}=O$$

Fig. 14.32 The structure of dolichyl phosphate.

Dol
CTP ⤵
CDP ⤴
       These steps occur with the oligosaccharide oriented to the cytosolic face of the endoplasmic reticulum

P-Dol
UDPGlcNAc ⤵
UMP ⤴

GlcNAc-P-P-Dol
UDPGlcNAc ⤵
UDP ⤴

GlcNAc (β1-4) GlcNAc-P-P-Dol

5 Mannose residues are then transferred from GDPMannose to give the structure shown boxed in structure below

Reorientation of the oligosaccharide in the membrane

4 Mannose residues are transferred from Man-P-P-Dol

3 Glucose residues are transferred from Glc-P-P-Dol

These steps occur with the oligosaccharide oriented into the lumen of the endoplasmic reticulum

Man-(α1-2)-Man-(α1-6)
Man-(α1-6)
Man-(α1-2)-Man-(α1-3)
Man-(β1-4)-GlcNAc-(β1-4)-GlcNAc-P-P-Dol
Glc-(α1-2)-Glc-(α1-3)-Glc-(α1-3)-Man-(α1-2)-Man(α1-2)-Man-(α1-3)

Fig. 14.33 The dolichyl oligosaccharide biosynthetic pathway.

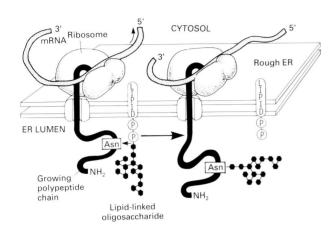

Fig. 14.34 The transfer of lipid-linked oligosaccharide to protein asparagine.

After the formation of this 14-residue chain, the oligosaccharide chain is transferred to an asparagine residue of a polypeptide chain that is being synthesized on a ribosome in the vicinity of the dolichyl diphospho-oligosaccharide, as shown in Fig. 14.34. As the nascent polypeptide chain passes into the Golgi apparatus, further processing of the carbohydrate chain can occur (see p. 45).

A key enzyme in the modification of the carbohydrate chains in the Golgi apparatus is *N*-acetylglucosamine galactosyltransferase. This ubiquitous enzyme is found in many types of cell bound to the membranes of the Golgi apparatus and is a marker enzyme for this organelle (see p. 45). It adds galactose in β1-4 linkage to the terminal residues of both core oligosaccharide branches:

UDP-galactose + *N*-Acetylglucosamine → *N*-Acetyllactosamine + UDP

Lactose is synthesized by lactose synthase, which consists of two proteins, A and B. The A-protein is *N*-acetylglucosamine galactosyltransferase and the B-protein is α-lactalbumin (see p. 59), a milk protein. B-protein modifies the substrate specificity of A-protein from *N*-acetylglucosamine to glucose so that we have:

UDP-galactose + Glucose → Lactose + UDP

B-protein interacts with A-protein, which is bound to the membranes of the Golgi complex and this event is the initiation of lactation. The B-protein (α-lactalbumin) is excreted in the milk.

Biomembranes, receptors and signal transduction

The plasma membrane consists of a lipid bilayer in which are embedded proteins, including glycoproteins, and glycolipids. The proteins can be integral proteins, which have helical regions passing through the lipid bilayer, or peripheral proteins, which are more loosely attached, often through fatty acyl or prenyl groups. Many of the proteins are receptors; two important groups of receptors include those that act through G proteins and those that have tyrosine kinase activity in their cytosolic domain. The G-protein-coupled receptors belong to a family having seven transmembrane domains. The receptors with tyrosine kinase activity are mostly involved with growth control. The receptors bind ligands and recycle through an endosome system. The effects of these receptors are mediated by cascades of signalling molecules, including other protein kinases, cyclic AMP, phosphoinositides and Ca^{2+}.

Transport of small molecules through the plasma membrane is mediated by transport proteins and may be passive transfer, facilitated diffusion or active transport. A diverse family of adhesion molecules mediates certain kinds of interaction between cells that are in contact with one another.

There is a cytoskeletal system within the cell, consisting of microtubules, actin microfilaments and intermediate filaments. Transport of molecules and cell organelles along these filaments occurs by a process similar to the mechanism of muscle contraction.

THE BASIS OF MEMBRANE STRUCTURE

THE ROLE OF THE PLASMA MEMBRANE

The plasma membrane forms a barrier between the cell and its external environment, thereby maintaining the interior of the cell as an enclosed, coordinated system. This membrane consists of a lipid bilayer, the structure of which is explained more fully below, within which are embedded proteins that act as receptors or transporters. These proteins enable the cell to engage in a dynamic interaction with its environment. Thus it receives signals from hormones and growth factors. Some of the receptors bind adhesion molecules that function as cell recognition agents and enable the cell to respond to contact with other cells. There is communication between the plasma membrane, which is the cell's sense organ, and the nucleus, which is a control centre for many cell activities.

STRUCTURE OF THE PHOSPHOLIPID BILAYER

The properties of phospholipids are such that they naturally form bilayer structures in solution, in contrast to detergents and fatty acids, which form micelles. Part of the driving force for the formation of bilayers is the fact that, as shown in Fig. 15.1, the phospholipid molecule has a hydrophilic headgroup and a hydrophobic tail. Such molecules will tend to form structures in aqueous environments such that the hydrophilic moieties face the aqueous environment and the hydrophobic moiety is orientated towards the centre of the structure, away from the water molecules. A detergent micelle has a more or less spherical shape, as shown in Fig. 15.2, but the two fatty acid side-chains of a phospholipid are too bulky to fit into such a formation, and a phospholipid thus adopts the bilayer structure. Not all phospholipids have strong bilayer-forming potential. Some, such as phosphatidylethanolamine, with a relatively small headgroup, can adopt the hexagonal phase in the membrane. As shown in Fig. 15.3, this has the form of an inverted micelle, with the hydrophilic groups in the centre. Phosphatidylcholine, on the other hand, strongly promotes bilayer formation alone or in mixtures with other phospholipids, with protein inserted as shown in Fig. 15.4.

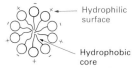

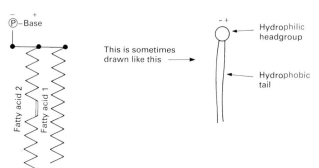

This is sometimes drawn like this ——▶

Fig. 15.1 The geometry of a phospholipid.

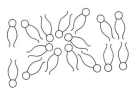

Fig. 15.2 Some lipids and most detergents form spherical micelles with a hydrophobic core.

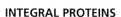

Fig. 15.3 An inverted micelle has a hydrophilic core.

INTEGRAL PROTEINS

Membrane proteins are of two main types: those that have, in addition to intracellular and extracellular domains, hydrophobic domains that traverse the membrane lipid bilayer one or more times, as sketched in Fig. 15.4, and those that are more loosely attached to the membrane, or are attached by lipid anchors. Proteins that have transmembrane domains are known as integral or intrinsic membrane proteins, and those attached by other means are termed peripheral (extrinsic) proteins. The hydrophobic transmembrane domains form a helical conformation. Each turn of an α-helix requires 0.541 nm, so the width of the hydrophobic span of the bilayer of about 3.5 nm permits six to seven turns. Examples of proteins having several transmembrane domains, and those that are anchored to the membrane by other mechanisms, are given later. It should be emphasized that, for most proteins, the identification of transmembrane domains is at present mostly based on predictions from amino acid sequences; the solving of membrane protein structures lags behind that for soluble proteins.

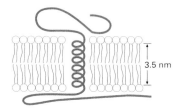

Fig. 15.4 Integral proteins traverse the bilayer and have cytoplasmic, transmembrane and extracellular domains.

The complete amino acid sequence is known for many integral membrane proteins. The sequence of one of these, glycophorin, is shown in Fig. 15.5. This red blood cell protein bears carbohydrates on its extracellular domain that have blood group specificity. The hydrophobic residues are shown in red, and it can be seen that the transmembrane domain has many of these. The points of attachment of carbohydrates are indicated by squares, for O-linked chains, and hexagons, for N-linked chains. In this case, the N-terminus is extracellular, but this is not the case for all integral plasma membrane proteins.

ANCHORING OF PROTEINS BY LIPIDS

Many peripheral proteins (and in some cases, domains of integral proteins) are anchored into the plasma membrane through linkage to fatty acyl groups or isoprenyl groups inserted into the membrane bilayer, as shown in Fig. 15.6. Linkage of fatty acids can be as esters or thioesters, or as N-acyl groups. Isoprenyl groups are attached to cysteine as thioethers. The discovery of the importance of isoprenyl groups resulted from investigations of the inhibition of cell growth that results from the use of inhibitors of HMG-CoA reductase. It was found that the inhibition could not be relieved by addition of cholesterol, and that the isoprenoids farnesyl diphosphate (see p. 167) and geranylgeranyl diphosphate

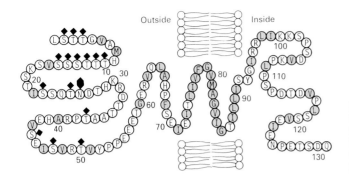

Fig. 15.5 Glycophorin has a domain structure typical of single-helix transmembrane proteins.

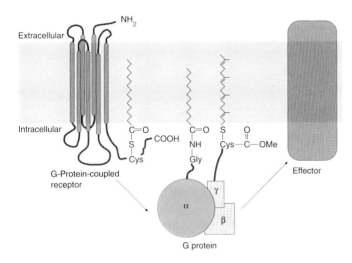

Fig. 15.6 Proteins or protein domains can be attached to membranes by fatty acyl or prenyl groups.

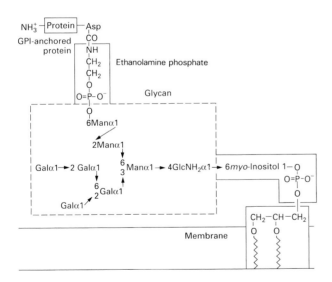

Fig. 15.7 Attachment of proteins to membranes by glycosylphosphatidylinositol anchors.

methylated. In such proteins, there is an amino acid sequence −CAAX at the C-terminus, which is involved in this attachment, the geranylgeranyl group being attached to the cysteine, and AAX then being removed with methylation of the cysteine.

Another method of attachment by lipids involves a glycosylphosphatidylinositol group. Such a structure is shown in Fig. 15.7. The protein is attached to the glycan moiety, and the complex is anchored to the membrane by the fatty acyl groups of the phosphatidylinositol.

PROTEIN DYNAMICS IN THE LIPID BILAYER

As indicated in Fig. 15.8, proteins can move laterally in the plane of the membrane, and can rotate around an axis vertical to the plane of the membrane. However, they cannot tumble through the plane of the membrane. The fact that they can move laterally is illustrated very well by the phenomenon known as capping. This is the name given to the effect seen when, for example, a lymphocyte is stimulated by a mitogen tagged with a fluorescent label. Initially, the fluorescent label is distributed over the entire surface of the cell. After a few minutes it starts to cluster, and after about 30 min has formed a cap, as shown in Fig. 15.9.

MEMBRANE RECEPTORS

RECEPTOR STRUCTURE

Plasma membrane receptor proteins have an extracellular domain that has the function of binding the agonist or other ligand that interacts with the receptor. In the case of some receptors, the main function is to bring about the internalization of the ligand to the cell interior. This is the case with the receptors for apoprotein B and for transferrin, illustrated in Fig. 15.10. Receptors of this type often have relatively small intracellular domains.

Other receptors have the function of transmitting the signal into the cell interior, and have intracellular domains that bear functionally active sites, such as those that interact with G proteins (see below), or have protein kinase activity (see p. 208). The detail of the structure of the β-adrenergic receptor, which activates a G protein, is shown in Fig. 15.11. This receptor, in common with many G-protein-activating receptors, has seven

were essential for the post-translational modification of certain proteins essential for growth. Geranylgeranyl diphosphate is a 20-carbon isoprenoid synthesized from the 15-carbon farnesyl diphosphate by reaction with isopentenyl diphosphate. It had previously been found that a number of proteins undergo acylation by fatty acids, such as palmitate and myristate, during

post-translational processing. Figure 15.6 shows a G-protein-coupled receptor with palmitoylation through a thioester linkage to a conserved cysteine. The G-protein α subunit (see p. 205) has myristate attached in amide linkage to N-terminal glycine, and the γ subunit is shown with a geranylgeranyl group attached to a C-terminal cysteine with its carboxyl

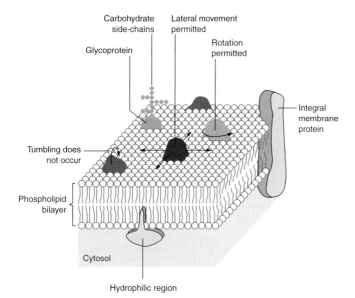

Fig. 15.8 Proteins can rotate and move laterally in the membrane but cannot tumble.

transmembrane domains (7-TMD). The figure illustrates the multiplicity of sites on the protein that are required for a variety of functions: Asn-6 and Asn-15 bear *N*-linked carbohydrate; Cys-106, Cys-184, Cys-190 and Cys-191 are required for

normal ligand binding and cell surface expression. As ligand binding is thought to occur in the hydrophobic region, these cysteines might actually stabilize the correct folded conformation. Asp-113 is conserved among all 7-TMD receptors

that bind biogenic amines. Its replacement by Asn causes a great decrease in the potency of agonists in stimulating adenylyl cyclase. Ser-204 and Ser-207 are required for normal binding and activation by catecholamine agonists. A palmitoyl residue is attached to Cys-341 and penetrates the bilayer, binding that part of the intracellular domain to the intracellular surface. Ser-260 and Ser-346 are sites phosphorylated by cyclic AMP-dependent protein kinase.

THE INSULIN RECEPTOR

The insulin receptor has been studied in some detail. It is a large transmembrane glycoprotein of about 350 kDa, composed of two 135-kDa α subunits and two 95-kDa β subunits, linked by disulfide bonds to form a β-α-α-β heterotetramer, as shown in Fig. 15.12. Both subunits are encoded by a single gene of about 150 kb pairs, with 22 exons (grey bars in Fig. 15.12) separated by 21 introns. Translation of the mRNA yields a proreceptor that is glycosylated and forms

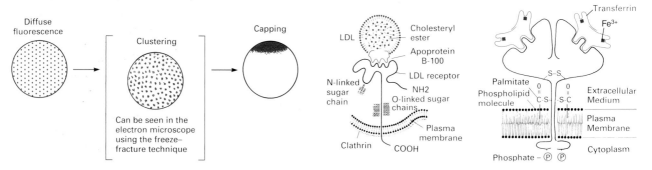

Fig. 15.9 Capping is characteristic of surface antigens that form aggregates.

Fig. 15.10 The LDL and transferrin receptors comprise single transmembrane domain proteins.

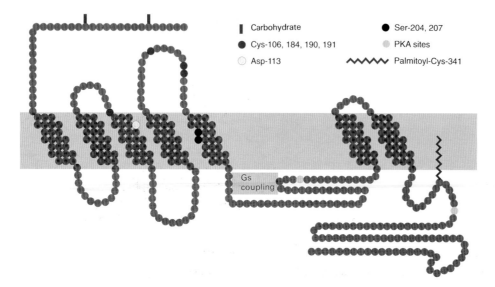

Fig. 15.11 The β-adrenergic receptor is a seven transmembrane domain protein.

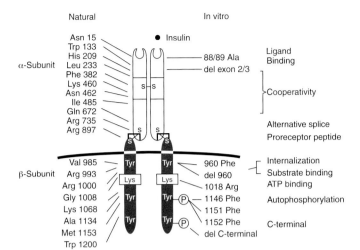

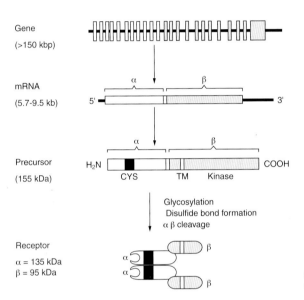

Fig. 15.12 The insulin receptor structure and the function of its domains.

Fig. 15.13 The insulin receptor mRNA leads to a single polypeptide that is cleaved to α- and β-chains.

that have been identified in diabetics with marked clinical resistance to insulin are shown; these patients required 10–1000 times the normal dose of insulin. On the right of the figure, several sites are indicated at which in vitro mutagenesis has assisted in identifying the functional domains shown on the far right.

The activated insulin receptor has a number of target proteins, two of which are named insulin receptor substrates IRS-1 and IRS-2. In Fig. 15.14, IRS-1 is shown being phosphorylated and, as a result, binding and activating other signalling proteins, one of the most important of which is phosphoinositide (PI) 3′-kinase. This leads to formation of PtdInsP$_3$, which activates a protein kinase cascade that phosphorylates GLUT 4, stimulating its binding to the muscle plasma membrane (p. 177), and phosphofructokinase-2 (p. 179), thereby stimulating glycolysis.

CLINICAL IMPLICATIONS – MUTATIONS IN IRS-1

Mutations in IRS-1 may be significant in the insulin resistance associated with type 2 diabetes. Polymorphisms of IRS-1 are significantly more common in patients with type 2 diabetes than in controls and include the G972R (glycine 972 to arginine), S892G, G819R, R1221C and A513P variants. Of these, the G972R polymorphism is the most common and has been studied most extensively. This polymorphism is found in Caucasian populations, with a prevalence of 5.8% in

disulfide links before cleavage to form the mature receptor (Fig. 15.13). This inserts into the plasma membrane by a short transmembrane domain in each of the β subunits. The cytosolic portions of the β subunits carry protein tyrosine kinase domains. In common with other receptor tyrosine kinases (see p. 209), these can phosphorylate tyrosines within the cytosolic domain of the receptor – a process known as autophosphorylation. This process is initiated when the receptor is activated by binding insulin. In addition, the tyrosine kinase activity can phosphorylate tyrosines in target proteins. Mutant receptors that have defective α subunits have activated tyrosine kinase activity in the absence of insulin, indicating that the α subunit acts as a regulatory subunit, inactivating the kinase activity of the β subunit; this inhibition is relieved by insulin binding. On the left of Fig. 15.12, a number of naturally occurring mutations

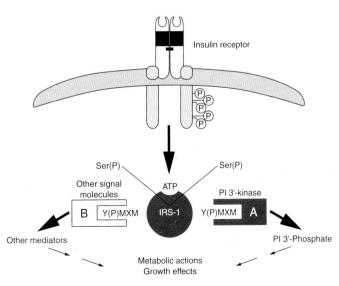

Fig. 15.14 Insulin receptor substrates mediate insulin action.

normal and 10.7% in patients with type 2 diabetes, respectively. In Caucasian populations, obese carriers of this polymorphism show decreased insulin sensitivity during an oral glucose tolerance test.

NEUROTRANSMITTERS

In certain types of synapse, transmission of the nerve impulse is mediated chemically, by neurotransmitters such as acetylcholine, serotonin (see p. 127) and the catecholamines adrenaline and noradrenaline (p. 125). The neurotransmitter is released from storage sites in the presynaptic terminal and then, after stimulating the postsynaptic terminal, is inactivated. Monoamine oxidase inactivates serotonin and plays an important role in degrading catecholamines. Acetylcholine is hydrolysed by cholinesterase to choline and acetate. Cholinesterase also hydrolyses a muscle-relaxing drug, succinylcholine, used in anesthesia. Individuals with abnormal cholinesterase can fail to hydrolyse the drug and consequently suffer prolonged paralysis.

ANALYSIS BY CLONING OF THE NICOTINIC ACETYLCHOLINE RECEPTOR

Receptors for acetylcholine, the neurotransmitter, are classified by their response to the agonists nicotine and muscarine. The two types of receptor are very different in structure, muscarinic receptors being of the 7-TMD type, interacting with G proteins, whereas the nicotinic receptors have four transmembrane domains and, when activated, function as ion-conducting channels across the membrane.

An illustration of the use of genetic engineering to analyse receptor structure is given by work on this receptor. The nicotinic acetylcholine receptor (AChR) has five subunits, two α and one each of β, γ and δ (see insert in Fig. 15.15). The genes of the four types of subunit have been cloned and the products expressed in *Xenopus* oocytes after injection of mRNAs transcribed in vitro. The oocytes were then found to bear functional AChR, which normally they do not possess. Modification of the gene for the α subunit by site-directed mutagenesis resulted in the changes to various functions of the a subunit shown in Fig. 15.15.

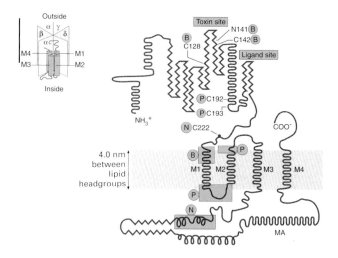

Fig. 15.15 The domains of the α subunit of the acetylcholine receptor. B,= acetylcholine binding affected; P, gating or permeation affected; N, no effect.

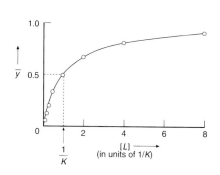

Fig. 15.16 The adsorption isotherm.

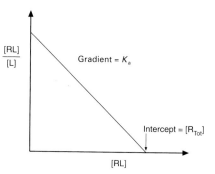

Fig. 15.17 The Scatchard plot.

ANALYSIS OF BINDING TO RECEPTORS: THE SCATCHARD PLOT

It is characteristic that binding phenomena exhibit saturation kinetics. If, in the binding of a ligand (L) to its receptor (R), [L] is the concentration of free ligand and [RL] is the concentration of bound ligand, then the ratio of [RL] to all forms (bound or free) of the receptor, i.e. $[RL]/[R_{Tot}]$, is known as the saturation fraction, and is given the symbol γ. A plot of γ against [L] is referred to as the adsorption isotherm, as in Fig. 15.16, in which K is the association constant of the complex.

The quantities most often needed to be extracted from binding data concern the dissociation constant, K_a, for the complex and the total number of receptor molecules $[R_{Tot}]$. These can be obtained from a plot of [RL]/[L] against [RL] as shown in Fig. 15.17. This is known as a Scatchard plot and it derives from the following analysis. The association constant $K_a = [RL]/[L][R]$, where [L] and [RL] are as defined previously, and [R] is the concentration of unbound receptor.

Because:

$$[R] = [R_{Tot}] - [RL]$$

then:

$$[RL]/([L][R_{Tot}] - [L][RL]) = K_a$$

This can readily be rearranged to give:

$$[RL]/[L] = -K_a[RL] + K_a[R_{Tot}]$$

which is the equation of a straight line with negative slope K_a and intercept on the abscissa $[R_{Tot}]$.

A linear Scatchard plot is obtained only if there is one binding constant. If sites with different binding constants are involved, a plot that is biphasic or more complex is the result. A plot of this type is shown in Fig. 15.18, from which it is possible to extract information as shown in the figure.

G PROTEINS

G-PROTEIN ACTIVATION

Many receptors activate adenylyl cyclase, the reaction of which is shown on p. 93.

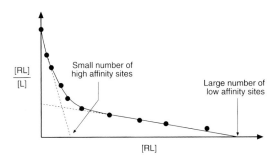

Fig. 15.18 The non-linear Scatchard plot.

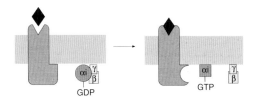

Fig. 15.21 Inhibitory G protein α subunits.

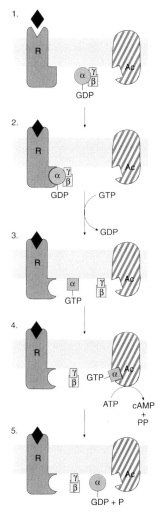

Fig. 15.19 The mechanism of action of G protein.

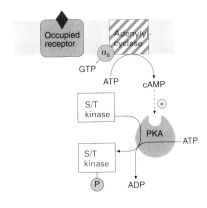

Fig. 15.20 The activation of PKA by adenylate cyclase activity.

1. In the non-activated state, GDP is bound to the α subunit of the G protein.
2. Occupation of the receptor by an activating ligand causes binding of the G protein to the receptor.
3. This brings about exchange of GTP for GDP on the α subunit, separation of the βγ subunit complex from the heterotrimeric complex, and release of the α subunit with changed conformation.
4. GTP-α then binds to and activates adenylyl cyclase, which catalyses formation of cyclic AMP from ATP.
5. The α subunit has GTPase activity, and hydrolyses GTP to GDP and P. This causes the α subunit to dissociate from adenylyl cyclase, deactivating it, and the

heterotrimeric GDP complex then reforms and is available to start the cycle again.

Activation of adenylyl cyclase by the α subunit results in synthesis of cyclic AMP, and leads to activation of PKA and thus its downstream target serine/threonine (S/T) protein kinases, as illustrated in Fig. 15.20.

THE G-PROTEIN SUPERFAMILY

Some heterotrimeric G proteins have a type of α subunit that inhibits rather than activates adenylyl cyclase (Fig. 15.21). The inhibitory α subunits are designated α_i, whereas stimulatory subunits are designated α_s. These subunits bind their complexes to receptors that function by inhibition of cyclic AMP formation. The monomeric G proteins are typified by the 21-kDa product of the *ras* oncogene (p21^{ras}; see below). The bacterial elongation factor EF-Tu is a monomeric G protein.

The structures of some of the G-protein superfamily are summarized in Fig. 15.22. These show the binding sites of two toxins that catalyse ADP-ribosylation of certain G proteins (see below), CT indicating cholera toxin and IAP islet-activating protein. In this superfamily, several highly conserved GTP-binding regions are recognized, as shown in Fig. 15.23. Much of what is known of their structure derives from the crystallographic structure of p21^{ras}. The numbering of specific residues (those underlined) in the following comments relates to the p21^{ras} structure. In G-1, the

This activation depends on the coupling of the enzyme to the receptor by G proteins, so named because they bind guanine nucleotides. There are two main types of G proteins: heterotrimeric proteins, which have α, β and γ subunits, and monomeric proteins. Activation of receptors as a result of binding a ligand activates adenylyl cyclase through heterotrimeric G proteins. The following description refers to steps in the mechanism of activation shown in Fig. 15.19:

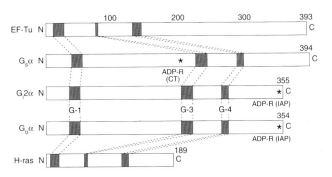

Fig. 15.22 The G-protein superfamily.

	Residues	G-1	Residues	G-3	Residues	G-4
EF-Tu	18-25	G H V D H G K T	80-84	D C P G H	135-138	N K C D
Gsα	47-54	G A G E S G K S	223-227	D V G G Q	289-295	N K Q D
Gi2α	40-47	G A G E S G K S	201-205	D V G G Q	270-273	N K K D
Goα	40-47	G A G E S G K S	201-205	D V G G Q	270-273	N K K D
Ha-ras	10-17	G A G G V G K S	57-61	D T A G Q	116-119	N K C D

Fig. 15.23 Homologies between G proteins.

amino acid sequence motif $GX_4GK(S/T)$ is involved in bonding through the ε-amino group of Lys-16 to α- and β-phosphates of GTP or GDP. The $\underline{D}X_2G$ motif of the G-3 region binds the catalytic Mg^{2+} through Asp-57 with an intervening water molecule. In the characteristic sequence motif of G-4, $(N/T)(K/Q)X\underline{D}$, Asp-119 hydrogen bonds to the guanine ring.

ADP-RIBOSYLATION

ADP-ribosylation refers to a complex of ADP molecules linked through their ribose moieties. A representative structure is shown in Fig. 15.24. Such a complex is built onto a variety of cell proteins, including nuclear proteins and some cytoplasmic proteins. It also forms part of the action of the toxins of the bacteria *Vibrio cholerae* (cholera toxin) and *Bordetella pertussis* (pertussis toxin), the causal agent of whooping cough. Cholera toxin brings about ADP-ribosylation of $α_s$, preventing association of $α_s$ with βγ subunits, and so persistently activates adenylyl cyclase. ADP-ribosylation of $α_i$ by pertussis toxin also activates the enzyme by deactivating the inhibitory action of the subunit. The ADP moieties are transferred to the protein from NAD^+ by ADP-ribosyltransferase, with release of nicotinamide.

CYCLIC AMP AND GENE REGULATION

One of the most important effects of cyclic AMP is exerted through gene expression. This is mediated through a cyclic AMP response element (CRE) in the promoter of many genes. CRE is constituted by an 8-bp palindromic sequence, TGACGTCA. Activator proteins such as CRE-binding protein (CREB) bind to CRE to induce transcription, after phosphorylation by PKA. Genes induced by cyclic AMP include those involved in the action of hormones, in cell differentiation and in cell proliferation. The system is outlined in Fig. 15.25.

CELL SIGNALLING SYSTEMS

PHOSPHOLIPASE C AND INOSITOL PHOSPHATES

Phospholipase C (PLC) plays a key role in activating the Ca^{2+}/calmodulin and PKC systems described in earlier chapters. Various members of the PLC family hydrolyse different phosphoinositides to diacylglycerol and the corresponding headgroup. The γ isoform of phospholipase C (PLC-γ) is particularly important in mediating growth factor signalling. The discovery of the importance of the hydrolysis of $PtdInsP_2$ to diacylglycerol and inositol 1,4,5-trisphosphate ($Ins[1,4,5]P_3$) was a breakthrough in this area. $Ins(1,4,5)P_3$ releases Ca^{2+} from intracellular stores, which are probably mainly in the endoplasmic reticulum. Then Ca^{2+} and diacylglycerol, acting together, activate PKC which in turn activates its downstream target S/T protein kinases. Ca^{2+} also binds to calmodulin and thereby activates other kinases, as shown in Fig. 15.26.

INOSITOL PHOSPHATE METABOLISM

The structures of D-*myo*-inositol 1-phosphate and D-*myo*-inositol

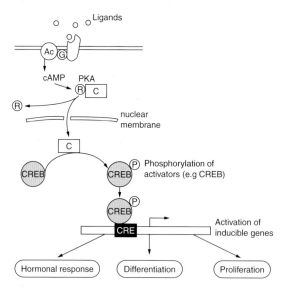

R = PKA regulatory subunit

C = PKA catalytic subunit

Fig. 15.25 Cyclic AMP is involved in gene regulation through CRE and CREB.

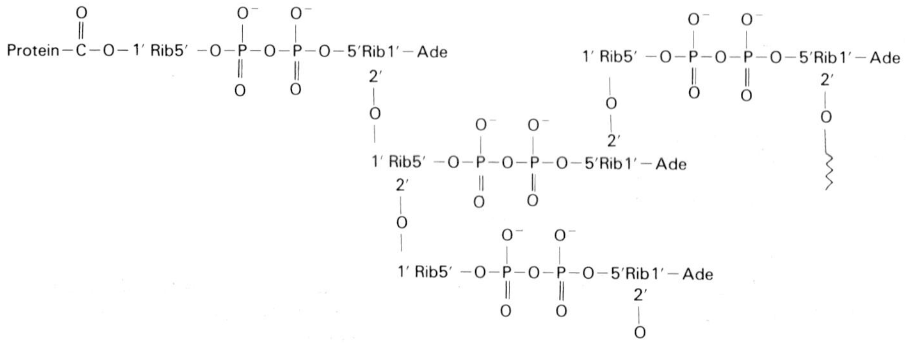

Fig. 15.24 The chemistry of ADP-ribosylation. Ade, adenine; Rib, ribose.

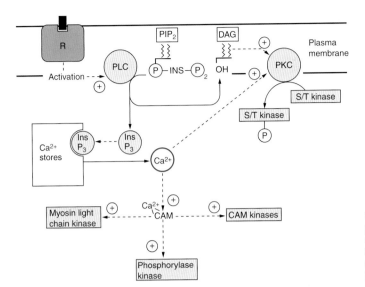

Fig. 15.26 The phospholipase C cell signalling system. CAM, Ca^{2+}/calmodulin; Ins, inositol.

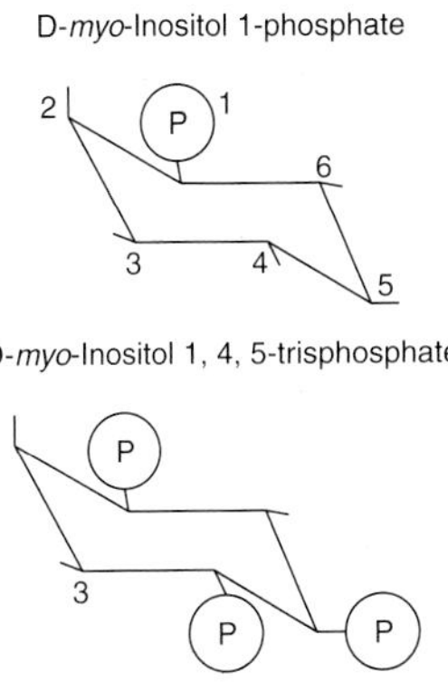

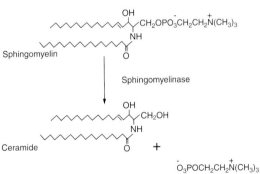

Fig. 15.27 The structure of inositol phosphates.

1,4,5-trisphosphate are shown in Fig. 15.27. In inositol phospholipids, it is the C-1 phosphate to which a diacylglycerol group is esterified. A considerable number of inositol phosphates can be formed from InsP_3. The products recycle to inositol, which then participates in resynthesis of PtdInsP_2. Some of the main reactions are shown in Fig. 15.28. After hydrolysis of PtdInsP_2 to InsP_3 and diacylglycerol (DAG), diacylglycerol is acted on by a kinase that phosphorylates it to phosphatidate (PtdOH), which then reacts with CTP to form CMP–PtdOH (alternative abbreviation CDP–DAG). Phosphatases of varying degrees of specificity convert InsP_3 to inositol (Ins), which can then react with CMP–PtdOH to form PtdIns, and thence other phosphoinositides. InsP_3 can be phosphorylated to Ins(1,3,4,5)P_4, which undergoes further metabolism as shown. Few of these inositol phosphates apart from Ins (1,4,5)P_3 have been assigned any role in cell physiology, though Ins(1,3,4,5)P_4 plays a role with Ins(1,4,5)P_3 in activating Ca^{2+} entry into the cell.

PHOSPHOINOSITIDE 3'-KINASE

Other phosphoinositides have been shown to originate from kinases that phosphorylate the 3' position. One of the most important of these reactions results in the formation of PtdIns(1,3,4,5)P_4 from PtdIns(1,4,5)P_3, a reaction catalysed by a phosphoinositide (PI) 3'-kinase. The phosphoinositides with a 3'-phosphate engage in cell signalling, but apparently not

by being hydrolysed by a phospholipase C. They appear to activate certain protein kinases, and form an important class of signalling molecules.

SPHINGOLIPIDS IN SIGNALLING

In addition to those described above, a number of other lipids act as signalling molecules; these include the sphingolipids, and prostaglandins already described. The most important signalling molecule derived from sphingolipids is ceramide. This is formed from sphingomyelin as a result of activation of sphingomyelinase (Fig. 15.29). This has been linked to activation of several cell surface receptors, including the

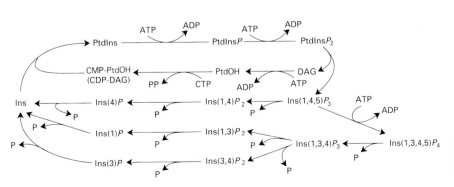

Fig. 15.29 The action of sphingomyelinase.

Fig. 15.28 The metabolism of inositol phosphates and phosphoinositides. Ins, Inositol.

tumour necrosis factor (TNF) receptor, the interleukin 1 receptor and the nerve growth factor receptor. Enzymes activated by ceramide include a protein kinase and a protein phosphatase. In the case of the TNF receptor, as illustrated in Fig. 15.30, protein kinases are a major target, and these include a protein kinase cascade that includes kinases that activate a cytosolic phospholipase A_2. This hydrolyses phospholipids containing arachidonic acid, releasing the arachidonic acid from which prostaglandins and other products that cause inflammation are produced. Sphingosine is also thought to act as a signalling molecule.

NITRIC OXIDE IN CELL SIGNALLING

Nitric oxide (NO), like the prostaglandins, is an intercellular signalling molecule, as opposed to the intracellular molecules we have mostly discussed previously. It is important as a cardiovascular regulator, decreasing blood pressure. It is produced by neurons and by macrophages, in the case of the latter as a weapon against pathogens. Although it has an odd number of electrons and is a free radical, it is chemically relatively stable but reacts rapidly with species containing unpaired electrons, such as molecular oxygen, superoxide anion and metals (see p. 142). It is formed from arginine by the pathway illustrated in Fig. 15.31. See p. 93 for the role of nitric oxide in the action of the drug sildenafil.

PROTEIN TYROSINE KINASES

The structure of a number of receptor tyrosine kinases is shown in Fig. 15.32. They can be divided into classes on the basis of their structures. Class I is typified by epidermal growth factor (EGF) receptor, comprising proteins having two extracellular cysteine-rich domains (red boxes) and a single intracellular kinase domain (pink). Class II includes receptors of the insulin receptor type – disulfide-linked heterotetrameric $\alpha_2\beta_2$ structures. These also have cysteine-rich repeats (shown in red) and intracellular kinase domains (pink). Class III receptors are characterized by five immunoglobulin-type extracellular domains (white blebs), with the kinase domain (pink) having a non-kinase insert. Class IV is similar to class III but with only three immunoglobulin-type domains (see also Fig. 5.19). The kinase domain not only phosphorylates other proteins but can also phosphorylate itself

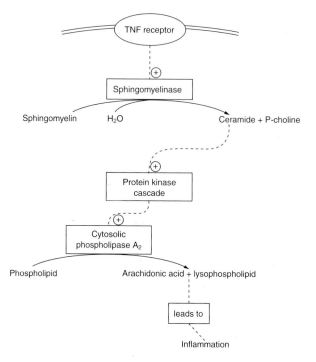

Fig. 15.30 Sphingolipids are involved in cell signalling.

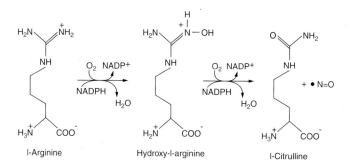

Fig. 15.31 The biosynthesis of nitric oxide from arginine. The mechanism is complex. In the first step the enzyme consumes 1 mol of NADPH to form hydroxy-L-arginine, which is an enzyme-bound intermediate, and then consumes 0.5 mol of NADPH to oxidize this to citrulline.

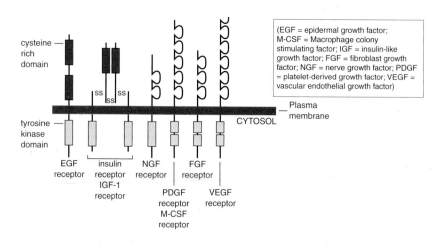

Fig. 15.32 Receptor protein tyrosine kinase classes.

(autophosphorylation), often at many sites, each site having a particular function in binding and activating different downstream signalling molecules. Figure 15.33 illustrates this for the PDGF receptor which mediates the signalling system that is activated by PDGF. Some associated proteins have been described. Grb2 and Shc are molecules known as adapter molecules that link other members of the signalling system and are discussed further in Chapter 16.

Signalling through these receptors normally involves formation of complexes. These complexes often include soluble protein tyrosine kinases, such as Src, the product of the c-*src* protooncogene, which in some cases become bound to the plasma membrane. In the case of Src, this binding occurs through attachment of a myristic acid residue to the N-terminal glycine, as shown in Fig. 15.34. The kinase domain of Src shows homology to that of the PDGF receptor, but does not have the non-kinase insert in the kinase domain. Src also has two domains found in many proteins that are involved in binding in the activation complexes. These are known as Src homology (SH) domains, because they were first found in Src. SH-2 binds to specific phosphorylated tyrosines. Figure 15.35 shows some typical interactions. Src is shown phosphorylating tyrosines in PI 3'-kinase and Ras-GAP (Ras-GTPase-activating protein), a protein that activates the GTPase activity of the product of the *ras* proto-oncogene. The phosphorylated proteins are shown binding to tyrosine phosphates in the PDGF receptor. Phosphoinositide-specific phospholipase C (PLC-γ, one of the isoforms of the enzyme) also binds as part of the complex.

RECEPTOR TRAFFIC

THE ENDOSOME SYSTEM

Ligands bound to surface receptors are internalized by a system of vesicles, as described for the LDL receptor on p. 168. The receptors cluster in areas of the membrane known as coated pits. These areas of the membrane are coated internally by a protein known as clathrin. On binding ligand, the coated pit invaginates and forms a coated vesicle (Fig. 15.36). The vesicles then lose clathrin, and enter the early endosome system. This appears to consist of a system of pre-existing vesicles or tubules with which the uncoated vesicle fuses. The early endosome

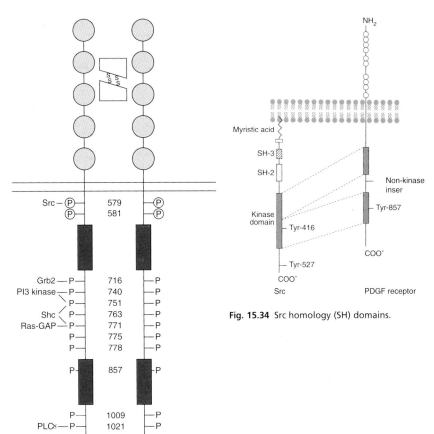

Fig. 15.33 The domain structure of the PDGF receptor and its phosphorylation sites.

Fig. 15.34 Src homology (SH) domains.

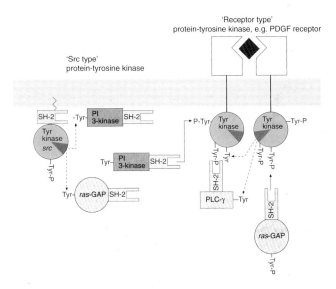

Fig. 15.35 Interactions between receptor tyrosine kinases and their substrates in cell stimulation.

compartment is acidic and causes ligand and receptor to dissociate, and then divides into a vesicle that recycles to the plasma membrane with the receptor, and a vesicle, known as a late endosome, that fuses with a lysosome, resulting in the processing of the ligand. There are variations of this scheme. For example, in the case of the transferrin receptor (see inset), transferrin and its receptor both recycle back to the plasma membrane, only the iron being dissociated by the low pH of the endosome.

THE ROLE OF CLATHRIN

Clathrin is a molecule that controls the formation of coated pits and coated

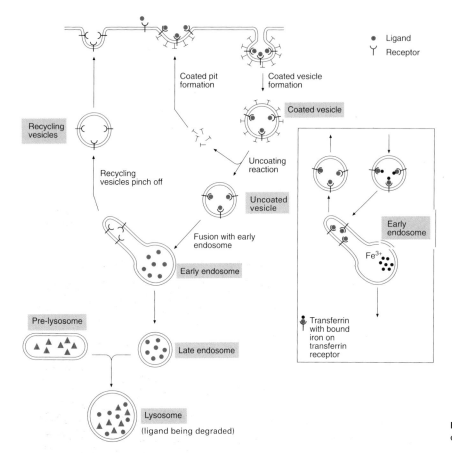

Fig. 15.36 The role of coated vesicles and endosomes in receptor cycling.

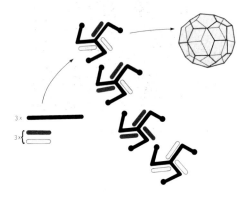

Fig. 15.37 Triskelions of clathrin form clathrin baskets.

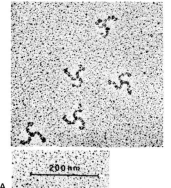

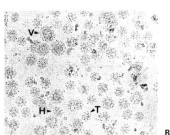

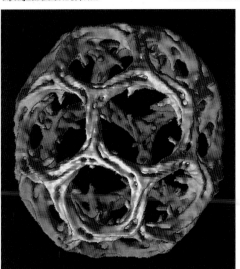

vesicles. It has heavy and light chains that assemble into structures known as triskelions (from triskele, a name for a three-legged figure) (see Fig. 15.37). In this figure, the red and pink light chains represent different isoforms that appear to associate randomly with the heavy chain (black). In vitro, the triskelions can be made to associate reversibly into structures known as baskets, shown as a three-dimensional model in Fig. 15.37. Figure 15.38 shows (A) an electron micrograph of individual triskelions, (B) unstained coated vesicles from human placenta, in which hexagonal barrels (H),

Fig. 15.38 Various levels (A, B, C) of clathrin assembly visualized by electron microscopy.

so-called tennis ball structures (T) and larger coats containing vesicles (V) can be seen, and (C) structure of a clathrin coat determined by electron cryomicroscopy, emphasizing the packing of individual clathrin triskelions.

THE CYTOSKELETON

THE RED CELL CYTOSKELETON

Within the cytoplasm there is a system of structural proteins that are implicated in the mechanical properties of the cell. These form an internal system of fibres known as the cytoskeleton. In the red cell, the prominent components of this system are spectrin and actin. As shown in Fig. 15.39, the α and β chains of spectrin interact through assemblies of actin and tropomyosin with ankyrin to link spectrin to the red cell membrane. The band 4.1 protein, so named because of its position on gels of red cell proteins, might also be involved in linkage to the plasma membrane.

ACTIN MICROFILAMENTS

Actin microfilaments are polymers of actin that perform a structural role in the cell. After treatment of the cell to remove most other proteins, actin filaments can be visualized by a technique known as freeze-etch microscopy, as shown in the electron micrograph of a fibroblast in Fig. 15.40. The majority of actin filaments are aggregated into stress fibre bundles, indicated by the arrowheads. Another component of the cytoskeleton, known as intermediate filaments (see below) are also seen (indicated by asterisk). Flaps of plasma membrane lying above (indicated by a) and below (b) the cytoskeleton can be seen. At position c, all of the lower membrane has been removed by the detergent used in making the preparation, revealing the underlying glass coverslip.

The way in which actin filaments are organized in a microvillus is shown in the sketch in Fig. 15.41. The filaments are arranged in bundles, held together by other structural proteins. The two ends of the filaments have polarity, and are denoted plus and minus ends.

MICROTUBULES

Throughout the cytoplasm, there also runs a network of microtubules (see Chapter 1). These are formed from the protein tubulin and, if a fluorescent antibody against

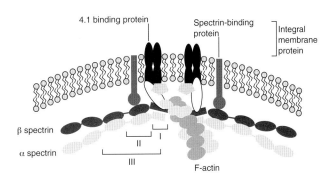

Spectrin sites for:
I: F-actin and protein 4.1 binding
II: integral membrane protein binding
III: interchain binding

Fig. 15.39 The components of the red cell cytoskeleton.

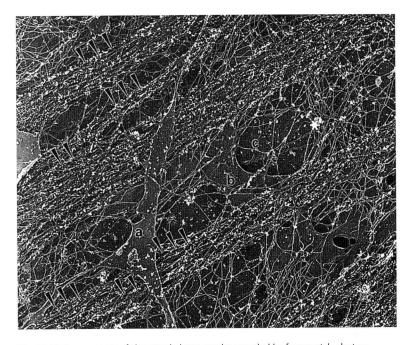

Fig. 15.40 Components of the cytoskeleton can be revealed by freeze-etch electron microscopy.

tubulin is used to stain a cell, this network can be visualized, as shown in Fig. 15.42. As can be seen, the microtubules tend to radiate out from the nucleus, around which the most dense fluorescence can be seen.

Tubulin consists of heterodimers of α and β subunits, that form cylindrical polymers as shown in Fig. 15.43 (α tubulin in pink, β tubulin in white). Polymerization of tubulin can be achieved in vitro. This requires the presence of GTP, which binds to the subunits, which have GTPase activity. As the tubulin filament grows, therefore, it consists of subunits with GDP bound, and a growing cap of subunits with GTP bound. The presence of GTP stabilizes the polymer, and the activity of the GTPase may regulate the rate of growth.

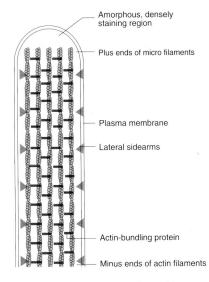

Amorphous, densely staining region

Plus ends of micro filaments

Plasma membrane

Lateral sidearms

Actin-bundling protein

Minus ends of actin filaments

Fig. 15.41 The arrangement of actin filaments in a microvillus.

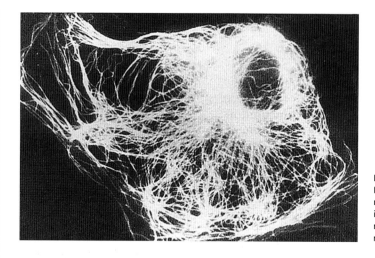

Fig. 15.42 Microtubules revealed by immunofluorescence microscopy.

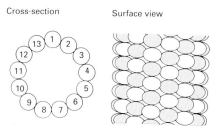

Fig. 15.43 Microtubules are polymers of tubulin.

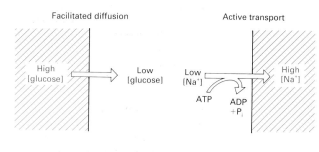

Fig. 15.44 Facilitated diffusion is concentration-dependent; active transport is energy-dependent.

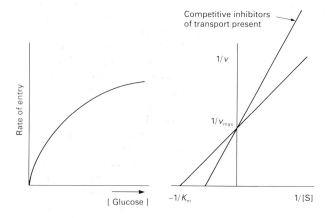

Fig. 15.45 The kinetics of transport are similar to enzyme kinetics.

Microtubules play a major role during cell division. Among other functions, they form the spindle fibres that separate the chromosomes during the M phase of cell division.

INTERMEDIATE FILAMENTS

Another component of the cytoskeleton consists of structures known as intermediate filaments. These are formed by polymerization of proteins such as keratins. Keratin can be of several types. The hard keratins form structures such as nails, hooves and feathers. Others, known as cytokeratins, are found within many cell types and exist in several isoforms. Other types of protein also form structures of the intermediate filament type. In the nucleus, lamins A, B and C are intermediate filament proteins that form the nuclear lamina and are important in maintaining the nuclear membrane (see p. 2).

MEMBRANE TRANSPORT

FACILITATED DIFFUSION AND ACTIVE TRANSPORT

One of the functions of the plasma membrane and other cell membranes is to regulate the passage of a variety of small molecules that need to be taken up by or extruded from the cell, or cell compartment. One type of transport is known as facilitated diffusion (see Fig. 15.44). This is energy independent and can only function down a concentration gradient. Another type of transfer, known as active transport (also shown in Fig. 15.44), has to be driven, often by including a reaction in which ATP is hydrolysed to ADP and P. This can occur against a concentration gradient.

A feature of transport systems, including facilitated diffusion, is that they exhibit saturation kinetics, as shown in Fig. 15.45. This indicates that a transport site exists that can only be occupied by a limited number of molecules. Inhibition can occur, and a K_m can be calculated by techniques similar to those used in enzyme kinetics.

ION TRANSPORT

In the nerve axon, the action potential is regulated by the influx of Na^+ through a gated channel. K^+ then leaves by other channels to return the membrane potential to normal (see Fig. 15.46). Ionic concentrations are eventually restored by a membrane transport system known as the sodium pump (see Fig. 15.47). This involves the action of an ATPase, isolated preparations of which hydrolyse ATP when stimulated by both Na^+ and K^+. As with all enzymes utilizing ATP, Mg^{2+} is also required. Transport can also be driven by an ion gradient, as shown in Fig. 15.48. In the system shown, glucose and Na^+ move in the same direction (hence the need to give glucose as well as NaCl in infant diarrhea). The term 'symport' is used to describe such a system, and the protein is known as a symporter. When molecules move in opposite directions, the term 'antiport' is used, the protein being known as an antiporter.

CELL ADHESION

THE EXTRACELLULAR MATRIX

The extracellular matrix is a complex macromolecular matrix of fibrous proteins, collagens, elastin, fibrillin, glycoproteins

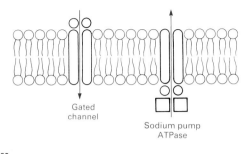

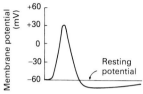

Gated channel

Sodium pump ATPase

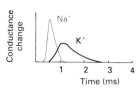

Resting potential

Fig. 15.46 The action potential results from a gated channel and the membrane potential is restored by the sodium pump.

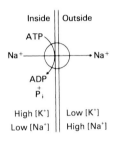

Fig. 15.47 The action of the sodium pump.

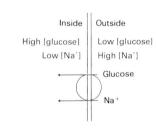

Fig. 15.48 Glucose transport is Na⁺-dependent and represents a symport system.

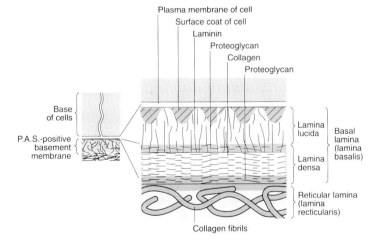

Fig. 15.49 The outer surfaces of cells are coated with a layer of glycoproteins and the basement membrane contains collagen and other proteins. PAS, periodic acid Schiff reaction.

and proteoglycans (see Fig. 15.49). It is secreted by connective tissue cells and also forms an extracellular layer surrounding most cells of the body. The extracellular matrix contains elastic fibres comprising a core of elastin surrounded by a mantle of fibrillin-rich microfibrils, elastin and fibrillin being large glycoproteins. The elastic fibres endow connective tissues such as blood vessels, lungs and skin with the critical properties of elasticity and resilience.

CLINICAL IMPLICATIONS – DISORDERS OF THE EXTRACELLULAR MATRIX

Disorders associated with this complex are multisystem and include Ehlers–Danlos and Marfan syndromes, pseudoxanthana elasticum, cutis laxis, osteogenesis imperfecta, osteopetrosis (as well as the more common disorder of osteoporosis), ageing and osteoarthritis. Clinical features include joint hypermobility, bony deformities, skin lesions including blistering, bruising and scarring, cardiovascular and gastrointestinal problems including aneurysms, gut perforations and hernias, impaired and unstable joints and occular and dental abnormalities.

There are at least ten subtypes of Ehlers–Danlos syndrome, in some of which genetic mutations in collagen structure and synthesis have been identified. Marfan syndrome is due to a genetic defect in fibrillin, a glycoprotein constituent of microfibrils, with bony deformaties, cardiovascular abnormalities including defective cardiac valves and aortic aneurysms.

There are at least four subtypes of osteogenesis imperfecta (brittle bone disease) due to genetic mutations in the type 1 collagen triple helix. Patients have fragile bones, which fracture readily, weak tendons, thin skin and abnormal teeth. Epidermolysis bullosa is a group of rare skin diseases with underlying molecular defects in keratin, laminin or type IV collagen structure.

Lathrysm is a multisystem disease due to impaired activity of lysyl oxidase, an enzyme involved in formation of the cross-links in collagen. This results in reduced collagen and elastin cross-linking accompanied by aneurysms, bone demineralization and deformation and unstable joints with hemorrhages. It may be due to a genetic defect in enzyme structure or acquired inhibition due to ingestion of β-aminoproprionitrile, an irreversible inhibitor of lysyl oxidase found in the seeds of the sweet pea. Therapeutic use of penicillamine, a selective chelator of Cu^{2+}, can similarly lead to impaired oxidase activity.

Osteoporosis is a metabolic bone disease with a major hormonal (estrogen) component particularly affecting post-menopausal women. Predisposing factors include Indo-Asian ethnicity, poor nutritional status (calcium, phosphate, vitamin D, protein), alcohol and tobacco misuse and immobility.

CELL ADHESION MOLECULES

The external surfaces of cells carry protein molecules that have the function of binding the cell to other cells or to substrates in the extracellular matrix (see Fig. 15.49). These protein molecules are

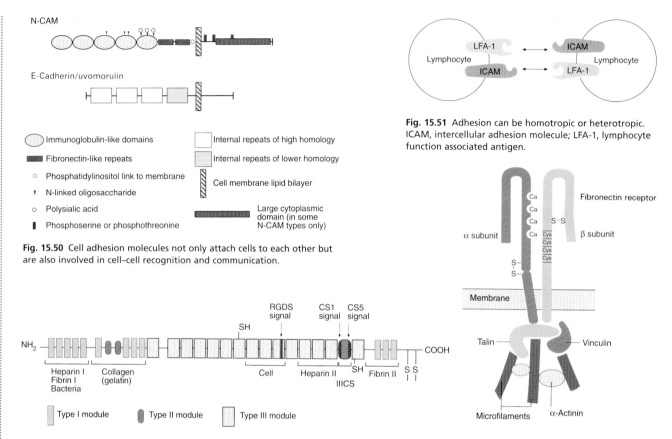

Fig. 15.50 Cell adhesion molecules not only attach cells to each other but are also involved in cell–cell recognition and communication.

N-CAM

E-Cadherin/uvomorulin

Immunoglobulin-like domains

Fibronectin-like repeats

Phosphatidylinositol link to membrane

N-linked oligosaccharide

Polysialic acid

Phosphoserine or phosphothreonine

Internal repeats of high homology

Internal repeats of lower homology

Cell membrane lipid bilayer

Large cytoplasmic domain (in some N-CAM types only)

Fig. 15.51 Adhesion can be homotropic or heterotropic. ICAM, intercellular adhesion molecule; LFA-1, lymphocyte function associated antigen.

Lymphocyte LFA-1 ICAM Lymphocyte
ICAM LFA-1

Fig. 15.52 The fibronectin receptor is an important integrin.

Fibronectin receptor
α subunit   β subunit
Ca   S–S
Cys
Membrane
Talin   Vinculin
Microfilaments   α-Actinin

Fig. 15.53 The function of many fibronectin domains is known.

RGDS signal   CS1 signal   CS5 signal
SH
NH₂   COOH
Heparin I / Fibrin I / Bacteria   Collagen (gelatin)   Cell   Heparin II   IIICS   SH   Fibrin II

Type I module   Type II module   Type III module

known by the general term adhesion molecules, and are of a variety of types. Two of the more important classes are typified, as shown in Fig. 15.50, by NCAM (neural cell adhesion molecule) and E-cadherin (epithelial Ca^{2+}-dependent adhesion molecule). Such molecules can bind like-to-like (e.g. NCAM to NCAM) when present on different cells. This is known as homophilic binding. Alternatively, heterophilic binding can occur, as shown in Fig. 15.51 for LFA-1 (lymphocyte function associated antigen-1) and ICAM (intercellular adhesion molecule) on lymphocytes.

INTEGRINS

LFA-1 is an integrin. The integrins are a widespread and numerous class of cell receptors that function in cell adhesion. They are typically heterodimers of α and β subunits, which are members of families of homologous proteins from which families of integrins can be formed, α subunits being numbered 1–8, or designated by letters referring to specific adhesion molecules (e.g. L for LFA-1, or v for vitronectin). Fibronectin, a large

(2500 residues) fibril-forming glycoprotein found in the extracellular matrix, binds to a number of types of integrin, such as $\alpha_4\beta_1$, $\alpha_v\beta_1$, $\alpha_v\beta_3$. A typical structure of an integrin is shown in Fig. 15.52. When an integrin interacts with a molecule that it recognizes, such as fibronectin, an intracellular system for informing the cell of these contacts is activated. Thus, the intracellular domains of fibronectin receptors make contact with proteins such as talin and vinculin, proteins associated with the cell cytoskeleton through actin filaments, and

these thus form a kind of signalling system in addition to their other functions.

FIBRONECTIN

The various binding domains of fibronectin are shown in Fig. 15.53. These are composed of three types of homologous repeating unit, known as modules and named types I, II and III. Thus, five type I modules near the N-terminus form a heparin-binding domain, and other binding domains are

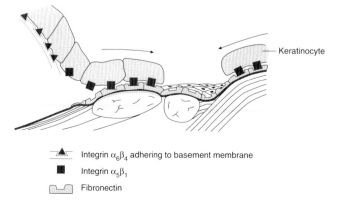

Integrin $\alpha_6\beta_4$ adhering to basement membrane

Integrin $\alpha_5\beta_1$

Fibronectin

Keratinocyte

Fig. 15.54 Involvement of integrins in wound healing.

indicated in the figure. Many integrins recognize the sequence motif –RGDX– (where X is S, V, A, T, C or F). The so-called CS1 and CS5 signals in the IIICS region are cell adhesion signals with different specificities, CS1 towards lymphoid and certain tumour cells, CS5 towards melanoma cells.

CLINICAL IMPLICATIONS – WOUND HEALING

The way in which integrins can function is illustrated by their involvement in wound healing. Thus, integrin $\alpha_6\beta_4$ is a component of the hemidesmosome, a specialized cell junction between epithelial cells such as keratinocytes and the underlying basal lamina. On wounding, integrin $\alpha_5\beta_1$, which is a fibronectin receptor, is expressed. Cells engaged in wound repair express fibronectin, and the keratinocytes migrate over this to cover the wound (Fig. 15.54).

The post-genomic era and its impact on the future of biochemistry and molecular biology

Having introduced the rationale for the subjects considered in this chapter, bioinformatics is discussed. Not only cell growth, but also in many cases cell death is a controlled process. Controlled cell death is termed apoptosis, in contrast to death that results from toxins or other damage, which is termed necrosis. Caspases play an important role in apoptosis. Certain genes known as tumour suppressor genes, of which p53 is one product, are implicated in the prevention of uncontrolled growth. It is thought that telomerases play a role in the ageing process. Growth factors and their receptors activate a cascade of protein kinases that are implicated in growth stimulation. The role of these systems in tumorigenesis is discussed.

INTRODUCTION

The aim of the biochemist is to understand all aspects of the function and reproduction of living cells in terms of the laws of physics and chemistry. The knowledge gained is valuable in furthering the understanding, prevention and treatment of tissue pathology. Since we learned that the information that governs the biosynthesis and function of all the components of living cells resides in the nucleic acids, in particular DNA, it has been a major objective to determine the structure of the genome of many organisms, including man. This has now been accomplished for the human (but see p. 223) and for a wide variety of organisms – mice, fruit fly, nematodes, plants, yeast. Two objectives can now be delineated, to continue the work on structure and, even more importantly, to determine the detailed functions of all components of the genome that go to determine the phenotype. A new discipline has arisen – genomics – which is subdivided into structural genomics and functional genomics.

Given the above background, it is clear that biochemists have been challenged to invigorate their subject, now backed by a knowledge of the structure of many genomes; hence the phrase the 'post-genomic era'. We hope that throughout this new edition we have shown the impact of our new knowledge, which has permeated all aspects of biochemistry, and have stressed how, in medicine, the knowledge that genetic polymorphism plays a major role in determining susceptibility to disease has resulted in a hunt to find linkage between gene loci and disease. In this chapter we are concerned with some examples of our thinking with respect to the control of cancer, growth and longevity.

BIOINFORMATICS

With the explosion in the knowledge of the structure of nucleic acids and proteins it has been natural to attempt to apply computational methods to interpret the data. There has arisen a new discipline 'bioinformatics'. Although this is now a commonly used scientific term it is difficult to define. A succinct definition may be as follows: 'The collection, archiving, organization and interpretation of biological data'. Areas that come within this definition are the identification of genes within the structural genomes, comparison of the primary structures of proteins with a view to discovering their function, models of molecular evolution, the prediction of protein tertiary structure from primary structure and approaches to protein–protein interactions.

GENOMICS AND PROTEOMICS

Bioinformatics has given rise to many new words of varying usefulness. We have already mentioned genomics, which can be defined as the comparative analysis of the complete genomic sequences from different organisms, used to assess evolutionary relations among species and to predict the number and general types of proteins produced by an organism. Such predictions are tested by proteomics, whereby the proteins that compose the proteome, defined as the complement of proteins expressed by a cell or organ at a particular time and under specific conditions, are characterized (see p. 78). The total number of proteins in the proteome can exceed the number of genes in the genome due to differential splicing and post-translational modifications such as phosphorylation.

BIOINFORMATICS AND DRUG DEVELOPMENT

The pharmaceutical industry is enthusiastic about the use of bioinformatics and computer graphics to assist in the design of putative drugs that will interact with the active site of an enzyme they wish to inhibit. Recent successes concern the inhibition of the protease essential for the propagation of HIV-1 (p. 29) and the neuraminidase of influenza virus. This technique is also very useful in the modification of lead compounds, i.e. compounds thought to have the potential to lead to the discovery of useful drugs, because they are known to inhibit enzymes, but that might not themselves be suitable as pharmaceutical agents. Such lead compounds might be synthetic chemicals that have proved to be toxic, or natural substances, many of which have come from plants. This hopefully is the age of 'rational drug discovery', which, especially in the case of cancer, will replace the use of rather brutal chemotherapeutic agents. One recent success has been the use of Glivec (imatinib mesylate, or Gleevec in US), which is effective in the treatment of chronic myeloid leukemia and also gastrointestinal tumours. The drug inhibits a number of tyrosine kinases, including the PDGF receptor kinase. Glivec has set a precedent for the approach of molecularly targeted therapy and has demonstrated that it is pivotal to identify the right target for the right group of patients. Mouse monoclonal antibodies have also been rendered suitable for use as drugs. Examples are Herceptin, which recognizes a protein found in breast cancer cells and Humira for the treatment of rheumatoid arthritis.

BIOINFORMATICS AND MEDICINE

Orthologs and paralogs

The structure of the human genome of some 3 billion nucleotides has revealed only about 30 000 genes, of which only about a third have been characterized and assigned a function. Bioinformatics will surely be important in furthering this work, especially in the pairing of genes in different species with respect to their common structure and function (such genes are known as orthologs, in contrast to paralogs, where genes with a similar structure have a function that differs between species). Such a process was used successfully in identifying the function of the protein expressed by the gene responsible for cystic fibrosis.

Polymorphism and disease

Throughout this book, attention has been drawn to the influence of gene regulation on metabolic processes. In addition, many examples have been given of the effect that gene variation, resulting in polymorphism in protein structure, has on human health. Very often, replacement of a single amino acid is involved. In the great majority of these cases in the past, the emphasis has been on adverse effects, leading to the use of the term 'inherited disease', but it is apparent that beneficial effects can also occur, as in the case of apo-Al (Milano), discussed on p. 172. It seems likely that the importance of individual characteristics, which can now more easily be examined at the level of the genome, will become a major factor in the study of human health. Whereas some diseases are clearly familial, in others genetic influences are more subtle. In polygenic disease (p. 51), association between polymorphism and disease is more difficult to define but serious efforts are now being made to make progress in this, as for example, in type 2 diabetes and asthma.

Pharmacogenetics

The application of genomics to pharmaceutics has been termed pharmacogenetics. With a knowledge of the structure of the patient's DNA it might be possible to select the most effective drug for the treatment of the disease in that particular patient; patients could also be advised concerning their life style. This is most appropriate in the case of polygenic diseases (see p. 173). For example, if the patient's DNA indicates a susceptibility to type 2 diabetes later in life, the patient could be advised to avoid becoming obese. If the DNA structure suggests an enhanced likelihood of breast cancer an appropriate drug such as tamoxifen, taken prophylactically, might be advised. In the case of a monogenic disease such as Huntington's disease (see p. 52), where the gene gives rise to a protein, huntingtin, of unknown function, an ethical problem arises because at present there is no cure, although family planning advice might be relevant.

Investigation of polymorphism

Gene function in the hereditary diseases can sometimes be found by reverse genetics (see p. 51) but in other cases it is more difficult to find genetic molecular markers. Because most of the human genome does not code for protein, a large amount of sequence variance exists between individuals. If these variations in DNA sequence, referred to as DNA polymorphisms, can be followed from one generation to another they can serve as genetic markers for linkage studies. Restriction length polymorphisms (RFLPs) were the first type of molecular marker to be used. RFLPs arise because mutations create or destroy the sites recognized by specific restriction enzymes (see pp. 25 and 49), leading to variations between individuals in the length of restriction fragments produced from identical regions of the genome. Other DNA polymorphisms have proved useful, particularly single nucleotide polymorphisms (SNPs, pronounced 'snips'). These constitute the most abundant type; a frequency of about 1 per kilo basepairs, which means some 3 million in the human genome. They are therefore useful for constructing high-resolution genetic maps to characterize human populations, migration patterns and evolution. They will be used to identify genes predisposing to common diseases that contribute to significant human morbidity and mortality, e.g. substance misuse, hypertension.

APOPTOSIS

There are two primary pathways by which cells die; necrosis and apoptosis. Necrosis can be described as accidental cell death that occurs when cells receive a structural or chemical insult, e.g. a toxin or anoxia, from which they cannot recover. In necrosis the cells swell and burst, which results in a damaging inflammatory response. In the adult human, millions of cells die in this way every minute; we only maintain a constant size because cell division exactly balances cell death.

In contrast to necrosis, apoptosis involves cell shrinkage, the main features being shown in Fig. 16.1. The dying cells lose their surface contact with their neighbours and shrink, but retain their organelles. Chromatin condensation occurs with eventual fragmentation of the nucleus and cytoplasm into multiple, small apoptotic bodies. These bodies can be lost from the epithelial surface and undergo extracellular degeneration or be phagocytosed by neighbours or macrophages and undergo phagosomal digestion. The term 'apoptosis' can be used broadly to encompass all forms of such normal or pathological cell death, encompassing regulated activity that is central to embryogenesis and homeostasis. Apoptosis begins with a signal that can come either from within the cell, e.g detection of radiation-induced DNA breaks, or from without, e.g. decrease in the level of an essential growth factor or hormone. The signal induces the cell to make a decision to commit suicide. The programmed cell death has a latent and execution phase.

THE ACTION OF CASPASES

The apoptotic bodies are produced as a result of the action of a group of proteolytic enzymes named caspases, all of which have cysteine at their active site and cleave their target proteins at specific aspartyl residues (name derived from *cysteine aspartase*). The caspases are made as inactive precursor zymogens (see p. 154 and Fig. 16.2), procaspases, and are activated by cleavage at an aspartyl residue to liberate one large and one small subunit, which associate into $\alpha_2\beta_2$ tetramers to form the active enzyme. In humans, there are 10 different caspases. In apoptosis, caspases are activated in an amplifying proteolytic cascade (p. 191), cleaving one another in sequence. Procaspases are made continuously by healthy cells, so the suicide machinery is always in place; all that is needed is the trigger to activate it. Procaspases can become activated in many ways, one of which involves the

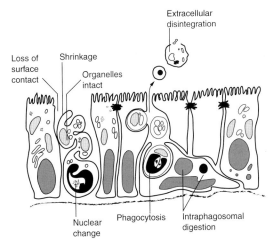

Fig. **16.1** Scheme of events in apoptosis within an epithelium.

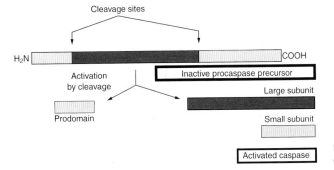

Fig. **16.2** Activation of a caspase.

mitochondria. Following a toxic insult, a member of the Bcl-2 family of proteins (see below) binds to mitochondria and opens a channel, which causes the release of cytochrome *c* (see p. 139) and other proteins. These proteins actively induce apoptosis. In the cytoplasm the cytochrome *c* binds to the scaffolding protein Apaf-1 and the complex causes the autoactivation of a procaspase.

APOPTOSIS AND DISEASE

Research on apoptosis has taken a central position in all cell biology research. In part, this is because aberrations in apoptosis play a role in the etiology of many diseases, such as autoimmunity, AIDS and cancer. It is also emerging as a key factor in neurodegenerative diseases, such as Alzheimer disease, and also in myocardial infarction and stroke. Many chemotherapeutic agents act by inducing cancer cells to undergo apoptosis.

APOPTOSIS AND CANCER

The action of p53

Normal cells can be transformed to cancer cells by oncogenes (see below), although this process can be prevented by the products of other genes known as tumour suppressor genes. One of these genes is p53, which produces a 393-amino-acid residue nuclear phosphoprotein that binds to DNA and activates transcription from some promoters. In over half of human cancers, p53 is deleted or inactivated by mutation. The majority of cases of the familial Li-Fraumeni syndrome is caused by germline mutations in p53. Another piece of crucial evidence is the high rate of tumour development in p53 knockout mice (transgenic mice lacking the p53 gene).

The p53 protein contains four main functional modules, as shown in Fig. 16.3. Amino acids 1–42 comprise an acidic transcriptional activation domain that mediates protein–protein interactions. The central region (residues 102–292) is the sequence-specific DNA-binding domain, which is most frequently mutated in cancer cells. p53 can bind DNA as a tetramer and oligomerization is mediated by a domain that is found at residues 324–355. The C-terminus (367–393) non-specifically binds nucleic acids. p53 is involved in the regulation of cell cycle progression (see p. 22) in response to DNA damage. When cells sense DNA damage induced by agents such as ionizing radiation, levels of p53 rise dramatically, which causes the cell to delay

entry into S phase until the damage has been repaired.

p53 and apoptosis

In addition to the above activity of p53, it also influences apoptosis. The crucial player is the Mdm2 protein, a 491-amino-acid residue nuclear phosphoprotein (in humans) that contains a p53 binding domain at its N-terminus. A small region of the N-terminus of p53 forms a tight protein–protein interaction with an N-terminal, hydrophobic pocket domain in Mdm2 (see Fig. 16.4(A)). When p53 is bound by Mdm2, it is targeted for destruction by the ubiquitin-dependent proteasome pathway (p. 48). The transcription of *mdm2* is dependent on p53. Consequently, p53 drives the transcription of the gene product that will target its own destruction and in tumour cells that lack Mdm2, p53 will be stable (Fig. 16.4(B)). In tumour cells with a mutant p53, the transcription factor, normal p53, is absent. When p53 function is lost, apoptosis cannot be induced and the accumulation of mutations required for cancer to develop becomes more likely.

The rise in the concentration of p53 results in a burst of the transcription of p53-regulated genes, which are involved in cell killing by apoptosis. One of these is Bcl-2, which is a member of a large family of related proteins, some of which are anti-apoptotic. The family is characterized by the presence of one to four blocks of conserved protein sequence called BH

domains. A Bcl-2 protein can form a complex with a pro-apoptotic family member called Bax, the effect of which on mitochondria has been described. The gene encoding Bax is disrupted in one class of human colon cancers.

TELOMERES AND TELOMERASES

Telomeres and telomerase have been given much attention because, as will be explained, they might be relevant both to cancer and to the problem of the longevity of an organism. The lagging strand of DNA is synthesized by means of a primase that produces an RNA primer for the DNA polymerase (p. 24). The primer is then normally removed, but there is no way to synthesize the lagging-strand sequence that is complementary to the small region at the end of the chromosome (which is at least as large as an RNA primer). So with continuing cell division, sequence is lost from the ends of linear chromosomes. Various problems are solved by packaging the chromosome ends into special structures called 'telomeres'. The cells must distinguish the ends of a chromosome from breaks in DNA. When a cell detects a DNA break, it stops its progression through the cell cycle and repairs the break by joining the ends together. Telomeres keep normal chromosome ends from inducing cell cycle arrest and from being joined to other DNA ends by repair machinery. Telomeres permit the chromosomal DNA to be replicated out to the very end. Telomeres

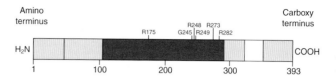

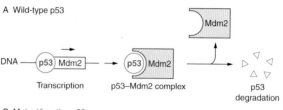

Fig. 16.3 The main functional domains of p53 protein.

Fig. 16.4 Action of p53 in tumour cells.

are composed of many repeats of short DNA sequences e.g. TTAGGG3′. These repeats are synthesized by an enzyme called telomerase (Fig. 16.5). Telomerase is a ribonucleoprotein in which the RNA and protein components are both essential for the synthesis of telomeric DNA. Telomerase generates tandem repeats of the short sequence encoded by telomerase RNA. For example, vertebrate chromosomes end in multiple copies of the sequence C_3TA_2/T_2AG_3. After telomerase elongation of the 3′ strand, a conventional DNA polymerase probably synthesizes the complementary strand. Most human and some mouse somatic cells do not express telomerase at detectable levels and, as a consequence, cell division results in telomere shortening. In contrast, most human tumours express telomerase. This led to the hypothesis that the replicative potential of mammalian cells might be determined by their amount of telomeric DNA. On this model, the ability to express telomerase and hence maintain telomeric DNA would be a crucial step in tumourigenesis. This hypothesis has been supported by experiments in which the ectopic expression of the catalytic subunit of the telomerase holoenzyme enabled human cells to multiply indefinitely. It is now clear, however, that telomere shortening is not the only stimulus to provoke senescence; control of the cell cycle certainly plays a part. Consequently, telomerase is under intense study in cancer research and offers a possible site for chemotherapy.

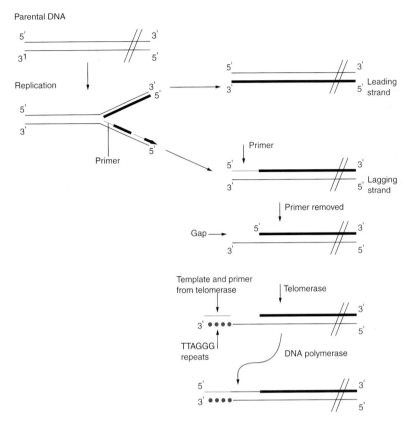

Fig. 16.5 The role of telomerase.

GROWTH CONTROL AND CANCER

BACKGROUND

Genomics has had a profound impact on our understanding of growth control. The realization that certain viruses cause cancer resulted in the discovery that the source of the oncogenicity lay in specific genes, which came to be called oncogenes. Further work revealed that the oncogenes were in fact mutated forms of normal genes that are involved in the control of cell growth. In many cases, the mutation enables the gene products to escape the normal controls that regulate their activity, so that they were, in effect, permanently switched on. As a result, they brought about the unrestricted growth associated with malignancy. A number of oncogene-related proteins have already been described, especially in Chapter 15.

ONCOGENES AND CYTOKINES

The work on oncogenes led to a much greater understanding of the mechanisms by which cells normally regulate growth, and allowed elucidation of the pathways by which the growth control mechanisms function. The main components of these pathways are:

- compounds known as cytokines, secreted by a variety of cells to act on other cells by interaction at the cell membrane;
- cytokine receptors in the cell membrane, many of which have a cytosolic domain with tyrosine kinase activity (see p 208);
- downstream mediators of signal transduction, such as soluble tyrosine kinases, protein kinase C and the phosphoinositide system;
- transcription factors that are acted upon by the downstream components.

Some oncogenes, and their activities, are listed in Table 16.1. The homologues of the viral (v-) oncogenes found in normal cells are called cellular (c-) oncogenes, or protooncogenes. It transpires that many protooncogenes are cytokines.

The number of cytokines now known to exist is very extensive. Some examples are epidermal growth factor (EGF),

platelet-derived growth factor (PDGF), fibroblast growth factor (FGF), transforming growth factors (TGF-α, TGF-β), vascular endothelial growth factor (VEGF). The names often reveal the system in which the cytokine was first defined, but they are secreted by a variety of cells under appropriate conditions. For example, PDGF was discovered during investigation of the growth-promoting activity of platelets but has subsequently been found to be secreted by other cell types.

SIGNALLING AND GROWTH CONTROL

In the normal situation, cell growth is under strict control and the unrestricted growth characteristic of tumour cells does not occur. Normal cells are subject to contact inhibition and when they come into contact with other cells their growth is inhibited. It is a characteristic of cancer cells that they are not subject to this restriction. Although the mechanism of contact inhibition is not understood, there are indications that it involves signalling pathways similar to those described above, in which tyrosine kinase regulation and associated events are involved.

Table 16.1 Oncogenes and their activity

Virus of origin	Oncogene	Protooncogene	Mutation in oncogene
Simian sarcoma virus	v-sis	Platelet-derived growth factor	Minor amino acid replacements
Avian erythroblastosis	v-erbB	Epidermal growth factor	Lacking domains normally involved in regulation
Rous sarcoma virus	v-src	Src (existing protein was not known before oncogene discovery)	Change in residues at the C-terminus; as a result phosphorylation of tyrosine important in regulation does not occur
Rat sarcoma	v-ras	Ras (existing protein was not known before oncogene discovery)	Point mutation results in failure of Ras to hydrolyse its bound GTP, so it remains permanently active

The control of cell growth has mostly been studied using cells in culture. The system can be illustrated in outline using PDGF as a typical example. PDGF binds to its cell surface receptor, which activates its tyrosine kinase (p. 209) to self-phosphorylate tyrosines in its cytosolic domain (Fig. 16.6). A number of proteins then bind to the receptor at these phosphorylated sites. They include phosphatidylinositol 3′-kinase (PI3K), phospholipase C-γ (PLC-γ) and Ras, together with an adaptor protein Grb2 (growth factor receptor-bound protein 2). Grb2 was identified as a protein that binds to activated EGF and PDGF receptors. It

forms a complex with two other proteins, Shc (for SH-containing protein, found by screening DNA libraries for genes encoding SH2 domains; see p. 209) and Sos. Grb2 and Shc are non-enzymic adaptor molecules containing the SH and other binding sites required to link other molecules together. Sos was originally found in so-called *son of sevenless* fruitfly (*Drosophila*) mutants (see below). Sos is activated by Grb2-Shc and, in turn, stimulates GDP release from and GTP binding to Ras, resulting in activation. Ras then activates a serine/threonine kinase, Raf, which phosphorylates downstream kinases MEK and MAPK, and these then

activate transcription factors (TF) which regulate gene expression. PLC-γ products activate protein kinase C, whereas PI3K products activate protein kinase B (PKB/AKT) and thereby c-Jun, which forms a transcription factor complex known as AP1.

SIGNALLING AND COLORECTAL CANCER

Many examples of the impact of genomics on cancer research can be found. One such concern is colorectal cancer. Although several oncogenes and oncosuppressor genes are known to be involved in colorectal carcinogenesis (see p53/Bax above), mutation of the adenomatous polyposis coli gene (*APC*) is regarded as being particularly crucial as an instigator of this process. In these tumours, a protein, now named APC protein, was found in a mutated form arising from a frameshift mutation. Normal APC protein participates in a signalling system with β-catenin. β-Catenin is found in the cell membrane-bound adherens complex with E-cadherin and α-catenin, but also in the cytosol, where binding with glycogen synthase kinase-3β (GSK-3β), APC and axin promotes ubiquitination and, hence, degradation (GSK-3β, although first identified as a kinase for glycogen, has many other roles in cell metabolism). In the nucleus, β-catenin promotes transcription of

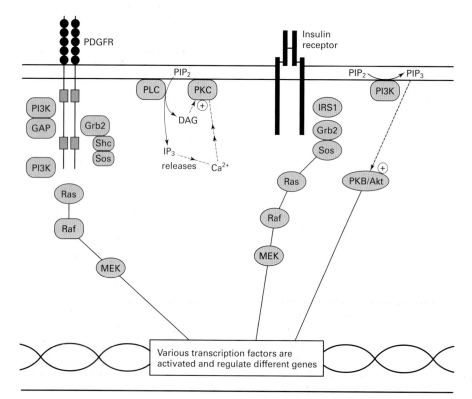

Fig. 16.6 Protein kinase signalling in growth stimulation.

a number of potentially tumorigenic genes by activating the transcription factor, T-cell factor (TCF). In cells with mutated APC, β-catenin does not undergo ubiquitination, and thus its effect on transcription is not regulated (see Fig 16.7).

INSULIN AND GROWTH CONTROL

The above schemes, although complex enough, nevertheless offer only limited insight into a highly sophisticated system for control of cell behaviours that, in addition to growth control, include differentiation, chemotaxis and epithelial plasticity such as could be involved in metastasis. More than one cytokine could be acting on a cell at any one time, each activating related but different systems that can interact with each other. For example, the insulin receptor, in addition to its role in regulating energy metabolism, can activate a mitogenic process and has important functions in growth control in many cell types. Its cytosolic tyrosine kinase domain, after binding insulin, undergoes self-phosphorylation, and binds IRS1 (p 203)/Grb2/Sos and this, in combination with other adaptor molecules, activates the Ras-Raf-MEK system in mediating the mitogenic actions of the hormone (see Fig. 16.6). When more than one agent acts on a cell, their effects can be synergistic or, in some cases, antagonistic. Moreover, although there are similarities in the downstream pathways used by different agents, there are also significant differences. Thus insulin activates IRS-1, whereas PDGF does not. The limitations in present knowledge leave much to be explained. For example, insulin is thought to translocate GLUT4 (p. 177) to the membrane to mediate glucose uptake as a result of the activation of PI3K by IRS-1. However, PDGF also activates PI3K but does not enhance glucose uptake in insulin-sensitive cells. It is thus supposed that IRS-1 has effects specific to glucose uptake.

The numbers of proteins involved in these pathways, many of them having been discovered as oncogenes, continues to increase. The essence of the system, however, lies in the principle that cascades of protein kinases and adaptor molecules are activated, leading to activation of transcription factors and other effector molecules that bring about the variety of effects observed.

FUTURE WORK ON THE STRUCTURE OF THE HUMAN GENOME

Reference has been made in this text that the structure of the human genome is

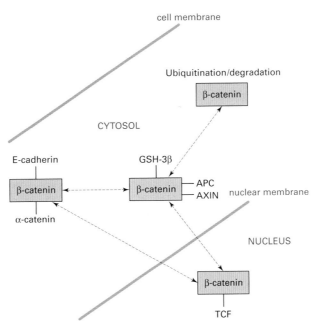

Fig. 16.7 The APC/β-catenin system

known. This statement needs to be qualified for two reasons. First, while a 'draft' sequence was published in 2001 this has been superseded by a second analysis in 2004 based on a laborious 'finishing' process in which each gap in the draft was re-examined. Even now some gaps remain in the sequence of 38 million base pairs but great progress has been made.

Second, the sequence is that of the euchromatin portion of the genome, which contains almost all of the genes that are both actively transcribed and quiescent. A typical cell nucleus has both euchromatin and heterochromatin which is transcriptionally inert and more condensed than the euchromatin. A future task is, therefore, to sequence the remaining 20% of the genome that lies within the heterochromatin. However, the repetitiveness of this chromatin means that it cannot be tackled using current methods even though the task remains important since these repetitive sequences are implicated in the processes of chromosome replication and maintenance.

GENOMICS AND EVOLUTION

Even before the determination of complete structures of genomes spanning organisms as diverse as yeast and man, it had become clear that there was a biomolecular thread linking the most sophisticated organisms with their primitive forebears, the earliest example

being the work on hemoglobin. These early results have been amply confirmed by work on genomes. The genomic DNA of a species can be cut into lengths of DNA of manageable size, which are then stored as what are known as gene libraries. These can be probed using cDNA of one species to search for similar sequences in another species.

Many recent developments derive from work on mutations in *Drosophila*. For example, the *sevenless* mutant, a gene product of which features in the pathways above, is so called because it involves a mutation in a gene that forms part of a system for differentiation of R7 photoreceptors in *Drosophila*. The product, Sev, is a receptor for an extracellular signal; it has tyrosine kinase activity and belongs to the insulin receptor family. Related mutations have been named as part of this family. For example, *boss* (*bride of sevenless*) codes for a protein expressed by R8 photoreceptor cells that is internalized by binding to Sev. *Son of sevenless* (*sos*) was found as a gene that encodes a guanine nucleotide-releasing protein required for the Sev receptor tyrosine kinase to activate Ras. This system was subsequently found to be present in many organisms, including man, and is just one example of the universality of many fundamental biomolecular systems. As more and more genome structures are determined, the elements of the evolutionary grand design will be progressively revealed.

Further reading

USEFUL GENERAL TEXTBOOKS

Alberts B et al. Essential cell biology, 2nd edn. Garland Science, 2004. ISBN 0-8153-3481-8.

Alberts B et al. Molecular biology of the cell, 4th edn. Garland Science, 2002. ISBN 0-8153-4072-9.

Becker WM, Kleinsmith LJ, Hardin,J. The world of the cell. 5th edn. Benjamin Cummings, 2003. ISBN 0-8053-4852-2.

Berg JM, Tymczko TL, Stryer L. Biochemistry, 5th edn. WH Freeman, 2002. ISBN 0-7167-2009-4.

Devlin TM. Textbook of biochemistry with clinical correlations, 5th edn. Wiley-Liss, 2002. ISBN 0-4711-5451-2.

Elliott WH, Elliott DC. Biochemistry and molecular biology, 2nd edn. Oxford University Press, 2001. ISBN 0-1987-0045-8.

Epstein RJ. Human molecular biology: An introduction to the molecular basis of health and disease. Cambridge University Press, 2003. ISBN 0–5216-4481-X.

Gaw A et al. Clinical biochemistry, 3rd edn. Churchill Livingstone, 2004. ISBN 0-4430-7269-8.

Nelson DL, Cox MM. Principles of biochemistry, 4th edn. WH Freeman, 2005. ISBN 0–7167-4339-6.

Lodish H et al. Molecular cell biology, 5th edn. WH Freeman, 2003. ISBN 0-7167-4366-3.

Mathews CK, van Holde KE, Ahern KG. Biochemistry, 3rd edn. Addison Wesley Longman, 2000. ISBN 0-8053-3066-6.

Pollard TD, Earnshaw WC. Cell biology. Saunders, 2002. ISBN 0-7216-3997-6.

Reed R et al. Practical skills in biomolecular sciences, 2nd edn. Pearson Prentice Hall, 2003. ISBN 0-130-45142-8.

Roitt I, Delves DJ. Roitt's immunology, 10th edn. Blackwell Science, 2001. ISBN 0-6320-5902-8.

Smith AD et al. Oxford dictionary of biochemistry and molecular biology. Oxford University Press, 2000. ISBN 0-1985-0673-2.

Turnpenny P, Ellard S. Emery's elements of medical genetics (with STUDENT CONSULT), 12th edn. Elsevier Churchill Livingstone, 2005. ISBN 0–4431–0045–4.

MONOGRAPHS ON SPECIFIC SUBJECTS

Branden C, Tooze J. Introduction to protein structure, 2nd edn. Garland Publishing, 1999. ISBN 0-8153-2305-0.

Franklin TJ, Snow GA. Biochemistry and molecular biology of antimicrobial drug action, 5th edn. Kluwer Academic Publishers, 1998. ISBN 0-4128-2200-8.

Frayn KN. Metabolic regulation – a human perspective, 2nd edn. Blackwell Science, 2003. ISBN 0-6320-6384-X.

Hardie DG. Biochemical messengers – hormones, neurotransmitters and growth factors. Chapman and Hall, 1991. ISBN 0-4123–0350-7.

Latchman DS. Eukaryotic transcription factors, 3rd edn. Academic Press, 1999. ISBN 0-1243-7177-9.

Lewin B. Genes VIII. Prentice Hall 2004. ISBN 0–1314–3981–2.

Murray A, Hunt T. The cell cycle – an introduction. WH Freeman, 1993. ISBN 0-7167-7046-6.

Orengo CA, Jones DT, Thornton JM. Bioinformatics, genes, proteins and computers. Bios, 2003. ISBN 1-8599-6054-5.

Primrose SB, Twyman RM. Principles of genome analysis and genomics, 3rd edn. Blackwell Publishing, 2003. ISBN 1-4051-0120-2.

Primrose SB, Twyman BM, Old RW. Principles of gene manipulation. 6th edn. Blackwell Science, 2003. ISBN 0-6320-5954-0.

Prusiner SB. Prions prions prions. Springer, 1996. ISBN 3-5405-9343-8.

Prusiner SB. Prion biology and diseases, 2nd Edition. Cold Spring Harbor Laboratory Press, 2004. ISBN 0–8796–9693–1.

KEY ARTICLES AND REVIEWS

CLINICAL IMPLICATIONS OF THE NEW GENETICS

Bentley DR. Genomes for medicine. Nature, 2004; 429:440–445. (This is one article in a Nature Insight supplement on human genomics and medicine.)

Fraser A. Human genes hit the big screen. Nature, 2004; 428:375–377. (At last, RNA interference makes large-scale screens possible in mammalian cells.)

Seymour AB et al. SNPs. A human genetic tool for the new millennium. In Annual Reports in Medicinal Chemistry 2003; 98:249–259, Elsevier, 2003. ISBN 0-12-040538-5.

225

Small DH et al. Alzheimer's disease therapeutics: New approaches to an ageing problem. IUBMB Life 2004; 56:203–208.

Weatherall DJ. Genomics and global health: Time for a reappraisal. Science 2003; 302:597–599. (The views of one of the UK's leading physicians.)

PROTEIN STRUCTURE, FOLDING AND DISEASE

Ciechanover A, Iwai K. The ubiquitin system: From basic mechanisms to the patient bed. IUBMB Life 2004; 56:193–201.

Dobson CM. Protein folding and misfolding. Nature 2003; 426:884–890. (Several articles in a Nature Insight collection.)

Ellisdon AM, Bottomley SP. The role of protein misfolding in the pathogenesis of human diseases. IUBMB Life 2004; 56:119–123. (A useful summary and source of references.)

Noble MEM, Endicott JA, Johnson LN. Protein kinase inhibitors: Insights into drug design from structure. Science 2004; 303:1800–1805. (A useful review of present and potential drugs.)

Ranson NA, White HE, Saibil HR. Chaperonins. Biochemical Journal 1998; 333:233–242. (A description of these amazing structures.)

Rockwell NC, Thorner JW. The kindest cuts of all: Crystal structures of Kex2 and furin reveal secrets of precursor processing. Trends in Biochemical Sciences 2004; 29:80–87. (See treatment of propeptides.)

Thornton JM et al. Protein folds, functions and evolution. Journal of Molecular Biology 1999; 293:333–342. (A review by the leaders in the field. See also their book (Orengo et al. 2003) above.)

PARKINSON'S DISEASE

Greenamyre JT, Hastings TG. Parkinson's – divergent causes, convergent mechanisms. Science 2004; 304:1120–1122.

MEMBRANE TRAFFICKING

Schekman R, Rothman JE. Dissecting the membrane trafficking system. Nature Medicine 2002; 10:1055–1062. (A review by the leaders in the field.)

RIBOZYMES

Steitz TA, Moore PB. RNA, the first macromolecular catalyst: The ribosome is a ribozyme. Trends in Biochemical Sciences 2003; 28:411–418. (The implications of the finding re the ribosome are relevant to ideas about evolution.)

REVIEWS DEALING WITH THE METABOLIC SYNDROME, DIABETES AND INSULIN RESISTANCE

Berger J, Moller DE. The mechanism of action of PPARS. Annual Review of Medicine 2002; 53:409–435. (Some information on a system now thought to be fundamental to problems of obesity and cardiovascular disease.)

Pessin JE, Saltiel AR. Signaling pathways in insulin action: Molecular targets of insulin resistance. Journal of Clinical Investigation 2000; 106:165–169. (Some more thoughts on mechanisms of insulin resistance.)

Tenenbaum A, Fisman EZ, Motro M. Metabolic syndrome and type 2 diabetes mellitus: Focus on peroxisome proliferator activated receptors (PPAR). Cardiovascular Diabetology 2003; 2:4. (A general survey of a modern plague.)

Virkamaki A, Ueki K, Kahn CR. Protein-protein interaction in insulin signaling and the molecular mechanisms of insulin resistance. Clinical Investigation 1999; 103:931–943.

Winer N, Sowers JR. Epidemiology of diabetes. Journal of Clinical Pharmacology 2004; 44:397–405.

CARDIOVASCULAR DISEASE

Stephens JW, Humphries SE. The molecular genetics of cardiovascular disease: Clinical implications. Journal of Internal Medicine 2003; 253:120–127.

REGULATION

Fell DA. Beyond genomics. Trends in Genetics 2001; 17:68–682.

Jope RS, Johnson GVW. The glamour and gloom of glycogen synthase kinase-3. Trends in Biochemical Sciences 2004; 29:95–102. (The enzyme is a key component in a large number of cellular processes and diseases.)

Klug A. Zinc finger peptides for the regulation of gene expression. Journal of Molecular Biology 1999; 293:215–218. (A review by the discoverer.)

Papin JA et al. Metabolic pathways in the post-genome era. Trends in Biochemical Sciences 2003; 28:250–258.

SIGNAL TRANSDUCTION

Kyriakis JM, Avruch J. Mammalian mitogen-activated protein kinase signal transduction pathways activated by stress and inflammation. Physiological Reviews 2001; 81:807–869. (Gives amplifying detail on protein kinase systems.)

CANCER

Vassilev LT et al. In vivo activation of the p53 pathway by small-molecule antagonists of MDM2. Science 2004; 303:844–848. (The first indication that drugs might be used to interfere with the action of p53.)

BLOOD LIPIDS AND THERAPY

Chiesa G, Sirtori CR. Apolipoprotein A-I(Milano): Current perspectives. Current Opinion in Lipidology 2003; 14:159–163. (Thought-provoking results concerning plasma cholesterol.)

Davignon J. Advances in lipid-lowering therapy in atherosclerosis. Advances in Experimental Medicine and Biology 2001; 498:49–58.

Kennedy MA et al. Characterization of the human ABCG1 gene. Journal of Biological Chemistry 2001; 276:39438–39447.

Index